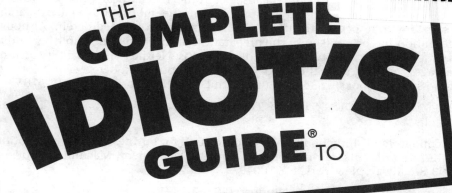

THE COMPLETE IDIOT'S GUIDE® TO

Beating the Blues

by Ellen McGrath, Ph.D. and Marcela Kogan

alpha books

A Division of Macmillan General Reference
A Simon & Schuster Macmillan Company
1633 Broadway, New York, NY 10019

Contents at a Glance

Contents

Introduction

Have you ever gone through a complete day without feeling bad about something?

Maybe you tried on a bathing suit and you were so repelled by your body that you wanted to run off to Alaska until summer was over. Or you had another fight with your spouse over whose turn it was to bring up the toilet paper from the basement. Maybe your child asked that you drop him off two blocks from the school so nobody knows you are related to him. Or your boss told you that the organization is "downsizing," but you won't be getting a pink slip—at least, not that day.

The fact is that everybody gets the blues sometimes. It's estimated that at any given time, nearly 90 to 95 percent of the population in this country feels bad about something. Almost anything in your work and personal life can give you the blues—your relationships with your spouse, parents, and children are a big source of blues for many people. Most of us get into a funk when we try to do too much for too many people and don't take enough care of ourselves. Sometimes rainy days and Mondays—and other days too—do get us down, and for very good reasons!

But whatever the source of your blues, once you understand where the bad feelings come from, you can take control over them, make more independent decisions, and feel better about your life. We've identified four categories for the everyday blues that everyone gets at least sometimes: Work, Relationship, Body, and Culture. Each category covers four types of blues. *The Complete Idiot's Guide to Beating the Blues* will help you identify in which category you are most likely to experience the blues and which of the 16 kinds of blues you may be facing at this moment!

Say, for instance, you feel unhappy because you are single and have no dates. Turn to Chapter 17 on the Home-Alone Blues to figure out why you are having trouble finding dates—there is usually a very legitimate reason—and what you can do to increase your chances of meeting people and maintaining a relationship. If you're in a funk because you just turned 40 and feel like you're over the hill—at least society seems to think so—you'll benefit from reading Chapter 12 on the Age-Rage Blues, which includes tips on seeing the positive aspects of aging.

This guide is packed with proven action strategies and exercises you can do that will uplift your spirit and enhance your self-esteem. I know they work because thousands of clients, students, or workshop participants I've seen over a period of 25 years have used them and recovered from the blues!

What You'll Find in This Book

The Complete Idiot's Guide to Beating the Blues is divided into six parts. You can read the book from cover to cover, or you can browse through the Table of Contents to find the chapters that address the kinds of blues you are now experiencing. Here's how the book is organized:

Part 1, "I Guess That's Why They Call Them the Blues," focuses on the differences between feeling blue and experiencing depression, describes how cultural expectations and standards adversely affect men and women, and points out the various types of blues we are likely to experience throughout the year.

Part 2, "The Moody Blues Learn to Sing a Happy Tune," shows you some quick strategies to beat the blues as well as the importance of physical activity in keeping the blues at bay. This part also covers the connection between food and mood and the different types of therapy available when your bad mood dips into a depression.

Part 3, "Easy Clues for the Ordinary Blues," helps you to create your own recipe for happiness and discover better ways to cope with feeling unattractive and getting older. You'll also pick up some tips on beating the blues when you're feeling burned out.

Part 4, "Beating the Blues in Relationships," deals with how to handle stressful situations with family members—spouse, parent, or child—and suggests ways of improving those relationships. We'll also address the unique problems singles face in our society today and how they can cope with them.

Part 5, "The Worker Blues: Monday-Morning Doldrums," highlights how the new corporate culture has changed the employer-employee relationship and what you can do to find a job you'll love. I'll also offer suggestions on what working parents can do to reduce the stress in their lives and improve their relationships with their families.

Part 6, "Mind Your Body to Mend Your Mind," shows you how the blues help create heart disease and slows recovery after heart surgery. We'll also tell the story of how one family successfully coped with cancer and turned the difficult experience into a positive one. The range of antidepressant medications on the market will also be highlighted, and we'll talk about the natural therapies (like St. John's Wort) that many people are discovering to beat the blues. You'll also find out what you can do to beat the blues over the long haul.

Blues Extras

To help you get the most out of this book, we've included the following helpful information boxes:

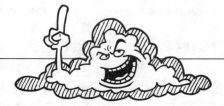

Funk-y Facts

In these boxes, you'll find bits of information including statistics, studies, anecdotes, and other interesting facts related to the blues and depression that may help you put your blues into perspective.

Dr. Ellen Says

These boxes contain practical tips on ways to beat the blues, suggestions on improving relationships, advice on how to handle difficult matters, and tidbits on where to turn for help.

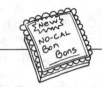

Guiltless Pleasures

Check these boxes for different ways you can reward yourself for taking positive steps to beat the blues and enhance the quality of your life.

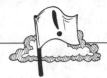

Blues Flag

These boxes contain warnings you should keep in mind and things you should avoid doing when dealing with anxiety-provoking situations that may increase your chances of getting the blues or experiencing depression.

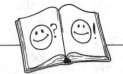

Terms of Encheerment

Check these boxes for definitions of useful terms, descriptions of each of the 16 types of everyday blues, the meaning of various therapies, and other explanations that are worth knowing.

Acknowledgments

For Ellen:

It takes a village to raise an adult and certainly to beat the blues. I would like to thank the members of my village for all of their inspiration, warmth, and wisdom. Thank you to my clients, students, family, and friends for helping me understand how complex the blues can be and how to beat them "one day at a time." The fact that even I learned to beat the blues is directly due to the safety and support the village has provided for me over many years. With a background like mine, I emerged with many skill deficits and a great deal to learn about how to be an effective adult. The village has taught me the essential lessons on how to work, love, and play, and for that I am immeasurably grateful to all of you. Your voices echo throughout the pages of this book.

Of course, as in every village, each member makes a unique and special contribution. Marcela Kogan was essential in making this book happen. She helped me organize into words the experiences the village has had in beating the blues. As I developed the material and we e-mailed chapter after chapter back and forth, the work grew in quality and clarity. She is a superb writer, interviewer, and synthesizer of vast amounts of information! It was a joyful and wonderful collaboration for which I will always be grateful.

To the Macmillan village, a large thanks for having the vision to do a book like this and make such important information available to so many. A special thanks to Gary Krebs, the talented and delightful Editorial Director of the book; Kathy Nebenhaus, Publisher, the warm and skilled mid-wife of the project; Development Editor Lynn Northrup, Production Editor Christy Wagner, and Copy Editor Susan Aufheimer, who cleaned up our copy and added many helpful observations we were able to incorporate in the text; and the rest of the Alpha Development Team for coming through for us.

Special thanks also to Margaret Durante, Publicity Director of Macmillan, for her guidance and gift for book publicity; and to my agent, Faith Hamlin, of Stamford Greenburger & Associates, for her very able assistance in successfully navigating the complex world of book publishing.

A number of dear friends were available for critical support and consistently helped me beat the blues when I was very tired. Mary Brewster astonished me by the quality of her ideas, her talent as a clinical psychologist, and her own success in beating the blues. Blair Brewster, her husband, taught me essential lessons about the psychology of men and how to be a business coach based on the success of his company, Electromark, in Wolcott, New York. The managers and staff at Electromark have also been wonderful teachers about coaching for stronger performance. Billy and Kate Brewster, their children, are a consistent delight in my life.

Dr. Alice Rubenstein, one of the most gifted psychotherapists in the universe, continues to grow in her wisdom regarding how to navigate the world, and I'm so grateful she continues to share it with me. Ginger Sherman and Dan Silverman gave invaluable advice and support about how to solve problems in the executive suite and how a high-energy, very successful couple can combine career success with having a beautiful new daughter, Eve.

Cynthia Graff, CEO of Lindora Medical Clinics in southern California, has taught me equally important lessons about how women executives can convert negative experiences and discrimination into personal and professional success and still feel great about themselves as women. Dr. Victoria Felton-Collins, a gifted financial advisor and coach to me in financial management, has proven to be a wonderful friend and model of success.

Joan Lunden, of *ABC/Good Morning America* fame, is another inspiration in learning when to hold and when to fold in the business world and how to move on to more satisfying pursuits when our needs change.

Other Family of Choice members who have provided much needed support during this process include: Steve and Gwenda Freeze, Mark and Nancy Bailey, Jeff Bolwell, Bruce Lippian, Rora Tanaka, Janis Smith, Dr. Robert Portman, David Booth, Jane Garnett, Barbara, Bill and Chris Everdell, Saundra Miller, Bill Arp, Jeanne Reiss, Dr. Carol Lindquist, Karen Bohan, Becky Guthary, Pascale St. Surin, and Karoly and Hank Gutman.

Pat Manocchia, my friend and the owner and director of La Palestra Center for Preventative Medicine in New York City, has a very special gift for inspiring us to become genuinely strong and healthy and to learn a rich lifestyle of preventative medicine. My trainer, Mark Tenore, helped me keep my body together as well as my mind, by his nurturance, wisdom, and high performance standards during this arduous writing process.

Thank you all!

Finally, and most importantly, the book would not have been written without the outstanding support of my own family, my husband, Dr. Harry Wexler, and my two sons, Joshua and Jordan. Harry offered outstanding creative ideas to enrich the work and expand the ideas to accurately reflect men's experience. And he and the boys did not hassle me about all the weekends and nights I was chained to the computer. Talk about outstanding men! Thank you to each of you from the bottom of my heart. Your love, who you are, and who you are becoming continues to help me beat the blues!

For Marcela:

When I accepted the assignment to coauthor a book on beating the blues, I thought, "Oh, I know all about this subject." After all, I had written dozens of feature stories about overcoming depression gone through individual and group therapy for many years. But as I approached each chapter, I realized that I had been slowly losing a grip over my life. I had become lazy about improving my intimate relationships, about thinking through my professional goals, and pursing my personal hobbies and passions.

So each chapter became a refresher course, and I, once again, felt excited about new possibilities.

I am grateful for having had the opportunity to work so closely with Dr. Ellen McGrath. Her attention to detail, sense of personal integrity, witty humor, warmth, and genuine care about the topic of this book pushed me up yet another notch as I stretched to enhance my understanding of the subject and improve my writing abilities. Our collaboration was truly a work in progress, a test of how well we both applied the conversation skills Ellen advocates through these pages. Through hours of telephone interviews, I was fortunate enough to catch a glimpse—just a glimpse—of how she shaped the storms and fires of her past into an honorable, hard-working, and heart-felt life.

Other people were also crucial in making this book happen. I thank Editorial Director Gary Krebs for encouraging me to take on such a challenging project and making this book such a high priority. Many thanks to Lynn Northrup, our Development Editor, who gave us helpful hints on how to improve our work as she read between the lines of each chapter, and to Christy Wagner, our Production Editor, who was a good sport in making last-minute corrections and put up with or frequent calls for "one more thing" before the book went to press.

I would also like to thank my father, who was way ahead of his time in advocating mind-body solutions to solve everyday problems and encouraged me to believe in my own healing powers, and my mother, who has shown me the importance of thanking God for what we have. Many thanks are also extended to my in-laws, who supported me throughout this project by watching our children during our vacations as I toiled away in hotel rooms, battling my own version of the blues for working during "family time."

Most importantly, I would like to thank my husband, Mitchell, whose support, enthusiasm, and reassurance sustained me through the difficult months of working on this book, and who was always able to stop my blues from getting black by bringing the picture back into focus with his clear, grounded perspective on life. I couldn't have seen this project to its completion if Mitchell hadn't been willing to shoulder more than his share of household responsibilities at a time when he was writing a book as well. Many thanks to my two sons, Ariel, 6, and Daniel, 2, who were a constant reminder of the challenge we all face to balance work and family in order to stay healthy. I hope they will read this book when they get older and find effective ways of coping with their blue moods.

Part 1

I Guess That's Why They Call Them the Blues

Do you flinch when you look at yourself in the mirror and notice wrinkles under your eyes? Do you feel bad that you can't pick up your child at school because your slave-driver boss won't let you out of sight? Are you in a funk when the holidays come around? Are you confused about your role as a guy in today's world?

If you answer "yes" to any of these questions, there is a good chance that you've experienced the everyday blues. But don't worry, everybody gets the blues sometimes. And feeling bad can be good if we understand where the bad feelings come from and take steps to fix what's wrong in our lives. The chapters in this section cover the 16 types of everyday blues most of us experience at some time, describe how societal expectations influence our moods, and spell out the differences between the blues and clinical depression.

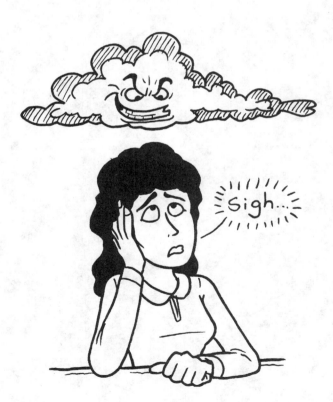

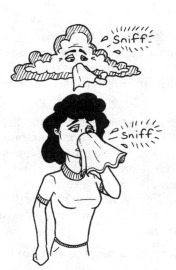

Chapter 1

The Blues: Common as the Common Cold

In This Chapter

➤ Why everybody gets the blues sometimes

➤ Code red! How the blues can signal a deeper problem

➤ How men, women, children, and seniors cope differently with the blues

➤ The four categories of everyday blues

➤ The blues aren't all bad!

➤ A six-step action plan to beat the blues

All of us get some form of the blues at one time or another. There are the Body-Image Blues and the Moody Food Blues, the Bedroom Blues and the Home-Alone Blues, the Bad-Boss Blues and the Monday-Morning Blues, the Age-Rage Blues and the Burnout Blues, the Cardiovascular Blues and the Cancer Blues…Whew! Seems like everywhere we turn these days, the blues are just waiting to get us down. Even worse, the blues are gaining strength while we're weakening in our ability and resolve to find and fight them.

I know this battle well. Blues territory is where I used to live and I still visit there too often. If some of these blues sound like you, then welcome to our Village of the Blues Brothers and Sisters! You're in good company, because it's estimated that at any given time in this country, up to 30 to 45 percent of the population struggles with the blues.

That's more than one-third of the country! And if we're speaking of the *everyday blues*—those sad, disheartening, ho-hum feelings that make us feel lethargic, sluggish, and bored—the percentage is closer to 90 to 95 percent of the population. These symptoms issue a warning that something is not right in our lives and that we better fix it before it gets worse.

If misery loves company, then we've got a great big party going on here! In fact, the blues are one of the most misdiagnosed of the mind/body conditions and a major public health problem in this country. It's easy for doctors to misdiagnose depression because depression is often masked by physical symptoms. Unresolved blues make our bodies sick, and sick bodies feed our unresolved blues. But while feeling blue is crummy, this upsetting emotion can give you energy and motivation to change. It's a warning sign to help steer you away from falling into a clinical depression, a much more serious condition that requires professional treatment.

In this chapter we give you an overview of the different types of blues so you can more easily decide where you are most likely to have trouble. These are the everyday blues, the ones all of us get at some point in our lives, We'll look at why we get them and what we could do to overcome these negative feelings that keep us from leading a more fulfilling life. The most important thing to remember from this point forward is this: Your blues are normal, and if you'll use the action strategies we describe in this book, your blues will be a source of power to change, inspire wisdom, and create deeper connections to others.

So Many Blues, So Little Time

You know when a cold is coming on. Your throat gets scratchy, your nose is stuffy, your head feels achy, and you have an overall feeling of malaise. If you're smart, you'll take it easy and give your body a rest before you start to feel worse. The symptoms are your body's way of telling you: "Ooohhhhh Charlie (or Charlotte), slow down, relax, or else I'll really give you something to worry about!"

The blues are your symptoms of a mental cold. Listen to them or pay the price. And if you think you're the only one who gets the symptoms, you can sigh with relief when you hear this: *Everybody* gets the blues sometimes, just like everybody catches a cold. We may not get them every day and not in every way, but feeling blue is a normal part of living. If somebody tells you they don't ever get the blues, check their pulse to see if they're alive.

People who have the blues can still function, although usually not as well as they would like. But just because you have the blues doesn't mean you have *depression*. No matter how hard they try, people who are clinically depressed *can't* function in one or more basic life areas, such as work, personal relationships, or body functions. We can't avoid the everyday blues, but we can avoid their cousins, the clinical depressions.

Not only does everyone get the blues, but the blues have grown to epidemic proportions. Research indicates we are 10 times more likely to have the blues than our grandparents and that the rate of the black blues (clinical depressions) is climbing at an alarming rate, particularly among young people. The blues continue to grow because our pace of living has accelerated so much. We have less and less recovery time and more and more emotional, physical, mental, and work demands loaded on us. Something has to give and it's usually our emotional health.

And the blues feed on themselves to grow. It's easy to see the world through blue-colored glasses when we're down. Everything seems like a big ordeal. Picking up our clothes off the floor seems like too much of an effort, never mind figuring out how we're going to dump that creep we're dating. When we're blue our problems appear insurmountable because our energy level is low and our negative thinking is high.

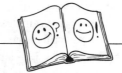

Terms of Encheerment

The *everyday blues* are those feelings of pain, sadness, and disappointment that stem from life's negative experiences, including normal losses, unfair treatment, and unresolved past sadness triggered by a current event. *Depression* is caused by changes in body chemistry, genetic vulnerability, and too many painful psychological experiences.

Why Does Everyone Get the Blues?

There are so many good reasons to get the blues, it's no wonder they're growing at such a phenomenal rate. We may feel that we don't measure up to society's expectations of what a man or woman should be. We may fall short of being the superparent we thought we'd become and feel that we can't provide for our families the way our dads provided for us. We're usually plagued by unrealistic notions of just how much we can do in one day. Or we compare ourselves to body builders or bathing beauties and gulp! It's not a pretty picture.

Everyone gets the blues for other reasons besides unfulfilled expectations or role overload. The blues are one of the best warning signals we have that we may be entering a danger zone. If the blues could speak, they would be shouting: "Code Red!" "Extreme Caution!" "Danger! Do Not Enter." "Act, Don't React!" The blues can be very helpful because they can serve as a warning beacon and give us a chance to think about what's wrong and fix it before it's too late. Here are two examples of how the blues work as life's warning system:

➤ You just got engaged and you suddenly feel insecure and blue. It makes sense that you would be nervous; after all, getting married is a big step. But these blues seem bigger than they should be. The blues are telling you that you need to think more carefully about whether you're making the right decision. Take some time alone to think. Seek the counsel of others. If you feel more resolved, then you'll feel stronger about the person you're going to marry and more committed to the marriage. If not, you can still get rid of that person without any legal hassles and divorce fees, so your blues helped you win either way!

5

➤ Every Monday you dread going into the office because you fear you'll find a pink slip on your desk. It makes perfect sense that you'd get the blues, since many of your colleagues have already been axed. But instead of letting your Monday-Morning Blues paralyze you, you think about what you can do to make yourself more useful to the company—and you take some computer courses. You feel more confident because you now have more skills and are in a better position to get a job elsewhere if the ax does come down. The boss notices your new positive attitude and is less likely to think of you when the next set of heads rolls.

But feeling bad is *really bad* if we just sit and sulk. Then our blues have the potential of getting worse and developing into a clinical depression. Because it's hard to tell whether you're blue or depressed since the symptoms can be similar and differ mainly in degree, I urge you to take the quiz in Chapter 2 to find out which one you have. You can beat the blues through the self-help exercises in this book, but if you are clinically depressed, you must get professional help as soon as possible.

Depression is a progressive illness and needs to be treated with psychotherapy and sometimes medication or it will typically get worse over time. But don't be blue about the black times! With current treatment technologies, we can successfully treat depression in about 90 percent of the cases. You just need to stop denying there's a problem and reach out for the help that's there for you.

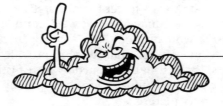

Funk-y Facts

Anyone, no matter how old they are, can suffer from depression. According to Harold Bloomfield, author of *How To Heal Depression* (Prelude Press, 1996), six million American children under 12 have clinical depressions and their parents don't realize it. Sometimes what is diagnosed as Attention Deficit Disorder (ADD), in which kids are easily distracted and can't sit still, is actually depression. One in 20 adolescents is also stricken with depression, and the suicide rate among teenagers has almost tripled in one generation. According to the American Psychiatric Association, up to 25 percent of people who are 65 and over have symptoms of depression or anxiety—and those numbers are expected to rise. A National Institute on Aging study of 1,862 people who are 71 and over showed that people who are depressed experienced a 55 percent greater decline in physical performance than those with no symptoms. The study appeared in a recent issue of *Journal of American Medical Association*.

I Guess That's Why They Call It (Anything But) the Blues

Despite the fact that the blues are as common as a sneeze, most people don't like to admit they have them. In our society, the blues or depression are viewed as a character flaw or a personal weakness, a way to shame and blame ourselves or an excuse for others to do it for us. People have not been taught to talk about their bad feelings, to acknowledge they feel vulnerable, or to understand that these bad feelings are common and appropriate. As a result, many of us are ashamed to admit we feel blue and blame ourselves for not being able to pull ourselves up by our bootstraps.

For these reasons, the blues often remain hidden and in disguise. They are more likely to be expressed in some of these ways:

> ➤ "I'm bummed out."
>
> ➤ "I feel crummy."
>
> ➤ "Life sucks."
>
> ➤ "I'm really ticked off!"
>
> ➤ "I'm too tired."

Dr. Ellen Says

Depression can make you physically sick. People who are depressed often produce too much of a hormone that suppresses their immune systems and increases their vulnerability to contracting diseases, including cancer and heart disease. But doctors treat patients' psychological symptoms of depression, less than the physical symptoms patients present. As a result, patients get trapped in the vicious cycle: Depression contributes to chronic illness and the illness contributes to depression.

Blowing Off the Blues Cover

Because it's such a bummer to be blue, many people cover up their sad feelings so these emotions come out looking like something else—anger, anxiety, recklessness, stomachaches, and other physical symptoms. Males and females of various ages tend to handle the blues differently because of how they were raised in our culture:

> ➤ *Women.* When women get the blues, they generally don't have to send out any smoke signals. They're quick to talk about how they feel to any good friend who wants to hear (usually other women) and will even buy you dinner if you're willing to sit with them as they re-examine every relationship in their lives to figure out why they're blue. In the end, though, many women assume everything is their fault and quickly accept blame for relationships going sour, projects going askew, and other miscellaneous disasters. They get so stuck in the bad feelings, their energy gets drained and they don't have any power left over to take action and solve the problem.
>
> ➤ *Men.* The way women deal with the blues is in direct contrast to how men handle such feelings, which typically is to deny they have any feelings of any kind and

do something, anything, to distract themselves. When men feel down they turn it outward and get mad, annoyed, and hostile. They drink too much, drive too fast, and engage in other self-destructive behavior that is often manifested in physical ailments—headaches, stomachaches, backaches. While men express their sadness through actions, women express their sadness through words and by showing sad feelings.

➤ *Children.* When kids feel blue, they aren't going to discuss their feelings over a Big Mac and an order of fries at McDonald's, especially to their guy friends who are wearing REALLY baggy pants, have long hair, look scraggly, and think COOL is never having to say you're sorry or feel sorry about anything. So kids often display the blues by breaking rules, withdrawing, or abusing alcohol, drugs, or cigarettes—scaring the hell out of their parents who are so concerned that their kids are heading toward skid row that they don't even consider the fact that the problem may stem from the kids not liking themselves and feeling blue.

➤ *Senior citizens.* Older people get the blues more often than many other groups. But too often, their complaints are written off as part of growing old. While certain physical and mental problems may arise due to aging, they may also be symptoms of depression and should be evaluated by a physician. When experienced by seniors, the blues are often called senility and they cause many a premature illness or death because they're overlooked or undertreated more than any other physical problem of aging.

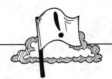

Blues Flag

People who feel blue experience short-lived symptoms of depression but continue to function in the basic areas of their lives. You are probably blue if you feel upset, sad, vulnerable, or angry over something that happened to you; anxious because of a recent loss; bad about yourself but still able to function despite feeling lousy; or you wish to be alone for hours or a day or two at a time.

The Blues for Every Season

The blues strike men and women, the old and the young, in surprisingly similar ways—often suddenly and unexpectedly. You could be standing by the water cooler at work really talking up a storm with your coworkers and all of a sudden you feel washed over by a wave of sadness and you don't know what hit you. Or you could be having hot and wild sex with your boyfriend when, out of the blue, you ask yourself—ever so fleetingly—"Is this all there is?" and you feel like crying.

Sometimes the blues come on more strongly during the holidays, anniversaries, at the start and end of the school year, and during certain seasons. About 35 million Americans get the winter blues when the weather gets dark and gray. And about 39 percent of Americans also suffer from the blues before or after the December holiday season. We give you more information on Seasonal Blues in Chapter 5.

Although it seems like the blues come from nowhere, they always stem from somewhere, even if it's hidden from your sight—a thought you had when you saw something, said something, or heard something. One of the strategies for beating the blues is to know which of the different kinds of everyday blues are most likely to get you, so when a blue feeling comes up, you know where to look for its source and what kinds of action to take to get rid of it.

Blues Brothers: The Four Categories of Everyday Blues

Almost anything in your work and personal life can give you the blues—and once we understand where they come from we can take control over them and make better decisions. There are four categories of everyday blues that everyone gets at least sometimes: Work, Relationship, Body, and Culture.

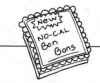

Guiltless Pleasures

Need a boost? There is more to beating the blues than sitting around racking your brain to figure out why you feel so bad. If you're not in the mood to think, take action: Go for a 10-minute walk, learn relaxation techniques, lift some weights, do sit-ups, or go for a jog. Physical exercise is a great mood booster and stress reducer because it immediately kicks in more oxygen to your brain, helping your body produce more endorphins, a chemical that makes you feel better.

➤ *Work blues.* I don't think I know a single person who doesn't have the Work blues at least sometimes. Getting up on Monday morning to put in a 60-hour week, after an exhausting weekend of taking care of kids, catering to in-laws, and working around the house is bound to put you in a funk. And if you don't like your job or don't get along with your boss…well…work isn't exactly a fulfilling adventure in learning and growth. (See Part 5 and Chapter 13 for help in coping with Work blues.)

➤ *Relationship blues.* Who doesn't have the Relationship blues these days, whether you are single or married? Many married couples moan that their marriage has lost its fizz, while singles groan that they can't find anybody decent to date. Not to mention the headaches we all get when we deal with our parents or our children. (See Part 4 for help in coping with Relationship blues.)

➤ *Body blues.* Do you like the way your body looks? Do you feel too old or too fat? Are you afraid of getting cancer or heart disease or living in such a way that you will probably attract one of them? Many of us get the blues when we think of our bodies not measuring up to the unrealistic standards of physical perfection our culture foists on us. (See Chapters 7, 11, 21, and 22 for help in coping with Body blues.)

➤ *Culture blues.* These are the blues men and women experience as a result of living in an outdated culture that demands too much and provides too little support for the pressures we face in modern life. Women get the blues because they are victimized by wage and social discrimination, and men are upset because they have lost their role as king of the realm—at home or at work. And it's real tough to live in a society where growing older is something to be dreaded because we lose our sex appeal, our intrigue, and our health. (See Chapters 3, 4, 5, and 12 for help in coping with Culture blues.)

WORK BLUES	RELATIONSHIP BLUES
➤ Monday-Morning Blues	➤ Bedroom Blues
➤ Bad-Boss Blues	➤ Parent Approval Blues
➤ Working-Parents Blues	➤ Pooped-Parent Blues
➤ Burnout Blues	➤ Home-Alone Blues
BODY BLUES	**CULTURE BLUES**
➤ Moody Food Blues	➤ My Fair Lady Blues
➤ Body-Image Blues	➤ Decoronation Blues
➤ Cardiovascular Blues	➤ Seasonal Blues
➤ Cancer Blues	➤ Age-Rage Blues

You Can Be Blue and Healthy Too

When most of us feel blue, we're too burned out to try to figure out why we're down. Typically, we just grab a bag of chips and plop ourselves in front of the TV, go out drinking with our buddies and drown our sorrows, or just sleep until the blues blow over. But while the blues may go away for a while, they are likely to come back with a vengeance, and we'll feel even worse unless we fix the reason they appeared in the first place.

But how do we figure out what's bothering us when everything seems kind of blah?

Are You True Blue?

Ask yourself what is your biggest area of vulnerability (and it may be more than one): Relationship ruins? Body betrayal? Work woes? Culture conflicts?

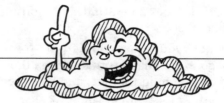

Funk-y Facts

"Over 100 million individuals worldwide suffer from some form of depressive illness," reports the psychiatric journal *Depression* in its 1993 debut edition. But don't think we all have the same *kinds* of blues or depressions. Depending on your ethnic background, you are likely to experience different kinds of depressions *and* even respond differently to antidepressant medication. For instance, African-American women in an outpatient setting studied by Dr. Nancy Russo of Arizona State University had a 42% higher rate of clinical depression than Caucasian women and were 20% more likely than white women to be prescribed drugs for their depression. Among Asians in America, Chinese women had greater rates of depression than Chinese men, partly because the women used accommodation rather than assertion, and this passive style increased their risk for depression. Suicide is over twice as high for Native American women and men as it is for the general American population. So, if you're not Caucasian, pick your depression specialist or beat-the-blues coach even more carefully to make sure she's up to date about ethnic differences in managing the blues.

To explore this problem, here are some sample questions you can ask yourself:

➤ Am I working too hard and have no time for my family?

➤ Do I genuinely like my job or my boss?

➤ Am I upset because I still let my mother get the best of me when I visit her?

➤ Do I hate my body? If so, why?

➤ Am I in a funk because my lifestyle has to change drastically as a result of a cardiac or cancer scare?

Name That Blue

As you are thinking about these questions, make a list of things that you have been feeling upset about in order of priority—and pick the three most important ones. Then over time try to follow this six-step action plan to beat your blues. The descriptions of each of the blues and their action strategies found in each chapter should offer you help and support along the way.

1. **Spot your favorite blue.** Figure out which quadrant your blues tend to fall under. If, for instance, you are so exhausted all the time from working too hard that you have no energy left to date—and that depresses you—your blues probably fit into two categories: Work blues and Relationship blues.

   Now take a closer look at each category and figure out which specific blue pertains to you. If you identify your blues as falling under work, you are probably experiencing the Burnout Blues. Under relationships, you may be going through the Home-Alone Blues.

2. **Understand where your blues come from.** Now that you've spotted your favorite blues, go to the chapters that address those blues to find out where they sprout from, how common they are, and how they are most likely to affect you.

3. **Rate the strength of your blues.** How severe are your own blues? Take the quizzes throughout this book to find out. If you prefer, you can also use your own 1 to 10 scale like the one we show here (with 1 being none to very little and 10 being a great deal) and circle the number that most closely gauges your blues level.

   Your Blues Scale: How Strong Are Your Blues Today?

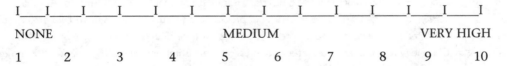

NONE					MEDIUM					VERY HIGH
1	2	3	4	5	6	7	8	9		10

   Check your Blues Scale daily like you would the fuel gauge in your car. See how much or how little of the blues you have and how much action you need to take to replace the energy the blues have used up.

4. **Check to see if the blues are turning black (beware of those clinical depressions).** If you find that you're coming up with many 8s, 9s, and 10s on your own scale, WATCH OUT! You could be in or headed for a clinical depression. Immediately take the *Are You Blue or Are You Depressed?* quiz in Chapter 2 to get a better sense of just how depressed you may be and *get professional help right away.* Also read Chapter 9, "When Self-Help Isn't Enough," Chapter 23, "Better Living

Through Chemistry," Chapter 24, "Let Mother Nature Help: Natural Therapies for the Blues," and Chapter 25, "The Blues Immunizations—Long Term Protection for Your Mind, Body, and Soul."

5. **Choose at least three favorite action strategies to beat the blues**. The chapters in this book all include some specific action strategies you can use to beat those particular blues. Or you can also turn to the more general blues-buster exercises in Chapter 6, "Quick Strategies for You to Beat the Blues," Chapter 8, "Beating the Blues: Let's Get Physical," and Chapter 25, "The Blues Immunization—Long-Term Blues Protection for Your Mind, Body, and Soul."

   From all of these action strategies, choose three favorite ones and practice them when you're not as blue so they become easy and natural for you. Then next time you start to feel the blues coming on, whip into action and try one or two of your favorite action strategies. You'll beat the blues before they've even had a chance to grow and get you.

6. **Review your progress and update your blues-buster skills**. Every few months, review your progress and evaluate which action strategies are working for you and which aren't. The blues change with each age and stage of life and so do the action strategies that work best to beat them. Sometimes you outgrow a strategy or sometimes it's not natural enough for you to continue to use it. If you're not sure how to evaluate this yourself, visit a coach or therapist who specializes in working with the blues. She can give you the feedback you need to make whatever adjustments are necessary.

Remember, beating the blues is a lifetime skill, so keep an eye on how your blues grow and change, and keep refining and updating your action strategies. If you commit to updating your emotional management skills, not only will you beat the blues, but you'll earn a higher return on this than on any other investment that you can make in yourself.

The Least You Need to Know

➤ At some point in our lives, all of us struggle with the everyday blues.

➤ People don't like to admit they have the blues because society still views depression as a character flaw.

➤ Feeling bad can be good if it causes us to pay attention to our feelings and take action to improve our lives.

➤ Men, women, children, and seniors react differently to the blues: Women blame themselves for being sad, men blame others, kids withdraw or break rules, and the elderly complain of physical pain.

➤ Americans get the blues year-round: Twenty-five million people get the winter blues (another 10 million are diagnosed with Seasonal Affective Disorder) and nearly 39 percent suffer from the blues during the December holidays.

➤ The four most common categories of blues are Work, Relationship, Body, and Culture blues.

➤ To beat the blues, identify one or two action strategies that work for you and use them!

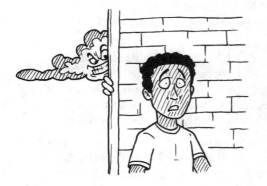

Chapter 2

The Big Bad Blues Can Get You Too!

In This Chapter

➤ Slipping from the blues into the black

➤ How the blues can signal danger

➤ Depressive genes, depressed minds?

➤ Quiz: Did you inherit depression?

➤ Protection for the depression-prone

➤ Quiz: Are you blue or are you depressed?

When many of us get the blues, we complain to our friends and family about how lousy we feel, we often see the world as unfair and unkind, and we mope around the house. Nobody wants to talk to us and the feeling's mutual. We would rather play solitaire, computer games, or stuff ourselves with fattening goodies. Usually, we have good reasons to feel down. Our bosses chewed us out for losing an account, the guys we date don't call us back, our wives are knocking us for not "communicating," we feel guilty planting our kids in front of the TV to watch endless *Barney* reruns, our lives are boring, or we're just overwhelmed by life's demands.

But feeling bad can be healthy and serve a good purpose if we take the bad feelings as a sign that something is wrong and we need to fix it to be happy. If our bad feelings continue to grow, however, if they grip us and won't let go, if our thoughts often flow from blue to black, then we're headed for something far worse than the everyday blues: a clinical depression, also known as the Big Bad Blues. This kind of depression is a serious illness that robs us of energy, joy, hope, love, and sexuality. In extreme cases, when depression is untreated, it can lead to even more severe ramifications, including death.

Sliding down the slippery slope from the everyday blues into this black mood is particularly risky for people who are predisposed to becoming sick when they're stressed or developing depression because it runs in their family. In this chapter, we'll take a look at who is prone to suffering depression and ways for you to gauge the level of stress in your life to reduce the likelihood of developing a clinical depression.

You can beat the everyday blues through the action strategies I have outlined in this book. But you'll need professional help to battle clinical depression. This chapter includes a quiz that will help you identify whether your bad moods are a healthy, realistic, and logical reaction to upsetting events, or if your response is unhealthy and an indication of serious depression.

Everybody Gets the Blues Sometimes

When we're in a funk, everything and everyone seems horrible. We may hate our jobs, question our parenting skills, or wonder why we married our husbands or wives. Many of us may even ask: "Is that all there is?" or "Is this as good as it gets? If so, I'm outta here!"

Usually, an upsetting event, a destructive action, or a negative thought triggers the bad mood. Here are some normal life categories I have come up with that may give you the everyday blues:

➤ *Nobody loves me.* Your college roommate—also the maid of honor at your wedding—didn't invite you to her wedding. You wonder whether she was really your friend after all. Come to think of it, do you have any real friends left when it comes right down to it?

➤ *Take this job and shove it.* Your boss told you to redo the proposal for the umpteenth time, and you're feeling like you just aren't cut out for this job (or maybe any other).

➤ *I'm a lousy mother (or father).* You got a call at the office from the principal that your kid's in trouble again for fighting with other children on the school bus—and you feel like staying at the office and never returning home again.

➤ *I feel like an unpaid maid.* Your husband fell asleep in front of the TV, leaving a sink full of dishes on the night it was his turn to clean up. This is the third time this week.

➤ *I'm a wimp.* You found out you are vastly underpaid for what you do and you wonder if you'll ever get the guts to ask for more money.

➤ *I'm such a bad son (or daughter).* You yelled and hung up on your mother when she asked: "So, met anyone yet?" You warned her not to ask you that anymore, and when she did again, you just lost it.

➤ *I'm so ugly.* You look at yourself in the mirror in the morning and see two new rolls of fat that weren't there yesterday.

These really are upsetting experiences, so why wouldn't you get the blues? It's normal to feel blue when life socks us with these challenges. Knowing you're not alone and that others go through the same thing can be a great relief in blues management. Paying attention to these blue periods also gives us an opportunity to do a quick inventory of our life: what's working and what's not working in our relationships and our jobs. What needs to change? What should stay the same? This inventory often results in reorganizing our priorities, making tough but crucial decisions we've been avoiding, changing our attitudes, leaving bad marriages, switching careers, or approaching our kids in a new way.

You may, for instance, call your newly married roommate from college to find out if the invitation got lost in the mail or if she is mad at you. Maybe you said something hurtful to her without realizing it and you decide you need to be more careful about what you say to people. Or you might tell that lazy husband of yours that if he doesn't start helping out you're dragging him into couples therapy (that'll usually get men going). Or you send your mother an apology note with a nicely worded request to avoid the topic of you dating unless you bring it up.

But if you're like most of us, you probably ignore the daily blahs and sneer at comments about the opportunity for self-growth that such misery invites. Instead, many of us slump in front of the TV watching reruns of *The Honeymooners*, raid the refrigerator for something half-way interesting (nothing qualifies as good enough when you're feeling blue), aimlessly surf the Internet, or call a friend to dump your blues on her. When you're done with the conversation, you feel better, she feels worse, but you figure: "Isn't that what friends are for?"

With these avoidance strategies, the blues usually go away—at least for a while. But they come back with more frequency and intensity because you didn't take care of the reason the blues were there in the first place. So, don't wait until your life is a total mess. You can train yourself to examine what's making you miserable and come up with creative ways to solve your problems.

The first step is to understand what depression really is so you can evaluate if you (or those you love) have it.

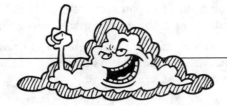

Funk-y Facts

According to the American Psychiatric Association, 5 percent of the population can be diagnosed as having major depression at any one point in time. At least 10 percent of the population will experience a major depression during their lifetime. You run a 20 percent chance of having a major or minor depression in your life.

What Is Depression?

Depression is an illness that affects your mood, thinking, bodily functions, and behavior. The National Institutes of Health came up with the following checklist for symptoms of depression:

➤ Persistently sad or empty mood

➤ Loss of interest or pleasure in ordinary activities, including sex

➤ Decreased energy, fatigue, feeling slowed down

➤ Sleep disturbances (insomnia, early morning waking, or oversleeping)

➤ Difficulty concentrating, remembering, making decisions

➤ Feelings of guilt, worthlessness, helplessness

➤ Thoughts of death or suicide, suicide attempts

➤ Irritability

➤ Excessive crying

➤ Chronic aches and pains that don't respond to treatment

You're probably thinking: "Hey, I get all of those! I must be depressed."

But don't get off labeling yourself so quickly. All of us get some of these symptoms sometimes, but that doesn't mean we're all depressed. To qualify as being depressed you must experience at least four of these symptoms for more than two weeks. Depressions are the Big Bad Blues, and they significantly interfere with your ability to function in at least one of your basic areas of life: For example, you sleep way too much or wake up too early and can't go back to sleep; you gain or lose a lot of weight in a short period of time; nothing is fun anymore; or you call in sick at work because you feel so lousy.

These things don't happen just once or twice. They keep happening for two weeks or more if it's a real depression.

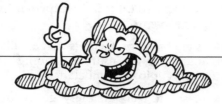

Funk-y Facts

Depression can occur from a chemical imbalance in the brain as well as psychological factors. Our feelings and thoughts, both pleasant and distressing, are the result of many electrochemical reactions that occur throughout our brains and bodies. Most depressions can be treated with chemicals called antidepressants, which correct chemical imbalances in the brain, replacing "feel-good" chemicals like serotonin that have been depleted because of stress, genetics, illness, or negative behaviors.

In contrast, people who feel blue experience short-lived symptoms of depression but continue to function in the basic areas of their lives. They're not at their best, they feel crummy, and sometimes it takes real effort to get through the day, but they get by. Soon they feel better. The blues fade due to their effort to keep going, or when the unpleasant experience stops, or when they find better ways to deal with the problem. But people with a depressive disorder can't "just shake it" no matter how hard they try. Their symptoms may go on for months, years, or even a lifetime. The worst advice to give a depressed person is: "Pull yourself together." Or, "Enough already! Pick yourself up by your bootstraps and get going." Or, "Uh, hasn't this gone on long enough? Look at the bright side and all the good things you have." Nobody can follow this advice, no matter how much they want to, because their bodies will be so physically exhausted and lethargic and their minds simply won't allow it if they're genuinely depressed.

Depressed people are also often filled with guilt because they can't figure out why they can't shake their bad moods, and the comments from friends serve only to deepen the depression.

The Blues/Depression Distinction

Blues refer to the bad feelings people get because of negative experiences such as losses, loneliness, discrimination, stress, and burnout. "Blue" people feel upset but can still function. *Depressed* people, by contrast, have bad feelings but *can't* function in the basic areas of life such as work, relationships, or managing their health—no matter how hard they try.

The following list highlights the differences between everyday blues and clinical depression.

Blues: Your bad feelings are based on real-life experiences. They are healthy, appropriate reactions to negative events.

Depression: Your moods are based on feelings that are bigger than life—exaggerations, delusions, denial, fantasy, or misunderstanding. They are unhealthy reactions to a chemical and psychological imbalance.

Blues: You have good reason to feel sad, angry, guilty, or anxious because of a loss or trauma, but you assume that eventually you'll get over it.

Depression: You figure that what's happening to you now is a harbinger of more losses in the future and there's nothing you can do to stop them.

Blues: You feel temporarily helpless, but, hey, it's not that bad and certainly not worth killing yourself over it.

Depression: You feel a sense of hopelessness, despair, and think about killing yourself to avoid the pain.

Blues: You just want to be left alone and don't want to see anyone for several hours or a day or two.

Depression: You are emotionally withdrawn and isolated for weeks or months at a time.

Blues: You feel hurt and upset, but you believe that you'll heal.

Depression: You feel that nothing you can do will ever make you feel good about yourself again.

Blues: You feel bad about yourself but don't blame yourself for your bad feelings.

Depression: You hate yourself and constantly feel bad about yourself.

Blues: Your bad mood is healthy because you can fix what's wrong and come out of it with wisdom, maturity, and creativity.

Depression: There is nothing productive about your mood. Your depression paralyzes you, and you feel physically and mentally worn down and sick.

Is It in Your Head, or in Your Genes?

Depression results from a chemical imbalance in the brain and a negative, distorted way of thinking. Like heart disease and hypertension, depression runs in many families.

Depression is almost always caused by a combination of one or more of the following factors:

➤ The disease runs in your family's gene pool.

➤ You lost a parent early on and never recovered from the trauma.

➤ You're having troubles at work or in your marriage.

➤ You have seasonal affective disorder (SAD).

➤ You aren't exercising or eating right.

➤ You have low self-esteem.

➤ You suffer from another medical illness.

➤ You grew up surrounded by people who were always negative and depressed.

You are more likely to develop depression if you inherited the depressive gene or if you were raised in an environment surrounded by people who always felt beaten down, hopeless, and powerless. But not everyone who inherits depression will succumb to the disease—or at least be depressed all the time. The disorder may skip a generation, or the depression may be triggered only when other factors are present—too much stress or the death of a loved one, for example.

If you are at risk, take extra care of yourself. Avoid high-stress situations if you can. But even if you can't avoid a high-stress environment, you can still reduce your risk of getting depressed by getting plenty of sleep, exercising, and eating healthy. When something gets you down, tend to it right away!

If you follow your doctor's orders and you still can't seem to lift your spirits, seek professional help to stop the symptoms from getting worse. Think of this depressive illness as being like cancer. If you know you are susceptible to breast cancer, you'll examine your breasts for lumps more regularly. If discovered early, the disease will be far more treatable.

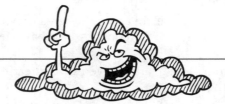

Funk-y Facts

If one identical twin has depression, there is a 70 percent chance that the other will also develop depression at some time. When children who inherit a depressive gene are adopted at birth by families without a history of depression, they are three times more likely to develop depression than the biological children of the adopted families.

Are You Prone to Inherited Depression?

The best way to find out if you're prone to bouts of depression is to ask your relatives. Like other traits, *inherited depression* can be passed down through generations. But good luck getting anything out of Uncle Jack or Grandma Bertha. In some families, the word "depression" is enough to make people run for cover!

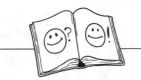

Terms of Encheerment

Inherited depression is the sad and bad feelings that result when biological, genetic, cultural, or psychological depressions grow in our families and are passed down to us as an increased vulnerability to both the blues and depression.

Some relatives may feel uncomfortable if you poke into the nooks and crannies of your family history—where all sorts of forbidden stuff lurks (like the uncle who ran away with the maid!). If it was your older relatives who suffered from depression, they might be more likely to simply say: "Life was hard back then."

Your family's depression was probably masked by other symptoms—alcohol abuse, eating disorders, chronic fatigue, and nervous breakdown. You may have heard, for instance, that Aunt Ethel "went off her rocker" and "took to her bed." Or that your grandpa just got into a lot of accidents, or Aunt Susy was a chronic complainer and had psychosomatic problems.

To determine whether you are more vulnerable to depression, take the following inherited depression quiz.

Did You Inherit Depression?

Answer "Yes" or "No" to the following questions.

1. Do you have any close relatives who often experienced nonspecific illnesses that may have been symptoms of disguised depression—like weakness, chronic fatigue, headaches, painful menstruation, constipation, sexual problems, obesity, appetite loss, or sleep problems)? ___

2. Do you have any close relatives who suffered nervous breakdowns, attempted suicide, or were unable to function in some basic area of their work, family, or social life? ___

3. Were any of your close relatives given shock treatments, antidepressants, or antianxiety drugs? ___

4. Is there a history of alcohol or drug abuse (including prescription drugs) in your family that may have been caused by or contributed to depression? ___

5. Did any of the women in your family consistently abuse food or have what would today be recognized as an eating disorder? ___

6. Did your mother, grandmother, or other close female relatives often seem visibly unhappy or discontented with their limited choice? Did they experience multiple traumas such as loss of children, accidents, natural disasters, or major financial setbacks? ___

7. Did your mother, grandmother, or other close female relatives work all or nearly all the time, caring for children, an ill relative, and/or working outside the home, so that they always seemed tired and rarely had any time for themselves? ___

8. Is there a history of physical or sexual abuse in your family? ___

9. Did any of your close male relatives exhibit the typical symptoms of male depressions like alcohol and substance abuse, violent behavior, preventable car accidents, being a workaholic, or denial of all sad feelings? ___

10. Did your close male or female relatives smoke enough to cause them disabling health problems or premature death from smoking? ___

Total number of questions answered "Yes": ___

You're probably vulnerable to depression if you answered "Yes" to more than one of these questions.

Just because you're vulnerable to developing depression doesn't mean you're doomed to suffer from this disease. So don't despair! Remember that you can learn to manage depression in ways your family could never know or teach you because they never had the tools. You're in a much better position to control your life.

Protecting Yourself From Inherited Depression

Leading a balanced life is key to feeling good about yourself. Having said that, let me add that most of us don't have a clue about what a balanced life feels like, although we read plenty of articles about people who've mastered the juggling act.

Let's look at a typical day in the life of a middle-aged father of two who is just trying to get by in today's hectic, confusing, cruel world. He rushes out of the house in the morning without eating breakfast, drops the kids off at school, and spends the next eight hours yelling at employees, getting yelled at by clients, and tracking down rumors about possible company layoffs. At dinner that night, his vegan daughter glares at a platter of fried chicken and tells dad he may as well be eating Dewey, the family dog.

His wife growls at him for not talking to anyone at dinner, and announces she is going out with her girlfriends to "get away from everybody." The dining experience is so unpleasant that he actually looks forward to retiring into the study to put in another four hours of work before his head hits the pillow.

If this poor guy is prone to developing depression, he is probably heading down to the pit because the

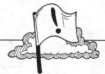

Blues Flag

Be prepared to feel worse before you feel better after you start digging out family skeletons. Recognizing that you come from a long line of depressed people is hard to deal with, and you'll probably resent the family members who "made" you that way. But these feelings will go away when you learn to accept your past and move on to a better future by incorporating the positive parts of the past and detaching from the negative.

stress in his life is out of control. But he could avoid depression—or at least get treatment early on—if he slowed down, took better care of himself, and gained better perspective on his life.

If depression runs in your family, keep an eye on how you are feeling and try to avoid getting too stressed out. The following exercise will help you track your mood. Write down events or situations that tend to make you depressed. Rate each event from 1 (for lowest stress) to 10 (for highest stress). Take a look at the following example.

In the past six months, I've experienced:

My mother's death	10
Being fired from my job	8–10
My 40th birthday	5–6
A failed relationship	7–8
Moving	6–7

If you have inherited depression to start with and have experienced more than one or two events with a score of 5 or more, watch out! You are likely to get depressed unless you are careful. So take better care of yourself. Attend workshops on stress management, and cope with depression by following the exercises in this book.

But remember, if you've inherited this nasty condition from your family, you may be experiencing depression even if there is no apparent reason for it.

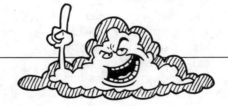

Funk-y Facts

If you find depression symptoms like alcoholism, sociopathy (operating without a conscience), or drug abuse among your close relatives, you're eight to 10 times more likely to develop similar symptoms. But by simply being female—regardless of your background—you have at least a one-in-four chance of experiencing major depression. The odds for men are one in eight.

Self-Help or Seek Help to Perk Up?

If your life gets out of hand and you neglect your health, relationships, responsibilities, and work for weeks, there is a good chance you'll fall into a depression, whether you are prone to it or not. Many people are suffering from depression right now but don't know it, and assume that their bad mood is just part of their personality.

But remember, depression is curable with the right treatment. If you are depressed, you must see a professional. The self-help exercises in this book won't help you. It's essential for you to determine whether you've got the blues or you're depressed. The following quiz will help you sort that out.

Are You Blue or Are You Depressed?

Answer "Yes" or "No" to the following questions.

1. I sleep more than eight hours on many nights, or I find it difficult to sleep at all. I often wake up very early in the morning and then typically can't go back to sleep. ___

2. I often feel lonely and isolated and find myself withdrawing from relationships. I have no relationship I would consider successful. ___

3. I often think about how I would kill myself, or I have attempted suicide. ___

4. I often use drugs, alcohol, cigarettes, and/or food to numb my feelings and escape reality and have experienced destructive consequences, such as health problems or endangering myself or others. ___

5. I truly believe something is wrong with me and it can't be fixed. ___

6. I sometimes feel totally overextended and get very frustrated and edgy when asked to do more than I'm already doing. ___

7. I often feel that I'm giving more than I get in my relationships. I have too few quality relationships to feel satisfied, or too many to maintain without feeling depleted. ___

8. I have been sick quite often over the last year with illnesses that are usually stress-related (for example, colds, headaches, stomachaches). ___

9. I often feel I'm a victim; I keep struggling to overcome feeling victimized although I haven't been particularly successful. ___

10. I am still depressed over having been treated badly as a child. I blame my parents, but we tolerate each other and/or I've grown to accept what has happened. ___

Now let's check your answers:

You may be experiencing depression if you answered "Yes" to two or more of the first five questions. When there is a major change in your sleeping ability, when you withdraw from people, have suicidal thoughts, use drugs or food to drown your pain, and feel hopeless, chances are you're experiencing depression.

You may just have the blues if you answered "Yes" to two or more of the last five questions. It makes perfect sense that you'd feel overwhelmed from trying to do too much, trying to be everything to everybody, and not feeling appreciated. You're okay so long as these feelings are not taking over your spirit.

You may be drifting from the blues to depression and back if you answered "Yes" to one or more of the questions from both the first and second section of the quiz. This means that you should keep tabs on your mood and be on alert.

If you think you are experiencing depression, first accept that you've got a disease which has a cure and that you need help. Remember, depression is not a weakness, it's a disease. Don't try to treat it yourself. (For more information on professionals who specialize in treatment of depression, see Appendix B, "Resources.")

If you've got a case of the blues—and it happens to all of us at one time or another!—the self-help exercises in this book can help you resolve your feelings. In the next chapters, I'll discuss why women and men get the blues and what they can do to break out of their cultural stereotypes so they can feel better about themselves and fulfill their potential.

The Least You Need to Know

➤ Feeling bad can be good if it motivates us to make positive changes.

➤ When the blues get out of control we fall prey to depression, which is a disease—not a weakness—that affects mood, thinking, bodily functions, and behavior.

➤ Alcoholism, accidents, psychosomatic symptoms, and other problems are often cover-ups for depression.

➤ It's crucial to determine whether you are experiencing the everyday blues or depression.

➤ Self-help exercises can help you beat the blues, but you need to see a specialist if you are experiencing depression.

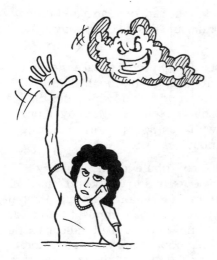

Chapter 3

I Am Woman Hear Me Roar... My Fair Lady Blues

In This Chapter

➤ How women need to unlearn some of life's lessons

➤ How a woman's inner voice guides her actions

➤ The 10 cultural commandments women are often expected to live by

➤ The six shades of women's blues

➤ Stick with good traditions, ditch the bad

➤ Quiz: How much are you influenced by others?

Do you flinch when you look at yourself in the mirror and notice that your eyelids are drooping so much you now look like a basset hound? Do you feel you're doing a lousy job balancing work and family, no matter how many new time-saving techniques you try? Are you down because you can't find a decent guy to date, your house is a pig sty, or you are too wimpy to ask your boss for a raise?

Have you lost your sex appeal or never found it in the first place? If the answer is "Yes" to any of the above, join the crowd! The growing crowd, I should say, since most women and an increasing number of men feel they are failing in some aspect of their lives and disappointing others BIG TIME. These days women have plenty of good reasons to get the My Fair Lady Blues.

Society places enormous responsibility on women to take care of hearth and home, excel professionally, look great, stay youthful-looking, and ensure everybody around us is happy.

Whenever anything goes wrong, women are trained and expected to take the blame—and honey, do we! We're the gold-medal winners at "taking it personally." And, of course, then we feel bad that we feel so bad! Is it any wonder that two to four times as many women as men get the blues? But don't listen to the counsel of many of our mothers who tell us to "learn to live with" such awful feelings, or resort to making excuses for being in a funk by blaming a "bad hair day" or PMS.

In this chapter, we'll look at the societal factors that contribute to why so many women get the blues and why we shame and blame ourselves so easily and effectively. Blues, shame, and blame are part of a rich and ruthless cultural prescription for women that has been around and active for hundreds of years. It's nearly impossible to escape this prescription unless you understand the grip and power of our cultural conscience. Then you can decide which aspects of your traditional upbringing you want to pre-serve because they make you strong and which rules need to be ditched because they get in the way of self-growth. By taking control of your life instead of letting the sick aspects of our culture lead you, you'll feel and be stronger and more confident—qualities that will help you keep the blues at bay. Although the chapter is directed toward women, men will also benefit from reading it because it will give them a greater understanding of the women in their lives.

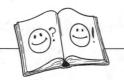

Terms of Encheerment

A *cultural conscience* is a person's core of traditions, the set of sanctioned values and thinking that exists deep within all of us that dictates how we must behave and what roles are "right" and "wrong" for us to fulfill. These prescriptions are taught to children as soon as they begin to grow, so the cultural conscience is very hard to change in an adult because it feels so natural and was planted so early.

Lady Sings the Blues

"The first problem for all of us, men and women, is not to learn, but to unlearn." —Gloria Steinem, author and feminist.

For centuries we've been taught to be ladies—speak when spoken to, go along to get along, smile and look pretty, and be the hostess with the mostest. These rules dominate our *cultural conscience*—that voice inside of us that tells us what is right, wrong, feminine, masculine, appropriate, and inappropriate for us as women and men.

Despite the sweeping social changes that have earned women positions as corporate executives and planted some men in the kitchen, deep down, most of us still live by the traditional rules. Let's take a look at the cultural code of conduct drummed into nearly every woman's brain from the time she's born. No matter how liberated you think you are, these behavior codes influence you more than you might like to admit because they're an inescapable part of being in our society.

I call them the 10 cultural commandments because they seem to have been written in stone a long, long time ago. These cultural commandments are the ancient laws directing women's behavior down through the ages. Beware if you dare violate these laws, because shame and blame and the blues will be your consequence for being a "bad" woman.

Lisa knows the kind of blues that come from violating the cultural conscience. A 34-year-old single woman, she looks like the complete modern woman. Lisa is a successful salesperson for a software firm. She owns her own condo, drives a sports car, and dates men with "a future." But at night, she feels lonely and blue and worries about when she'll find the right man to share her future and have a family. Lisa desperately wants to believe that it's terrific to be single and free, but her cultural conscience haunts her with the opposite message: Unless she's married, with kids and the proverbial white picket fence, there's something deeply wrong with her as a woman.

What kind of cultural commandments put women like Lisa in such a classic lose/lose situation?

The 10 Commandments of the Female Cultural Conscience

I.	Thou shalt be of service to all but yourself.
II.	Thou shalt not take the name of men in vain.
III.	Thou shalt not threaten abandonment no matter how bad it gets.
IV.	Thou shalt be seen (and thou better look good!) and not heard.
V.	Thou shalt be emotionally dependent on men, no matter how much more money thou makes than he.
VI.	Thou shalt always be thin.
VII.	Thou shalt never grow old.
VIII.	Thou shalt serve men sexually whenever they wish.
IX.	Thou shalt never consider thy work more important than a man's.
X.	Thou shalt not assume any rights beyond what men have bestowed on thee.

In other words, thou might as well be a doormat!

These rules are so rigid that there is no way we can nurture our creativity, fulfill our dreams, enhance our self-esteem, or have any fun! But dare to challenge these rules and you'll be slapped with guilt and insecurity. And who said women don't have choices?

But these rules haven't held us back completely.

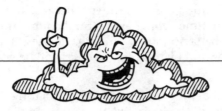

Funk-y Facts

About 25 percent of women experience depression at some time in their lives—more than twice as many as men. But specialists warn that these estimates may be too low because they are based on the number of people who seek treatment. Men are more reluctant than women to admit they feel depressed so they are less likely to seek help but may be just as depressed.

The traditional rules we've abided by have given us a chance to cultivate many useful talents and traits that can make us strong if we use them to our advantage.

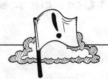

Blues Flag

If you ever catch yourself saying: "Nothing I do is ever good enough," or "I can't make the right choices," stop to think about which commandment you are violating. Then remind yourself that these cultural expectations don't have to determine your behavior anymore.

Because we were raised to take care of others, we know how to be intimate, compassionate, patient, sensitive, and good communicators. We know how to juggle many demands at once and be flexible as the needs of those around us change. These skills are key to becoming leaders, succeeding in any job, forming good relationships, fulfilling our potential, and leading a balanced and meaningful life.

Don't Throw Out the Baby with the Bath Water

Many of our traditions are worth keeping because they've served us well. Because of our cultural background, we tend to be intuitive, we know how to empower people, and we can keep communities together.

Can We Talk?

Because we haven't been able to speak out (that's not ladylike!), we've developed a keen intuition and ability to read expressions, body language, and other nonverbal cues. These skills are crucial in the business world, and men who generally are clueless about these nuances are finally realizing this is an area they need to master too.

More Power to You!

Women know how to make people feel strong, powerful, and confident. This ability to nurture makes us feel good and brings us closer to others. But sometimes in the process of bolstering other people's self-esteem, we neglect to pay attention to our own needs. Nurturing ourselves—reminding ourselves of our good qualities and potential—is key to successful blues management.

Home Sweet Home

Our cultural conscience reminds us that no matter how much we achieve, we are nothing without our families and close relationships. We organize birthday parties, family celebrations, and other activities to make friends and family members feel special. The drive to be connected to those we love helps us slow down when our lives get too hectic, forcing us to focus our attention on what's really important: people.

We Help Build Our Communities

Community connections enrich our lives and keep us healthy, and our traditional core tells us that taking care of the less fortunate is the right thing to do. That's why we volunteer at the local shelter, help out at the school fair, and make calls for charity donations. Feeling connected to a community makes us feel we are part of something larger than ourselves and keeps our lives in perspective.

All these traits can serve us well if we pay attention to our feelings and take care of our needs, too. The cultural conscience has taught us that one of the quickest ways to help ourselves is to help others. But whenever we give too much to others and don't get enough in return, our lives fall out of balance—and we get the blues.

How We Got Here

How did women get such a deal?

Women's cultural conscience flourished for centuries because the traditional roles worked well in those societies. The understanding was simple and clear-cut: Men controlled the power and resources and women supported the men in return for protection, food, shelter, and sometimes status.

But the 1960s changed all that.

For the first time since World War II more women were needed in the job market to meet service demands. So they flooded the market as secretaries, waitresses, and clerks—jobs they didn't necessarily find exciting but definitely more exciting than vacuuming, cooking, and cleaning. In her shockingly honest ground-breaking book *The Feminine Mystique* (Dell Publishing, 1989), Betty Friedan came out of the closet revealing that the lives of housewives were boring and full of emptiness.

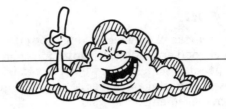

Funk-y Facts

Until the 19th century, the prevalent thought for why more women than men were struck with depression was that women were being punished for Eve's sin. The 19th-century rationalists dumped this theory, posing instead that women (upper-class women) got depressed because they were pursuing intellectual interests. Their cure: Devote more time to their husbands and children. And get plenty of rest.

Damned if You Do, Damned if You Don't

Today, traditional sex role expectations have reached crisis proportions. Most women have to work—yet our cultural conscience (as unmoving as the rock of Gibraltar) reminds us on a daily basis that we should be home with the kids baking cookies on rainy days, reading stories by the fireplace, and harvesting Kodak moments.

There are other mixed messages—in some cases outright lies—perpetuated by our cultural conscience:

Dr. Ellen Says

Having a job plays an important role in fighting the blues. A 20-year study by the Institute for Social Research and the National Center for Health Statistics revealed that employment outranks marriage and children as the most consistent tie to women's health. What keeps us healthy is having many sources of self-esteem. Women who have never worked outside the home have the highest levels of depression because all their self-esteem is usually based on one role: homemaker.

➤ We grow up with this illusion that our knight in shining armor will slip into our lives, knock us off our feet, and take care of all of our needs. But the fact is that the knight has got better things to do, since some men are opting for divorce rather than staying married. One-half of married women will get divorced when their knight's armor rusts and he bites the dust.

➤ Staying married doesn't fulfill us either, despite what society has taught us. A 25-year longitudinal study of college-educated women found that wives had the lowest self-esteem, felt the least attractive, and had little confidence in their abilities to do anything, including raising kids. The key reason housewives suffer from such low self-esteem is that their work is devalued by society.

➤ Working outside the home—a no-no according to society's traditional values—actually makes us feel better about ourselves because it creates multiple sources of self-esteem and achievement.

The bottom line is this: The more we stray from the script that society has written for us, the more distressed we're likely to feel because we are challenging the status quo and putting ourselves on the line. But sticking to the letter of the law offers us no relief either, since the rules are outdated and have little relevance to today's world.

It's a no-win situation. So it's no surprise that women get those Culture Blues!

Sexual Abuse, Tummy Tucks, and Other Social Downers

Let's take a look at the six types of blues that can stem from the conflicts caused by our cultural conscience. Most women will relate to some, if not all, of these. In upcoming chapters, we'll discuss how women can beat the blues in specific situations involving relationships, work, family, and other issues.

The Victim Blues

Many women haven't been trained to assert themselves in a conflict; they are taught to be nurturing and accommodating at all costs. So they often become victims of unfair and abusive treatment and assume that this is the price they have to pay just for being women.

Relationship Blues

Women feel bad for not having relationships or for having lousy ones. They tend to define themselves through their relationships, rather than their achievements, as men do. So when something goes wrong with a partner or friend, women blame themselves—and feel it's their responsibility to fix it at any emotional cost.

Because women are trained to think they are nothing without a man, they often feel incomplete without a relationship and then desperately seek one.

Age-Rage Blues

The blues really take off for many women when they realize they're growing older in a society that discounts anyone who isn't young and attractive. The cosmetic industry, media, and health-care system conspire to make women feel as if aging is a dreadful process that marks the beginning of the end.

Depletion Blues

Women are experiencing greater role overload than ever before. Society still expects them to be the primary caregiver of the family, but it also requires them to go out and make a living. As a result, women feel stressed out from trying to be in too many places at one time.

Body-Image Blues

Women put themselves down because they don't look like magazine cover girls—an impossible task since these images speak more to men's ideals of female beauty than any real depictions of women's bodies. These standards are set by multi-million dollar industries that benefit from women buying into diets, make-up, fashion, and cosmetic surgery.

Mind-Body Blues

Many women blame their blues on hormonal changes that take place during menstruation, after childbirth, and at menopause. While women do have some mood changes during these times in their lives, these don't fully account for the depression they experience. As women, we are raised to believe that our bodies are frail, that we can't take care of ourselves, and that somebody else must be in charge. Not taking charge of our bodies has various consequences: We blame ourselves for not feeling well when there is actually a physical problem that is making us sick. And when our stress is manifested in physical symptoms we don't realize that our bad moods are making us sick.

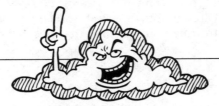

Funk-y Facts

Your hormones do alter your moods, but not enough to cause a real depression in most cases. According to a 1990 report issued by the American Psychological Association's National Task Force on Women and Depression—a task force I once headed—60 to 80 percent of women have some mild postpartum depression but it typically lasts only one to seven days. Most women don't plunge into depression after menopause, and, in fact, many experience what anthropologist Margaret Mead has called Post Menopausal Zest (PMZ), a surge of energy realized in part by the sense of freedom many women experience why they stop menstruating, when their kids are out of the house, and when they finally get to say what's on their minds. The women who experienced PMZ are those women who have resolved their Age-Rage Blues (see Chapter 12) and have broken free from society's stereotypes of aging as being a time of decline. And studies report that while 20 to 80 percent of women have some form of PMS, only 5 percent of them experience significant discomfort that requires treatment. So what looks like physical symptoms caused by hormonal imbalance are often untreated signs of depression.

Is the Culture Getting You Down?

To determine how much you are influenced by what others expect of you and whether this bothers you, take the following quiz.

How Much Are You Influenced by Others?

Answer the following questions "Yes" or "No."

1. When someone screams at you during a conflict, do you just sit there and take it or crawl into the nearest hole? *no*

2. Do you depend on someone else (parents, partners, relatives, or friends) to foot your bills? *no*

3. Do you feel significantly anxious and/or depressed about looking older and not looking as good as you once did? *no*

4. Do most of the compliments you get revolve around you being a great home-maker, hostess, volunteer, or other traditional role? *no*

5. Do you hold back your anger toward people instead of telling the person directly how you feel? *no*

6. Do you believe that by being a homemaker, you're not living up to your potential or doing enough with your life? *no*

7. Do you spend most of your time nurturing and caring for others and little on your own personal growth and achievements? *no*

8. Do you see your job as a burden that gets in the way of your marriage or raising your children? *no*

9. Are most of your relationships unequal in power, with you in the one-down position? *no*

10. Do you consistently put your partner's sexual pleasure ahead of your own? *no*

Total number of questions answered "Yes": ___

How did you do?

0–2 "Yes" answers: Congratulations! Your cultural conscience has made you a stronger person. You've chosen what you want from your life—rather than letting that choice be dictated by others—and you refuse to bend over backwards for others at the expense of yourself. This is the range we all want to attain! Keep tabs on yourself to make sure you continue to be at the helm of your future.

3–5 "Yes" answers: Your cultural conscience has taken a hold of you in ways that are not helpful. Your inside voice tells you what you should do but the inner voice clashes with outside demands and this conflict gives you the blues. Women in this group have their average share of problems because traditional expectations are placed on them in an increasingly nontraditional world.

6–8 "Yes" answers: Your traditional core is likely to get you down. Watch out! People in this group usually feel very conflicted about what they want out of life versus what they think they should want. The inside voice will probably win out, and you'll restrict your choices to accommodate others' wishes—an accommodation that will keep you in a vulnerable and dependent position. In that position, you are highly susceptible to the blues.

9–10 "Yes" answers: You're in trouble! If you don't tackle your conflicts with the cultural conscience and start taking control of your life, you're headed toward depression. This score indicates that you'll probably float in and out of depression most of your life because you let others take too much control. It's important that you see a mental health professional for treatment to resolve the conflicts. If you go it alone, you'll go down.

Guiltless Pleasures

To stop obsessing over a problem, take yourself to lunch, go for a walk in the park—do anything that will distract you from your thoughts. Studies show that women actually feel worse when they ruminate about their concerns. My advice: Wait until you cool down and can think more clearly before you tackle your problem and, in the meantime, go have a blast!

Don't Deny Who You Are

Maybe you thought you were free and pretty hip, but after doing these exercises, you discovered that you're more like the "good girl" you were raised to be. Here's one key piece of advice: DON'T DENY IT. If you do, you'll rob yourself of the chance to grapple with the conflicts that are holding you back from experiencing life more fully—and you won't be able to shake off the blues.

Confronting your fears is risky, but once you become more aware of how your past influenced you and learn ways to think more positively about yourself and your potential, you'll be faced with opportunities you've never imagined. And that's what freedom is all about!

Ditch Traditions That Chain You

Now that you know where you stand, you need to figure out which traditions work for you and which ones stand in the way of your progress.

Make a List, Check It Twice

Make a list of good things that are brought about by your cultural conscience (you know how to take care of people, you bring your family together, and so on). Then put the list someplace where you can see it so you can remind yourself of all the good qualities you have. Remind yourself every day about the good things you do because of the good values you have from those traditions.

Chart Your Pattern

To see where you stand on the continuum between traditional and nontraditional roles, draw a role line from 1 to 10, and make a list of what you've done for people over a one-month period. Evaluate each activity to determine the degree to which you played a traditional or nontraditional role and place a number nest to the activity.

Traditional   Nontraditional

1 _____ 2 _____ 3 _____ 4 _____ 5 _____ 6 _____ 7 _____ 8 _____ 9 _____ 10

Which end of the spectrum do you fall under on this chart? Did you fulfill more traditional or nontraditional roles?

If you clocked in at either end of the line you are likely to face more conflict, and you are more prone to getting the blues because your life isn't balanced. You want to fall somewhere between 3 and 7.

If you like this exercise, don't stop. Give your friends a copy of the chart and have them rate you on where they think you and they fall—and then talk about their perceptions (don't be mad if they pegged you as being traditional even though you've got green nail polish!). Also note in which direction your roles evolve over time. Are you becoming more traditional or nontraditional as you grow older? You may find that you are increasingly doing more of the house chores and taking on more of the expected traditional role. If that's the case, you need to figure out whether that's making you blue, and if so, take steps to share the load with other family members.

List Conflicts

Make a list of the conflicts you feel when your cultural conscience bumps up against pressures of daily life so that you can see when you get down on yourself and why. You'll feel more in control of your life after you write these feelings down because you'll understand where they come from. A few examples:

➤ *I'm never happy with my choices.* Many of us feel we've made the wrong decision regardless of whether we stay home or pursue a career or try something in between. We feel this way not because the choices we've made are bad, but because our culture tries to deny freedom of choice to women.

Dr. Ellen Says

On August 13, 1998, *USA Today* reported the findings of a new study of eighth-grade girls, which showed that the more girls endorse conventional femininity for women, the higher they scored on depression scales. According to Wellesley College psychologist Dr. Deborah Tolman, who reported the study's findings at the 1998 American Psychological Association conference in San Francisco, the notion of rigid sex roles squelch children's true identity. "Depression is about loss," Dr. Tolman says, "and what greater loss can there be than your self?"

➤ *Nothing I do is ever good enough.* When we do well at work, we feel guilty about not spending time with our kids. When we take too much time off from work to get involved with our kids, we feel we should be advancing our careers. We can't win because our culture expects us to be everything for everybody all at once.

➤ *My traditional voice won't let up.* No matter how much we disagree, we still hear voices deep inside saying things like "Who do you think you are?" or "Bad girl for not taking better care of her (mother/daughter)" or "You'll end up old and alone."

These conflicts create and maintain self-doubt and drain our energy because we're often fighting with ourselves.

What else is on your list?

These exercises and others in the book will put you more in touch with how you feel about your life and why those bad feelings are there. They are an example of how examining bad feelings can reap good results. If you are a woman living in today's society, you WILL get the blues at some time or another. It's unavoidable. But it's how you cope with them that makes all the difference in the world. And when you learn to convert the Culture Blues into new energy and wisdom, you have a new source of power that will help you achieve your goals.

The Least You Need to Know

➤ Women can beat the blues by learning how to undo ancient cultural commandments that still rule their choices in everyday life.

➤ Women get the blues because society encourages them to feel like victims and depend on others for their happiness. They become worn out, feel unattractive, and feel like prisoners to their hormones.

➤ Their cultural conscience taught women how to communicate, empower others, build communities, and maintain families; women must learn to use these traits to help themselves, too.

➤ Women need to identify which traditions serve them well and which ones get in the way, and then take action to remove the barriers to their fulfillment.

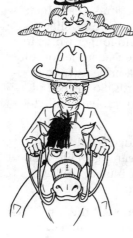

Chapter 4

Decoronation Blues: Even Jocks, Kings, and Cowboys Get the Blues

In This Chapter

➤ Masculinity in crisis

➤ Everyday blues in men's lives

➤ How some men suffer from "Alexithymia"

➤ How men may mask blues with physical symptoms

➤ The great things about being a guy

➤ The changes ahead as men learn to talk about their feelings—and listen

As we saw in the previous chapter, life for women hasn't exactly been a picnic as they fight to free themselves from the traditional chains that continue to restrain their potential. But men haven't exactly had it easy, either. Although it seems like they've got it made—they still control most of the world's institutions and much of its resources—guys are just as confused by the shifting roles and societal changes as the women they befriend, date, live with, or marry.

Many men today feel they're losing their "masculine" identity and they don't have anything to replace it. Society may be telling them that being "manly" is nothing to brag about. In addition to being the rational, strong, and protective guys they were raised to be, men are now expected to be emotional, empathetic, and communicative as well. Bred to be breadwinners, many men are now expected to leave the office early to do car pool while their wives are away on business trips.

These changes are confusing, disruptive, and disconcerting—and they form the basis of a new kind of blues which many men are experiencing for the first time. I call them the "Decoronation Blues" because the old male traditional role—the strong, silent, competent cowboy role that so many men have learned so well—no longer works in our Information/Interaction Age. And one of the worst parts of the Decoronation Blues is that many men can't even express their bad feelings and confusion because they don't have the emotional vocabulary to put their feelings into words. So instead of talking about what's bothering them—the healthy way to begin to resolve conflict—they just keep their problems bottled up.

By so doing, men are losing their opportunity to gain a deeper understanding of themselves, find out what they really want, and pursue a more meaningful life. And if the tension builds up inside for too long, men slide from feeling blue to feeling depressed, the serious condition that needs professional treatment.

And remember, the blues don't stay silent, no matter how often you tell them to "Shut up!" Over time silent blues evolve into mental and physical sicknesses, which can, in extreme cases, lead to death in the form of suicide or unnecessary heart attacks for a number of these unfortunate men.

The good news is that many men are fighting the Decoronation Blues and actively working to redefine what it means to be a man. They're doing major soul-searching to figure out what "male" traits are worth keeping and which ones should be discarded. In the process, they're learning to communicate better with themselves and others. In this chapter, we'll look at societal changes that have upset men's sense of self and what men can do to "get with the program," start talking, and develop their own practical action strategies to beat those Decoronation Blues! Although this chapter is directed toward men's concerns, women can benefit from reading it too so they can see where their guys are coming from when they react a certain way.

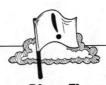

Blues Flag

Research shows that depression is twice as common in women than in men. But don't be fooled by the statistics. Many men who are depressed don't know they are suffering from this condition or aren't likely to admit it because such emotions are not considered manly. As a result, they never get professional help. Be smart and get a start: If you think you are depressed (take the quiz in Chapter 2), or someone else has suggested you are, get help!

Why Manly Men Get Mad

In the TV show *Leave It To Beaver*, which gave us a slice of 1950s America, Ward Cleaver came home after a long day at work to his wife, June—a thin, attractive, perky homemaker (a woman whose image feminists later used for target practice). June welcomed her husband into his palace with a hot meal on the table (never a TV dinner), a sparkling clean house, and a wide-open heart. June never asked Ward to babysit the Beaver, or vacuum the living room, or do car pool. His role was well defined: breadwinner. His success at it made him a happy man.

He and the Beaver never did do much hugging or talking about anything but sports. Guys just didn't do that type of thing back then. But that doesn't mean that Ward had no feelings. He was just trained not to show his emotions—and June never expected him to. The rigidity of these traditional male roles were limiting in so many ways, but the fact is that the roles worked well for a very long time. The economic needs of the Industrial Age demanded strict division of roles and labor between women and men.

It was very simple back then: The men brought home the bacon, and the women cooked it.

But the 1960s changed all that. The feminist movement and the influx of women into the work force shook up men and women and their image of themselves. Men were expected to help out with household chores, take a more active role in raising the children, and be more communicative. They were told to stop being so silent, protective, controlling, and aggressive, and to begin valuing relationships as much as they do achievement.

As a result, some men today are confused about what it means to be a man.

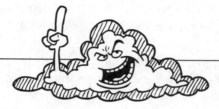

Funk-y Facts

Traditionally, research on gender differences shows that men and women exhibit depression in different ways. Although the lines between the way men and women react are becoming more blurred, and there are exceptions to the rule, when women get depressed, they generally show the typical signs of depression, like lethargy, loss of appetite, inability to concentrate or sleep through the night, crying, and hopelessness. But most men show their depression through actions, not words or exhibiting sad feelings. For example, depressed men tend to be angry or irritable, watch too much TV, drink, smoke, use drugs, overwork, overeat, or engage in other self-destructive activities.

What Lurks Behind the Facade

Men today have it tough in many ways—and they often get little sympathy from women or other men. Let's look at the sources of men's everyday blues:

➤ *Relationship blues.* Some men have trouble relating to women. They aren't sure how to act around them. Will they be slapped if they tell their usual dirty jokes? Thrown in court if they tell a woman she looks nice? They are trained to feel ashamed of needing intimacy and feel they've failed the new test of manhood if a women says, "How do you feel?" and they really don't have a clue. Or they *do* express how they feel and their partner snaps, "What's wrong with you! You shouldn't feel like that!" Yikes! No wonder silence is golden and feels like the smartest response to so many men.

➤ *No-Control blues.* Women are often victims of physical and sexual assaults as well as emotional abuse. But men are victims too—they often have little control over changes at work and believe they are unjustly blamed for making the women in their lives miserable. Older men are shamed for being inadequate fathers who are not home enough for the kids and younger men are increasingly victims of physical assault.

➤ *Getting-Older blues.* Older men may seem distinguished, but deep down inside many feel exhausted and extinguished. Their sexual hormones are pooping out right at the time their wives are feeling more feisty. Many begin to feel useless and depressed before they retire, as they see younger professionals stepping in to take their place. They may feel even more depressed after they retire, when their most meaningful daily activity is accompanying their wives to the mall to watch them shop.

➤ *Burnout blues.* More than ever, men have to worker harder to keep up with the frantic pace of today's world, often trying to cram 48 hours into 24. They hustle and bustle from work to child-care facilities, then bring home more work to do at night. Or they're single and expected to work 12- to 14-hour days. Work demands at the office or factory have never been more intense, while the amount of leisure time consistently shrinks.

➤ *Biceps blues.* Body image problems are usually much stronger in women than in men. But the biceps blues are rapidly growing for some men, too. Balding men desperately search for hair; flabby guys dream about washboard stomachs. Men who feel physically unattractive are beginning to take it personally, just like women have for so many centuries. Men who feel ugly in even a tiny part of their body tend to feel defective and worthless as an entire person.

➤ *Provider blues.* Men, especially those over 35, are conditioned to believe they must be breadwinners for the family. Their self-esteem depends on how much they achieve through work. When

Dr. Ellen Says

Cowboys would feel a heck of a lot better if they acknowledged that they have good reasons to be confused in a world that has been turned upside down in terms of traditional roles. According to Gail Sheehy, author of the groundbreaking book *Understanding Men's Passages* (Random House, 1998), almost a third of the working wives in America today (a total of 10.2 million women) earn more than their husbands.

their wives slip on their pumps and race off to work in the morning, some men feel that they've failed to provide for the family. When she returns exhausted at the end of her work day and blames him for not making enough money, he feels defeated again.

➤ *Decoronation blues.* Men are no longer the king at home or at work. And they don't like it. Instead of making the rules, men increasingly have to abide by them. Women have been taught early on how to deal with change, especially role changes. But men haven't, so they are having trouble adapting to being treated like one of their former subjects. Some older men in moments of honesty will tell you how much they hate giving up being king, and they won't let go without a battle.

Given all these social changes, we'd be suspicious if cowboys *didn't* get the blues! But good luck trying to get them to admit it. Women often harp on guys for not expressing their feelings, but can you blame them? From as far back as they can remember, men have been told to keep their feelings to themselves or they were wimps. By the time they got to be grown-ups they forgot they had any feelings. So often, men who have the blues don't even know they're feeling bad! Which is why when their women ask what's wrong, guys mutter "Nothing." Guess what, gals: Guys aren't holding back juicy information. From their perspective, when they say nothing's wrong they are telling you the truth! They don't feel it so they can't say it.

A Horse with a Name, Finally

There is actually a clinical name for men being unable to identify and express emotions. According to Dr. Ronald F. Levant of Villanova University, author of *Masculinity Reconstructed: Changing The Rules of Manhood—At Work, In Relationships, And In Family Life* (Penguin, 1995), men suffer from a common condition known as *Alexithymia*, a term Levant resurrected, which literally means "without words for emotions." This condition, says Dr. Levant, is so common that men don't even think of it as a problem.

In fact, when harangued by women for not saying what they feel or for acting distant, men often bark back: "That's just the way men are." This comment disarms many women. How do you argue with that? But research shows that men aren't and haven't always been that way—and, in fact, baby boys are said to be a lot more expressive than girls when they are born.

So what happened? Moms and dads—prompted by social norms of what behavior is and isn't acceptable for men—made sure their boys learned to control their emotions.

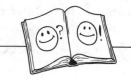

Terms of Encheerment

Alexithymia means "without words for emotions"—a condition that many men suffer from because they can't express their emotions.

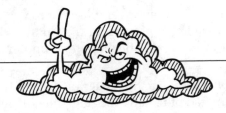

Funk-y Facts

The consequences of not knowing how you feel can be disastrous. Emotional numbness/ deadness often leads to physical health problems and clinical depression, and this can lead, in extreme cases, to suicide. Sadly, men are the leaders in the suicide department. Women try suicide three times more often than men, but men succeed at suicide three times more often than women. The reason: Men are more likely to complete the task with a more action-oriented weapon than, for instance, pills, which are what many women resort to, or a means to end their life. The highest suicide risk is the older man who uses a gun to end his life because he's sure there's no hope and no help.

Hey Mom, Quit Looking at Me Like That!

Earlier research has indicated, according to Dr. Levant, that when baby boys smiled at their mothers, their mothers smiled back at them more consistently than they did to their girls. For a long time, our culture favored male babies and catered to their needs. Mothers were afraid they would upset their temperamental boys if they didn't coo and goo with them, because their boys startled more easily, cried more often, and had more mood fluctuations. But something got screwed up because when their boy's expressions were unhappy, the moms didn't respond. Cowboy training to be alone and self-sufficient begins very early.

So boys learned that unhappy emotions are bad. Moms also didn't prompt their boy babies to have different emotional reactions but went all out for their girls, making all kinds of funny, sad, and mad faces.

As a result, baby boys grow up with a limited repertoire of emotional reactions.

Stand Up and Walk Tall, Son

Many dads, on the other hand, don't really notice they have a son until the kid turns 13 months and begins to stand on his own two feet, Dr. Levant points out. Then the dad sees a boy who will someday play ball, feed his family, and fix the porch window. He interacts with his son twice as much as he would with his daughter because he can identify so much more with another male and his potential helpful role.

Some dads also initiate their sons into the world of men by teaching them that fear and vulnerability are bad emotions that should be stifled. "Big boys don't cry," many dads tell their six-year-olds when they come home wailing from a scraped knee they got in soccer. "Don't be afraid, act like a man," is another bit of advice many dads pass along when being ridiculed at school creates misty eyes in their young sons.

If admitting you are scared or hurt is so bad—and if you admired your dad, the person who taught you these rules—why would you admit having these feelings? So it makes perfect sense that men just shut down! And when you're closed off like that, of course you aren't going to know you're having an emotional reaction, much less what words to use to describe how you're feeling.

Use It or Lose It

Being disconnected from yourself and others is one of the most damaging things you can do to your health and even your wealth. Men who don't realize they are feeling bad lose their jobs, mess up their relationships, and destroy their own self-image without knowing what's happening. Consider these examples:

➤ *Clueless at home.* A man who doesn't realize he said something hurtful to his wife, for instance, probably won't apologize. And if he keeps saying nasty things to her without saying he is sorry, he may lose her. A man who has a stronger relationship with his TV than with his wife will be abandoned by her first emotionally and then physically and not have a clue as to why.

➤ *Clueless at work.* A man who doesn't feel upset at the wrath of his boss may lose his job because he's ignoring the fact that the boss will fire him if he doesn't shape up his poor performance.

Simply put, a man who is unaware of his emotions can't live a meaningful life since he doesn't have the emotional compass to guide him on the path between health and illness and love and loneliness. If he doesn't recognize he is having an emotional reaction, he can't figure out what went wrong in the first place that made him feel so terrible. But just because he is unaware of his emotions doesn't mean that he isn't experiencing feelings. The feelings are very much there, but they are coming out in physical symptoms.

What he does feel, though, is pressure, in the heart, the head, and the gut. Over time, pressure builds up

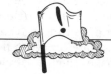

Blues Flag

Feel like you're about to scream at someone or hit them? Think, whisper, or yell: "STOP!!!" Take three deep breaths, take a five-minute walk, tell the person you'll get back to them later. Use the time out to gain control of yourself and your anger and figure out what's making you mad. Don't let your anger build up inside; if it does, pick out a strategic action plan to deal with the anger before you act, like hitting a basket of golf balls or going for a walk to let off steam.

until it explodes in some self-destructive act. On the other hand, some kinds of pressure can be good. If pressure gets him to think about what's wrong and pushes him to change the way he thinks or acts, he'll become healthier, stronger, and more skilled as a problem solver no matter what curve ball life throws him.

Real Men Mask Their Blues

When emotions are not verbally expressed, they get expressed internally. Men rarely talk about what's bothering them, but when something is making them anxious their hearts race, they get headaches, or they have other physical symptoms that signal there is trouble in paradise.

Not Tonight, Dear, I Have a Headache

When we get the everyday blues, we are likely to get the following symptoms:

➤ Headaches

➤ Stomachaches and gastrointestinal problems

➤ High blood pressure

➤ Back pain

Because many men focus on these physical symptoms when they are blue, they may worry that something awful is happening to them. If they have a small cyst, they're sure it's cancer. If they urinate too often at night, they're convinced they've got prostate cancer. A headache is a sign of a brain tumor. Their catastrophic thinking makes them so afraid and uneasy, they avoid the doctor and usually make their problems worse.

Men Self-Destruct Instead of Interact

When men feel down, they tend to distract themselves with an activity so they don't focus on their lousy mood. Sounds good to me! That's better than what women tend to do, which is obsess over why they feel so bad. According to Dr. Susan Nolen-Hoeksma, author of *Sex Differences In Depression* (Stanford University Press, 1990), the distractions can be helpful *if* they create energy and help people feel better first. Later on when they have more positive energy, they can figure out why they felt so bad in the first place.

But if men never investigate the origins of their bad moods and keep distracting themselves every time they feel miserable, they may be heading for trouble. The bad feelings may go away at first, but they are likely to keep coming back with more regularity and intensity, until they turn into depression.

Often, destructive behaviors become destructive behaviors. Consider these facts:

➤ More men than women are likely to smoke and use drugs and alcohol to medicate bad feelings.

➤ More men than women develop heart disease—the leading cause of death in this country—because they are more likely to overeat, smoke, and drink alcohol.

➤ Although they are aware of physical problems, many men put off seeing or refuse to see a doctor for a diagnosis. They ignore signs of something wrong with their health because they are not

trained to feel, think, or talk about problems. They've mastered cowboy lesson #1: Avoid vulnerability at all cost, even if, in some extreme cases, it means death.

Guiltless Pleasures

Call up a good friend to ask her out on a date or arrange for a romantic dinner for you and your spouse. Recent research in Dr. Dean Ornish's excellent new book *Love and Survival: The Scientific Basis For The Healing Power of Intimacy* (Harper-Collins, 1998) says that the number one factor in keeping us healthy is connection, love, and intimacy—not diet, exercise, or work.

➤ Many men feel that if they can't avoid vulnerability, they should head for the range, fast. This is cowboy lesson #2: Go herd some cows until you feel stronger but don't reveal your fears or tears to anyone along the way. When men feel vulnerable, they're trained to go off alone and not share their burdens with anyone but their horse, dog, or fishing pole.

Men Are a Changin'

Recent research (and our boyfriends and partners) report that all this turmoil has led to a good thing: Men are reassessing the values, duties, and roles they were raised with to figure out why they are catching so much flack from their girlfriends or wives, why they are so miserable at work, and why everything is going wrong when they thought they were doing it right. And what they're finding out is that, like women, they'll have to change or modify the way they think and act if they want to feel better about their lives. A lawyer who hates his job but feels he must keep it since he is the sole provider of his family, may, for instance, ask himself:

➤ If my wife also worked, could I try to find a different job that's more fulfilling?

➤ Would I really feel like I'm abdicating (that's a word a lawyer would use) my responsibilities as a man if my wife also made money?

➤ Do I really want to spend more time with my kids, or is work a good excuse to avoid the hassles of taking care of them?

He may, for instance, find out that his wife wanted to go back to work but thought he wanted her to stay home. And that having his wife work would take some pressure off him so he could look for a better job and come home in a better mood. He'd have to lose being a cowboy and accept that not being the sole provider doesn't make him less of a man.

But that's not so bad. While some traits may be worth abandoning, most characteristics that men were raised with are worth keeping and enhancing to fit changing circumstances. Men get bad press so often, it's easy for them to forget what's good about them.

What's Great About Being a Guy?

There are many traditional aspects of being a guy that are great and worth keeping. In his book *Staying the Course* (Fawcett Columbine, 1990), author Robert Weiss found that male professionals from the ages of 35 to 55 consistently demonstrated "resilience, determination, competence, and self-sufficiency as the basis of manhood." They were constantly struggling to be "good men" and "stay the course." Some women, of course, also possess these qualities, but it's more traditional for men. Besides these traits, here are some other qualities that are great about being a guy:

➤ *Action-oriented.* Guys are trained for action, and they're often great problem solvers. This is an important skill because they don't get stuck moaning and groaning about a problem as women sometimes do, but they focus on what can be done and then do it.

➤ *Provider skills.* Men futz around the house, fixing and building things because they want their partners to have "a good roof over their heads." They want to take care of their families—and this is a critical contribution to the health of our families and our society.

➤ *The Titanic response.* "Women and children first," men will shout at the scene of an accident, a fire, or some other disaster. Many men will risk their lives to save others, and in less dramatic situations, men often put the health and safety needs of others before their own. How's that for real courage and compassion!

➤ *He ain't heavy—he's my brother.* Men work their tails off because they've made a commitment to do their best and "no man breaks his promise." When the going gets tough, guys stick with it. This is critical to building trust and healing fears of abandonment loved ones may have.

What's Good About You?

To think about what being a man means to you, continue this list or write out your own to include other male traits that you believe are useful. If you just can't do it, ask a loved one to list what she feels are your strengths. Keep this list handy so you can refer to it when someone blames you for being a "typical guy." Frequent reminders of your good qualities will automatically lift your mood so that you can, later on, analyze what upset you in the first place and decide what you can do to fix it.

Feelings 101

Talking about figuring out why you are upset is putting the cart before the horse. Many men first need to identify when they are having an emotional reaction. Dr. Levant and a number of other psychologists, including Dr. William Pollack at Harvard Medical School, have developed a number of exercises to help men learn to feel and manage their emotions. They suggest that the first step for men is to pay more attention to their various physical symptoms. Dr. Levant suggests that men keep a daily log for a week listing each time they feel what he calls the "buzz"—the physiological component of emotion.

Log on Your Physical Symptoms

Log each "buzz" you experience that day, followed by a description of the physical sensation. After that, put down the time it occurred, the event that triggered it, or the context in which it happened (in other words what was going on when you became aware of that feeling). The event, Dr. Levant points out, could be "Boss slapped report on my desk," or "Colleagues talk about new Lexus."

The physical symptom that accompanies the buzz might be:

➤ Tightness in the throat, chest, or forehead

➤ Clenching your gut

➤ Grinding your teeth

➤ Feeling antsy

Once you can identify when you are having an emotional reaction, then you are ready to label what it is you are feeling.

Name That Emotion

The world of emotions has a language of its own and many men don't know it. The following exercises can help you develop an emotional vocabulary, which, in turn, will make you aware of different feelings and more able to express them and get support. Study the following emotional vocabulary words (listed in levels of intensity from strong to mild), adapted from Roger T. Crenshaw's book *Expressing Your Feelings* (La Jolla, CA, 1989).

Make a copy of this list and keep it with you when you need a reminder to pay attention to your feelings. Then try the "emotional management training" exercises listed on the next page.

Happy	Thrilled, fantastic, terrific, ecstatic, exhilarated, turned on, delighted, great, serene, wonderful, cheerful, glowing, jovial, neat, glad, good, satisfied, gratified, pleasant, fine
Caring	Tenderness toward, affection for, adoration, loving, infatuated, enamored, idolize, fond of, admiration, concern for, respectful, turned on, trust, close, warm toward, friendly, positive toward
Depressed	Desolate, dejected, gloomy, dismal, bleak, in despair, barren, grief, grim, upset, downcast, pessimistic, miserable, weepy, rotten, awful, blue, terrible, unhappy, down, low, bad, blah, sad, glum
Inadequate	Worthless, good for nothing, powerless, crippled, impotent, inferior, emasculated, useless, like a failure, defeated, incompetent, inept, deficient, insignificant, unimportant, no good, lacking confidence, uncertain
Fearful	Frightened, intimidated, terror-stricken, dread, vulnerable, paralyzed, afraid, shaky, risky, alarmed, awkward, defensive, nervous, anxious, hesitant, timid, shy, worried, ill at ease, jittery, on edge, uncomfortable, self-conscious

➤ After reading in the newspaper or seeing an upsetting story on TV, look at your emotional vocabulary list and decide which words apply to the story. Ask others how they feel about the story or a recent movie. Learn to connect the best word to the situation.

➤ Select three emotional words a day or week and see how many times you can use them appropriately.

➤ Study characters on TV or in the movies and watch people at home and work to see how and when they express feelings in words and body language. Try to increase your feeling words when you speak. Model and imitate how others do it.

➤ Use a golf counter or a tally sheet to count off how many feelings you have in an hour. Note what kind you tend to have and how you can expand your repertoire.

➤ Ask someone you trust to be a feelings coach. Just like a football game, have them tell you what feelings fit for what situation and how to move the emotional ball down the field.

➤ Talk to someone you trust—females tend to be better navigators here—and say, simply: "I'm trying to figure out how I feel. Can you help me do a reality check?" Sample questions could be: "Am I drinking too much?" or "Do I seem more irritable these days?" or "Am I showing enough love?"

➤ If you feel too self-conscious doing this, or if you can't stand the thought of saying these words to anyone, assess yourself. Ask yourself these questions in a feelings journal and write the answers as honestly as possible.

Other Blues-Busting Strategies

Everybody has a hard time changing the way they think and act, but for men, learning and using an emotional vocabulary can be a particularly effective way to beat the Decoronation Blues. Other strategies that help men beat the blues are:

➤ Get involved with sports to release steam at the end of a depressing or frustrating day. Hitting a bucket of golf balls after work has saved more than one marriage and turned many blue moods to bright colors.

➤ Discover creativity as a way to express how you feel. Most men in our society are cut off from their creativity at a young age because they're told it's irrelevant or sissy; but creative expression has always been a great way to convert blue moods into positive energy, increased productivity, and a satisfying release of feelings.

➤ Command respect from those around you, whether it's younger Generation-X workers or your spoiled children. Learn how to effectively communicate to let someone know he or she is being disrespectful to you. Suggest what they can say instead. Read books on positive communication or attend a class or workshop in how to set boundaries and say "Not okay!"

For men to break through these barriers, they must challenge their assumptions about how they are supposed to be and come to some satisfying definitions of strength and masculinity. This modernization of the old cowboy role is as much a part of the men's movement as feminism is to women's liberation and will lead to more freedom and health for both men and women.

The Least You Need to Know

➤ Men are in a state of crisis as they are forced to redefine "masculinity."

➤ Men often experience everyday blues because they no longer feel in control of their relationships and/or work.

➤ When men feel depressed, they often focus on physical symptoms such as headaches, high blood pressure, and backaches.

➤ Being a guy is great in many ways: Guys are trained to be problem-solvers, hard workers, and responsible.

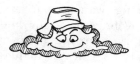
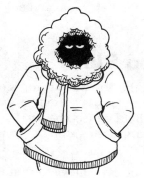

Chapter 5

Seasonal Blues Busters: One Month at a Time

In This Chapter

➤ With every season, there is a reason

➤ Bad news: Is it SAD or the blues?

➤ Brighten up your life with some light

➤ Sure-fire winter blues busters

➤ When the holidays bring you down

➤ Keep the Seasonal Blues away with action strategies for every month

January 2 brings the New Year for sure, but it also ushers in the season of the bear. A grizzly bear, in fact. And you don't have to visit the zoo to see this bear. You just have to visit me. I look more like a bear with those extra pounds from the holidays, and it's my season to be grumpy. The holiday cheer has faded, the light is low, and the work demands are high. School is starting again and the kids are grumpy too, from post-holiday recovery. All I want to do is make a big vat of lentil soup, turn off my answering machine, cell phone, and e-mail, and hibernate in my cave.

Do you have your own season of the bear? I call these blah moods the Seasonal Blues because these sad, gloomy emotions tend to emerge at the same time each season in reaction to what's happening with Mother Nature, in the culture, or as an anniversary reaction. Birthdays, Mother's or Father's Day, the holidays, the beginning or end of school—all can bring on the Seasonal Blues because they may remind us of failed relationships, family strife, time passing, unfulfilled dreams and dashed hopes, or a time that someone we loved died.

But you can learn to cope with the bear inside of you by being aware of your Seasonal Blues and recognizing that it's normal to have these funky feelings at certain times of the year. You can take steps to reduce the stress that usually accompanies the many seasons of your life. In this chapter we identify the various types of Seasonal Blues—and describe the action strategies that will help you overcome these blues and enjoy all the seasons of your life!

The SAD Story: Why Gray Makes You Blue

Right about the beginning of April, the weather warms up, the flowers start to bloom, and New Yorkers regain their sunny disposition (joke, joke…I know we aren't exactly known for our pleasant dispositions *any* time of the year). But I do feel the bear lumbering out of her cave, stretching and smiling in the warm spring sun. I'm coming alive again. YES!

To see what has happened to the world while I've been in the cave, I love to climb up to the roof of our brownstone. It's a special place for an urban dweller because we have a 360-degree view of downtown Brooklyn, downtown Manhattan, Staten Island, and the Hudson River. Gazing at the towering Manhattan skyline and the powerful Statue of Liberty in the harbor, I'm reminded again of the beauty and importance of freedom (especially from the blues).

Less lofty than these mental musings is the fact that I'm probably up there because of my basic biology. Like a hibernating grizzly bear, I've been stuck in semidarkness for the past four months and my body craves the light of the open sky.

There's no question that the change of weather affects our moods, thoughts, and behavior much more than most of us realize—and each person has a different reaction to the seasons. For most people, though, the transition to winter seems to be the toughest adjustment, and that's when they are most vulnerable to getting the Seasonal Blues, a sad, gloomy mood brought on by cold weather and the knowledge that a long, dark, often lonely winter is approaching.

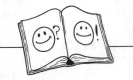

Terms of Encheerment

Seasonal Affective Disorder (SAD) is a form of clinical depression that starts in the autumn and lasts until spring, typically affecting people on gloomy winter days.

Thirty-Five Million Americans Can't Be Wrong

Nearly 25 million Americans fret and kvetch when the weather starts getting cold, but they can still get up in the morning and go to work, according to the National Institutes of Mental Health. But another 10 million people are so upset by the change of weather that they become quite dysfunctional and fall into a clinical depression—a condition that's now diagnosed as *Seasonal Affective Disorder (SAD)*. The depression usually starts in the autumn (October or November) when the light starts to diminish and lasts until spring when the light brightens and lengthens. This seasonal depression is usually accompanied by a craving for carbohydrates and sweet foods, weight gain, lethargy, and irritability. The depression can be so crippling that it may prevent people from going to work or taking care of their families; but usually it's just a sad and bad feeling that makes life more difficult until the person is exposed again to adequate amounts of light. A small percentage of people also get Summer Blues.

In *Winter Blues* (Guilford Press, 1993), Dr. Norman E. Rosenthal, a pioneer in the field of seasonal studies and the foremost authority on SAD, describes the lives of people afflicted with this form of depression. In the following quote, excerpted from his book, a woman describes the transformation of her mother's personality when the seasons change. Her elderly mother had suffered from SAD her entire life:

> *In late spring or early summer she is full of energy, requiring only five or six hours of sleep. She talks incessantly and tries to do too many things. Then in late fall (occasionally she makes it to Christmas), her personality takes a complete turn. She sleeps 12 hours at night, cries all morning, and then takes a nap. She won't drive the car, seldom leaves the house, and won't answer the telephone.*

It makes me sad to think of how many people suffer from SAD and don't know that shedding a little light into their life can brighten up their perspective.

When SAD Symptoms Surface

SAD is four times as common among women than men, but it afflicts people of all ages. The degree of seasonal difficulties varies from one person to the next, Dr. Rosenthal says. Someone may feel SAD symptoms in September, where others won't get hit with any powerful emotions until after Christmas, like the kind I experience. A severely affected person may come out from the winter slump in April, where someone who is only mildly affected may fully recover by mid March.

If you get into a funk when the days get shorter and the nights get longer, it's very important to distinguish whether you are experiencing a bout of the Seasonal Blues or a case of SAD. Look out for the following SAD symptoms:

➤ Extreme fatigue and lack of energy

➤ Inability to focus and concentrate for long periods of time

➤ Increased need for sleep or sleeping much more than usual

➤ Carbohydrate craving and increased appetite

➤ Weight gain

➤ Feelings of depression (see Chapter 2, "The Big Bad Blues Can Get You Too!" for a complete list of the symptoms of depression to see if you're a candidate)

If you are experiencing these symptoms daily for more than two weeks, you may be suffering from SAD, and I encourage you to seek professional help. See Appendix B, "Resources," for a list of resources for SAD diagnosis and available treatment.

All You Need Is Light (Most of the Time)

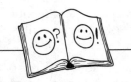

Terms of Encheerment

Light therapy involves daily exposure to a bright light, which can help alleviate or cure SAD symptoms. One theory for why light therapy works suggests that a person with SAD has something wrong with his or her biological clock in the brain that regulates hormones, sleep, and mood. As a result, the clock runs slower in the winter. Exposing the person to bright light helps to reset their clock and restore normal functioning and energy levels.

The happy news for SAD patients is that this form of depression is the most easily curable of all. Usually all you need is light and a chance to talk out your problems. Many patients who suffer from SAD can improve their moods with *light therapy*, which involves being exposed to a bright, artificial light of a certain intensity.

As little as 30 minutes per day of sitting near a light box made especially for beating the blues can make a huge difference in 60 to 80 percent of SAD patients, and this light can be purchased through companies which make products that simulate natural light. The side effects of light therapy are mild to nonexistent. But if you have other medical conditions or are taking medications, you need to check with your doctor about whether light therapy is safe for you.

If light therapy doesn't work, or if it lifts your mood only slightly but not enough so that you're functioning normally, you need to talk to your doctor about it. He or she may refer you to a psychiatrist who may suggest you also take antidepressant medication—at least during the season—to alleviate the symptoms of SAD and the underlying depression you're probably experiencing.

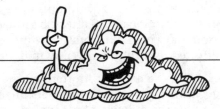

Funk-y Facts

Treatment with artificial light can also help children with SAD, according to the *Journal of the American Academy of Child and Adolescent Psychiatry*. In one recent study, 13 children and teens with SAD were exposed to low-intensity light for two hours each morning, and to high-intensity light for one hour a day in the afternoon or early evening. They sat about 18 inches from the light box while playing, reading, or watching TV. The results: 80 percent of the children reported feeling better while on light therapy. So if you have a gloomy winter child who has a positive personality transformation in the spring and summer, see a doctor and consider giving a light box to the little one as a gift for the holidays.

Other Cures for the Winter Blahs

Whether you've been diagnosed with SAD or are just experiencing Seasonal Blues, there are many things you can do in addition to light therapy to boost your mood. In his book, Dr. Rosenthal suggests that you brighten up your environment—ranging from trimming the hedges around the windows to putting in skylights to buying cars with sunroofs. (You guessed it—our van has a sun roof *and* a moon roof. The most impractical luxury for New York City, but a necessity for me to get more light so I can fight those Seasonal Blues and bear tendencies.) He also suggests that you consider the following options:

➤ *Keep warm.* Cranking up the heat along with shining a bright light has helped many patients combat symptoms of SAD. There are even fashionable visors available with a light inside so your therapy is portable and you look cool.

➤ *Forget the ski vacations.* During winter, head down south for a week or two where the weather is warmer and the sun is shining.

➤ *Exercise outdoors as much as possible when it's sunny.* In addition to improving your mood, exercise will help you keep your weight down—a problem for many people stricken by the winter blahs. If you can't exercise outdoors, you must, must, must exercise indoors. Lift free weights, ride an exercise bike, do push-ups, or jump rope, but whatever you do, MOVE! If you don't, the bear will take over your body and your mind for the entire winter season and you'll feel grizzled and grizzly by spring.

➤ *Manage your stress.* Avoid having to make important decisions—such as buying a house or picking a new career—during the winter months, when you are at your lowest point. Save big decisions for the warmer months, when you can think more clearly and more optimistically and with more energy.

Holiday Blues: 'Tis the Season to Be Grumpy

The winter weather produces one type of Seasonal Blues that we try to overcome by spending more time in the sun. Holidays can trigger another type of Seasonal Blues as we grapple with sad thoughts about our troubled families, bad memories from our youths, or other disappointments. And we are all supposed to be having such a great time!

Just preparing for the holidays is stressful enough. If you're a working parent, your work demands double or triple during this time of year and you just know that your biggest present of all will be a whopping case of the Burnout Blues (see Chapter 13, "Battling the Burnout Blues"). We fight the crowds at the malls, wait in long lines at the supermarket and post office, spend hours cleaning our homes and cooking huge dinners—in addition to working all day and taking care of our children. By the time the guests and family arrive, we're ready to smash the sleigh bells, strangle Santa, and stuff him back in the chimney!

Are we having fun yet? And then there's dealing with your family of origin: never easy and seldom fun. We all want to have a perfect, idyllic holiday like the families in Norman Rockwell paintings. And sometimes it starts out that way, but things deteriorate quickly. Instead of telling your mother how much you love her, you get mad at her for criticizing your child-rearing methods. You want to declare a truce with your brother, but you lose it when he starts bragging about his annual income again. And you want to enjoy your children's company, but you are horrified when, after opening up 20 presents each, they whine: "Is this all there is?"

If this scenario describes your feelings around the holidays, you couldn't be more normal. Even many of the people who are normally calm, happy, and content get all frazzled during the holidays and eat too much, sleep too little, and generally feel despondent. How did the holidays get to be this way?

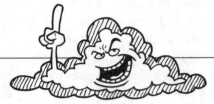

Funk-y Facts

I consulted on a research study during the 1997 holiday season for Pacific Health Laboratories, the makers of ProSol Plus, a natural therapy containing St. John's Wort, ginkgo biloba, and four essential vitamins. Pacific Health Laboratories wanted to know if the holiday blues were a media myth or a time for real Seasonal Blues. Results, which were published in *USA Today*, found that nearly 40 percent of Americans do suffer from the blues during or after the holiday season. The main reason: financial worries and separation from family. About 34 percent of the men and 44 percent of the women who responded to the survey said they got the blues. Take a closer look at the findings and you'll see that men and women do not have the same holiday blues. Men have more money blues and women have more relationship blues:

Reasons Cited	Women	Men
Financial concerns	10%	28%
Missing family/friends	13%	12%
Loss of loved ones	17%	3%
Post–holiday letdown	12%	6%
Stress	9%	4%

But you don't have to live with the Seasonal Blues forever. There is a lot you can do to manage your stress so you don't have to banish your family from your property forever or remain in permanent exile from the family campfires!

Santa's Tips for a Stress-Free Holiday

Holiday depression can happen during any holiday, but it strikes particularly hard in December when the world seems to be celebrating Christmas and Hanukkah. Typically, the holiday blues are short-lived, lasting anywhere from a few days to a few weeks prior to or just after the holiday. Symptoms of the holiday blues may include headaches, inability to sleep or sleeping too much, changes in appetite causing weight loss or gain, agitation and anxiety, excessive feelings of guilt, less ability to think clearly, and decreased interest in activities you once enjoyed, including food and sex.

Here are some suggestions that may help you manage the holiday blues. They are based on what has worked for me and my clients and gotten all of us through the holidays so we could live to tell the tale!

➤ Get organized so you don't leave all the chores for the last minute. If you celebrate Christmas or Hanukkah, start buying the presents in advance when the stores aren't crowded. In the spring and summer, when you see something for Aunt Sarah, buy it and save it. Wrap the gifts and store them in the closet until the time comes.

➤ Several weeks before the holidays, make a list of everything you need to do and prioritize it in order of importance. Can something wait until after the holidays?

➤ Ask yourself what you can delegate to others. Usually one-third to one-half of what we think must get done (and that we are the only ones who can do it) can either be forgotten or delegated to someone else during the holidays. Let go of the need to control and your holiday blues can disappear along with your list of "shoulds."

➤ Keep expectations reasonable by not trying to make this holiday "the best ever." Also be realistic about what you'll be able to do (in terms of cooking, entertaining, and so on) so you don't set yourself up for failure. For example, instead of bringing a homemade goodie to the holiday party, bring a store-made delicacy you pick up after work. Say "Yes, thanks, how about...?" when someone asks if there's anything they can bring to your dinner party.

➤ If you're feeling sad that your life isn't going right or if you're lonely because you don't have a partner or you're without family, don't get bogged down in the blues. Loneliness is a major source of stress, so I strongly advise you to get involved with the church, synagogue, or other volunteer organizations during the holidays. Volunteer to help at a soup kitchen, wrap presents for the Salvation Army, take a kid out who lost a parent to divorce or death and is sad. Helping others is the fastest way to help yourself, especially during the holidays.

➤ Don't expect that your holiday will be like it used to be when you were young, whether that was good or bad. You have changed, family members have changed, and so have circumstances. If you're craving the familiar feelings of childhood, look at your photo album, dig out the home videos, or work on developing your own traditions in your current family or among your friends.

Dr. Ellen Says

Want to lift the holiday blues? Put on a happy face. Really, just smile—a nice, full-faced grin will make you feel happier. Why does this happen? According to psychologist Robert Cooper, smiling transmits nerve impulses from the facial muscles to the part of the brain that controls emotions. Smiling tilts the body's neurochemical balance away from depression and toward mood elevation. So "act as if," and soon your mood will follow your behavior. You'll be smiling more on the inside too!

➤ Try your hardest to stay in balance in terms of eating, drinking, and sleeping. We deplete our reserves during the holidays and don't take time to fuel up again so we're less able to say no to holiday treats and drinks. They look mighty good when we're so tired. Instead, give yourself permission for a nap and then take it!

➤ Find time to do something for yourself—treat yourself like a special holiday guest. Offering a bath, a piece of special fruit, a good book, or the chance to sleep late one morning are all ways to treat a guest well...so give that holiday gift to yourself.

Many of these tips are common sense, and I'm sure you've heard them before. But it's easy to forget the obvious. That's why when the holidays roll around I take out this list and put it on my refrigerator door so I won't make the mistake of leaving everything to the last minute, and expecting that everything will be wonderful this year!

For Every Season Turn, Turn, Turn

Believe me, I'm not trying to dig up more types of Seasonal Blues just for the fun of it. But the fact is that there is something coming up on our calendars every month that can trigger bad moods, and set us off on a downward spiral to the blues. Mother's Day, Father's Day, birthdays, and other occasions can be wonderful opportunities to celebrate our lives—but they can also be the source of discomfort and pain.

Every celebration has potential downfalls, and we can avoid these letdowns if we know ahead of time what to expect and take steps to solve the problems that get in the way of our happiness. Consider the following calendar that describes our various moods as we celebrate special events throughout the year. Make a calendar of your own with each of the months, and list potential events that can trigger the Seasonal Blues for you.

As you're reading this calendar, think about your own feelings during the various holidays, commemorations, and celebrations, and consider what actions you can take to beat the Seasonal Blues and take more control over your life.

Blues for Every Season

January This is the month when the Post-Holiday Blues kick in. Depression rates go up in January, as people feel burned out from the holiday and let down by relationships. This is the most active month of the year for new therapy clients; but unfortunately, by the end of January, the commitment to change has usually faded into a distant memory, just like those New Year's resolutions to lose weight.

What you can do: Whenever I feel down after the buildup of the holidays, I try to get as much exercise as possible. January becomes a very active month with a variety of exercises even if I'm having trouble sticking to that diet. By February, I always feel better and stronger and actually have more success dieting in February than in January.

February   The blues rage across the singles community on Valentine's Day, as unattached people are reminded that they don't have Mr. or Ms. Right in their lives. People in relationships may also feel down when they look at how far from right their current partners are, or they may just feel disappointed in their partners if they don't come home laden with flowers, candy, or a card.

What you can do: Come up with your own new definition for a successful relationship and a happy Valentine's Day. Get together on February 14 with a group of friends and make a list of all the relationships you have seen that each of you consider successful. Together, you should be able to throw out the old ideas of relationships and construct a new model. Don't let Hallmark rule how you're going to feel on certain days! Make a commitment to each other about what you will do in the coming year to build better, stronger relationships to really celebrate next year's Valentine's Day.

March   Nothing much happens this month in terms of national holidays or traditional celebrations—and many people get the blues simply because they feel disconnected and empty. Winter is hanging on when it should have gone and there's nothing to look forward to.

What you can do: Recognize that this is down time, so use the lack of distractions to really connect to people. March is Relationship Building Month. Hang out at a bookstore, visit old friends, or go to concerts with new friends you have been meaning to call all year. Some people actually like this down time because they feel everyone is bored so they're more available to get together. Your relationship inventory will be well stocked for the year, if you build and harvest relationships in March.

April   The birth of spring, when lovers locked arm in arm stroll through the park, workers eat their bag lunches by the park fountains, and people begin to make plans for Easter and Passover. People who don't have partners or families to share the holidays with are vulnerable to getting the Seasonal Blues.

What you can do: If you're single, get outside and meet people. Join a hiking or biking club and go for nature walks with other people. Don't sit around by yourself watching reruns of the Easter Parade or munching on matzoh. Find out what community events are taking place locally and participate in them so you aren't alone during the holidays. If you have a partner, take time to plan how to spend the holidays in the most meaningful way to you, not to your parents. This is a good time of year to separate more from families of origin and develop your own traditions, since spring represents new beginnings.

May   Parents experience the End-of-the-School-Year Blues, as they desperately try to keep up with all the scheduled school functions. And then there is the anxiety that goes along with transitioning their children from school to summer activities and all the extra activities and child care to plan. Singles are often desperately planning their summer activities so they're not left behind, And Mother's Day falls in this month, so every unresolved issue with our moms is highlighted (see Chapter 15, "Coping with the Parent Approval Blues").

What you can do: Trying to keep up with the end-of-the-school-year activities is impossible, so don't try. My husband and I have learned to become military strategists and make our plan of attack in advance. For some activities, we do the divide-and-conquer routine, where he takes one kid and I take the other. For the most important events, we prioritize our work demands and accept that during this month we may get less done than usual at work. If you're single, commit to doing something new this summer that involves adventure and challenge. Push yourself with an Outward Bound survival course, bike the wine country of Napa or France, climb a mountain, or raft a river. You'll be stronger and more in control for the rest of the year. And Mother's Day? Read every chapter of this book twice and maybe you'll get through it. No, seriously. Mothers are so overwhelmingly important to our lives that every improvement in new relationships with them has a rippling effect, enhancing other relationships in our lives. So on Mother's Day, make an effort to take small steps toward getting closer to your mother—it's worth it.

June Hallmark doesn't let you forget it—June 20th is Father's Day—a great day if you are on speaking terms with your dad and can visit him. But people who don't talk to their fathers, or those who can't be with them because their fathers live far away or have passed away, or those who don't even know who their fathers are, will probably fall prey to the blues.

What you can do: It's better to try to make amends with your father (see Chapter 15) if at all possible. If you aren't talking to your dad, the first step toward repairing the relationship might be sending him a card. Even a small step toward him rather than away from him will make you feel better. If you live too far away, then phone home, pull out an old photo album, and tell your dad which pictures you're looking at so at least you can share the past even if you can't share the present. If your father has passed away, honor his memory by some ritual you construct for the day, such as lighting a candle for him, planting a flower in his name, making a donation to a charity he would have liked, or any gesture that connects you to the best part of him.

July If you can't afford a fun summer vacation, you're bound to get the blues during this month. Fourth of July only reminds you of how much independence you don't have from a crummy job, a rotten relationship, or a boring life.

What you can do: Survey people you know at your income level and ask them what type of vacations they are planning. This may give you a new way of thinking about leisure time and getting good ideas of places to go that you can afford. Think about trading places and about new destinations. Break out of your routine so you assert your independence and individuality. Try a new sport, wear a new style of clothing, listen to a different type of music, or go to some of the summer concerts you may have missed because you weren't organized enough to plan in advance.

August What could be worse than staying at the office, inputting data to a software program, while everyone else is throwing their cares to the wind at the beach? When the dog days of summer grip your heart, you have the summer blues, which tend to peak in August.

What you can do: Console yourself with the thought that everyone else's summer vacation will be over soon!

September   Going back to work after the summer and getting the kids ready to go back to school can be nerve-racking and overwhelming—especially if you also tend to feel down when the weather starts to change and begins to get cold. There is a letdown in returning to work after all the pretend or real fun in the sun from the summer, so many people experience fun withdrawal in this month.

What you can do: Planning ahead will make you healthy, wealthy, and wise. I usually buy my kids' clothes and school supplies in late July or early August to avoid the rush at the stores and ruining our August vacation. If you feel the winter blahs coming on, follow the action strategies suggested in this chapter. Plan a fun activity for September so the fun withdrawal is not so abrupt and doesn't stop just because summer is over.

October   This month is usually the beginning of the holiday jitters because we know what's coming. It's also usually a more intense time at work to make up from the lull in the summer. If workplace changes are going to occur, it's often during this month before the holidays move into full swing.

What you can do: Plan, plan, plan ahead. Print out a separate three-month (October, November, and December) calendar on your computer and begin to fill it in for the whole family. Begin and complete holiday shopping and travel so you're more in control when the stress begins. Work harder, smarter, and more visibly during this month because you're more likely to be noticed and appreciated now than at many other times. Plan a costume party and come as "Your Dark Side" if you're feeling the Seasonal Blues, or as "Your Dream Come True" if you're feeling pretty good this month.

November/December—the dynamic duo   If you're going to get the Seasonal Blues around the holidays, this is the span of time when you'll feel pretty lousy.

What you can do: Follow the action strategies set out in this chapter to beat the holiday blues. Practice and practice. In a few years, you'll avoid the holiday blues and actually have a great time during the dynamic duo season.

English poet John Keats captured the link human beings have to nature when he said in a poem: *Four seasons fill the measure of the year; There are four seasons in the mind of man.* Our thoughts, feelings, and moods have been shaped by the seasons, but we are not season slaves and can use the seasons to guide us through the stages of change and growth.

When the winter cold chills us to the bone, we can turn to the sun (or our new light boxes) for help and emerge from our caves. And when the sound of sleigh bells ringing taunts us with dark memories of days gone by, we can turn to ourselves, acknowledge the past, and own our power to improve the present, regardless of the season.

The best way to beat the Seasonal Blues is to take control of your feelings. Don't let Hallmark determine when you'll celebrate certain occasions, and don't wait until the last minute to buy presents for the holidays or purchase your child's back to school clothes. Make the purchase during off-season. You may not be in the spirit, but you'll save yourself a lot of headaches and problems.

Blues Calendar at a Glance: Chart Your Moods a Month at a Time

Month	Blue	Action Strategies
January	Post-Holiday Blues	Make a one-month post-holiday exercise plan and stick to it.
		Make a list of three major things you want to do and figure out what you have to do to carry them out.
February	Valentine's Day	Focus on what you've got by going out with a great group of friends for dinner instead of staying home alone.
		Connect, connect, connect!
		Reach out to an old friend by phone, fax, e-mail, or in person.
March	Boredom Blues	Open yourself up to new experiences by going to three places you've never been before.
		Broaden your mind by taking a class in something you've always wanted to study but never had time to.
April	Spring/Easter/ Passover	Embark on a mental "spring cleaning" adventure by making a list of negative things you say to yourself and sweeping them away.
		Stay in touch with people by getting involved in community activities during the holidays.
May	Mother's Day	Let yourself feel close to your mother by thinking back to her good qualities—and how you benefited from them.
	End of School Year	Learn to set limits and avoid burnout by just saying "No!" to some end-of-school-year bashes.
June	Father's Day	If you aren't talking to him, acknowledge your father in some way by sending a card, writing a letter, or just expressing your feelings in a journal.
		If your Dad has passed away, celebrate his day by looking over old photos or home videos.
July	Summer Vacation	If you're stuck in town, buy a travel guide for your area to read up on the history and hot spots you may have missed and go sight-seeing as if you were a tourist.
August	Bathing Suit Blues	Challenge social notions of the "perfect body" and just focus on how great the warm sun feels beating down on your body.

Month	Blue	Action Strategies
September	Back-to-School Blues	Take control of your calendar and alleviate some stress by shopping for school clothes and supplies early in the summer.
	Weather Changes	Be aware of mood changes as winter approaches and stay out in the sun as much as possible or buy a light box.
October	Holiday Blues Kickoff	Think ahead to December, and do your holiday shopping NOW to avoid inevitable holiday stress.
		Embrace the cool, crisp feeling of autumn by going apple picking to an orchard and taking a hayride.
November	Thanksgiving	If you don't plan to spend Turkey Day with family or friends, call your local church or synagogue to find out whether they are sponsoring a Thanksgiving dinner—and sign up for it.
		When spending the holiday with family, avoid overstuffing yourself and get some exercise—even if it's just going for a walk around the block.
December	The Heart of the Blues	Keep holiday expectations "reasonable" by acknowledging that you'll be stressed out and that things may not go that well with family.
		Volunteering to help others will always make you feel better, so donate your time to get involved with the church, synagogue, or charities.

The Least You Need to Know

➤ Some 25 million Americans get the Seasonal Blues, and another 10 million have Seasonal Affective Disorder (SAD).

➤ SAD is four times as common among women than men, but it's the easiest depression to treat.

➤ As little as 30 minutes per day of sitting under a light box can make a difference in 60 to 80 percent of SAD patients.

➤ SAD symptoms include extreme fatigue, inability to focus, having trouble sleeping or sleeping too much, carbohydrate craving, weight gain or loss, and feelings of depression.

➤ Keeping warm during the cold months, vacationing in sunny environments, exercising outdoors or indoors, and managing stress are other cures for the winter blahs.

➤ Holiday blues, a form of Seasonal Blues, are common as people try to do too much in too little time and have unrealistic expectations that can't be met.

➤ Establishing action strategies for every month can help you beat the blues whenever they hit.

Part 2
The Moody Blues Learn to Sing a Happy Tune

If you want to lift your mood, DON'T JUST SIT THERE! Do something! Climb a set of stairs, go jogging, vacuum your living room, do some deep-breathing exercises, meditate, or write your feelings in a journal. When a bad mood hits, you don't have to put up with it! The chapters in this section will give you some quick strategies you can use to beat the blues, and offer you some ideas of longer-term plans you can follow to maintain your well-being. If none of these strategies help you perk up, however, you may be sliding into a depression and need professional help. Read about the different types of therapy approaches for treatment of depression in Chapter 9 and get help!

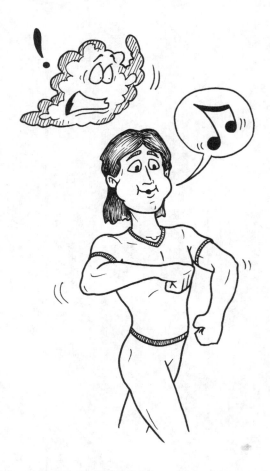

Chapter 6

Quick Strategies for You to Beat the Blues

In This Chapter

➤ Don't dwell on blue moods

➤ Beat the blues with the Action = Energy = Power formula

➤ Perk up with a 10-minute walk

➤ Rx for the blues: a goal a day

➤ How techniques such as deep breathing, meditation, and positive visualization can help you relax

➤ Journal writing: the ultimate self-help tool

The best way to beat the blues over the long haul is to figure out what you're feeling, determine why an event, comment, or thought upset you so much, and then take action. Do something productive that will make you feel better. But before you plummet to the depths of your soul (and believe me, it can get pretty deep and dark down there) you need to clear your head. You simply can't make any responsible, sound decisions about your life when you're sinking in a swamp of negative thoughts.

In this chapter, I'll focus on some quick action strategies you can take to improve your mood so you can do some serious thinking about why you were blue in first place. Taking a 10-minute walk, helping others, keeping a journal, learning relaxation techniques, and pursuing other strategies will help you regain perspective so you can more accurately reflect on what's getting you down and be more strategic in developing an effective response.

Life Can't Look Up When You're Down in the Dumps

When the blues strike, you can try to identify the specific factors that led to your bad feelings—someone said something nasty to you, you found out about a party you weren't invited to, you still can't decide whether to dump your boyfriend (or girlfriend), you can't seem to get pregnant. Don't worry if the upsetting incident or thought seems "stupid." Sometimes the smallest things can set us off on a downward spiral because they mean more to us than we know at first glance.

It's usually easier to wait until you feel better to figure out what you can do to solve your problem. Trying to analyze your feelings when you're down will make you feel worse because you'll dredge up all kinds of things you've done wrong in your life—every failure, flaw, and frailty—and say, "Well, no wonder I'm miserable! I'm such a jerk." The fact is when you're down in the dumps your thinking is distorted and you see yourself in a bad light, no matter how much you shine or how well you do.

Yet, many of us delve into self-analysis when we should be focusing on staying afloat. Why? Because when we're rummaging through our past for clues about our unhappiness we feel we are at least "doing something" to try to solve our problems, and that relieves our guilt. True, you'll shed some guilt, but you won't gain much useful insight either. And negativity breeds negativity. The more we think about negative things, the more we get stuck in a vicious cycle of doom and gloom, until not even a ray of light shines through the darkness our mind has created.

So try to put off figuring out why you're so gloomy until you feel better. The exercises suggested in this chapter will give you an immediate energy boost so you can get out of the negative thinking cycle that keeps you from finding creative solutions to your problems.

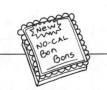

Guiltless Pleasures

When you can't stop obsessing over a problem, find something to do that makes you feel good. List 10 positive distractions—they can be as simple as going to buy flowers or as complicated as helping your son set up his Lego set. A distraction will help you regain perspective so you can figure out why you were bummed out in the first place.

Action = Energy = Power

You don't have to be a physicist to decipher this formula. The technical definition: Every action you take creates energy, and as your energy builds so does your power and your potential to meet your goals. In other words, once you get up and do something, you'll feel better and be in a better position to go after what you want and fight the negative thoughts that drain your energy.

To get a spark going when your battery is running low, go for a short walk, do relaxation exercises, write in your journal, or do something that will make you feel special.

Choose two or three action strategies from this chapter that most appeal to you. Write them down on an index card and keep the list in a place where you'll see it each day (your bathroom mirror, appointment book, billfold, car dashboard, or above the stove).

Practice your strategies several times when you feel less stressed until they feel natural and comfortable, then put them to work when the going gets tough.

This approach will protect you from getting down on yourself in a big way and generate more energy for the things that you really want to do.

A Goal a Day Keeps the Blues at Bay

Just like you take a daily vitamin for your body, take a vitamin every day for your mind. Each morning or evening, think of a daily goal and write it down in your appointment book, on a sticky note, in a notebook, or in your computer. Writing down one goal a day will give you the focus you need to accomplish something so that you feel in control. With writing, you're constantly reminded of the goal because you can see it, not just think about it.

You're probably thinking: "Just one goal? Now I can be even more blue because I'm an underachiever too. I've already got a hundred things on my current 'to do' list!" But here is the catch: "To do" lists often do us in. We may be so overwhelmed by everything we have to do (much of it being very boring) that it's easy to ditch the list and meet a friend for coffee instead. Then we feel even more like a failure for not "getting anything done." Focusing on one goal, however, is much more manageable. And after even the tiniest goal is accomplished, it creates positive energy to accomplish ever bigger and better goals.

The goal can be anything: getting out of bed, going to the market, taking the kids out for ice cream, calling up a friend. You can build up to larger activities, but avoid life-changing goals—such as "I'm going to look like a '*Baywatch* babe' as soon as I get off this couch and join a gym"—because these undertakings are destined to fail. The female lifeguards on *Baywatch* didn't get to look the way they do overnight—believe me, they work their buns off to get and keep in shape!

The 10-Minute Walk: One of the Best of the Blues Busters

It's 3:30 p.m. You're slouched over your desk in front of your computer, unaware of a message threatening to cut you off unless you push "OK," when a colleague throws a report on your desk and tells you to have a synopsis written in an hour. You're so tired it doesn't even faze you that you were caught snoozing. So what do you do? Charge to the vending machine to get a candy bar and hope it will give you the jolt you need!

Dr. Robert Thayer, a psychologist at California State University, Long Beach, conducted a number of excellent studies (described in his book, *Biopsychology of Mood and Arousal*, Oxford University Press, 1989), showing that even though we feel better right after eating a candy bar, we get more tired an hour afterward. Two hours later, we are even more wiped out than we were before we took that glorious first bite.

It's the same with smoking. After a cigarette, a smoker experiences an immediate reduction of tension. But within an hour or two the tension is back. And it feels worse. Consider the energy effects the next time you choose between energy boosters and energy busters:

➤ *Candy or cigarette.* After one hour: more tired; after two hours: no positive effect/ feel worse

➤ *Ten-minute walk.* After one hour: more energy/better mood; after two hours: still positive effect

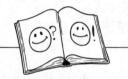

Terms of Encheerment

Endorphins are a group of substances formed in the brain that relieves pain and is thought to be involved in controlling the body's response to stress and determining mood. Endorphins have a similar chemical structure to morphine.

If you've picked up any magazine over the past three decades, you've read that regular exercise reduces depression and improves the quality of life. But you don't have to pump iron at the gym to perk up. Whenever the going gets tough, get up and walk at a normal pace for five or 10 minutes, counting your steps to yourself as you go: one, two, one, two, or one to 10 and repeat.

This kind of walk becomes a mood booster and a stress reducer. It feeds more oxygen to your brain right away, which produces *endorphins,* making you feel better and helping you think more clearly to relax and reduce your stress.

And it will save you from falling asleep at your desk— an especially important move when the boss walks by.

Some guidelines:

➤ Walk outside if possible; but if the weather is bad, take a walk inside your building, home, or apartment.

➤ Walk at a normal pace, not at an aerobic pace, and count your steps so you have the meditation effect at the same time you gain an exercise effect.

If you're too lazy to get going or you think that walking is boring, take a personal tape player with you so you can listen to music, books on tape, motivation tapes, or your bat mitzvah recordings—whatever turns you on! You may just end up loving this exercise. And if you do, consider adding some type of regular exercise to your life. You may want to get a gym membership, or start biking, hiking, or doing any other sport that will motivate you to keep healthy.

Remember: Exercise is one of the best protections from depression. See Chapter 8, "Beating the Blues: Let's Get Physical," on finding the right type of exercise program.

Helping Others Boosts Self-Esteem

When you're down, you naturally focus a lot on yourself and your misery. One way to beat the blues and realize you're not at the center of a miserable world is to reach out and help others. Just about everybody could use some help. You can cheer up friends by giving them a call. Make someone's day by smiling at them or telling them they look nice. You can take food, clothing, and blankets to the poor, help with organizing a party at work, or volunteer your time to an organization.

Find out what you enjoy and share it with others. If your first love is reading, you can volunteer with Literacy Volunteers, an organization that teaches people how to read. Or if you love animals, your local animal shelter or humane society is always looking for volunteers. Looking in the Yellow Pages under Social Service Organizations is a good place to start.

You will always receive more energy than you give. Remember, the quickest way to help yourself is to help someone else.

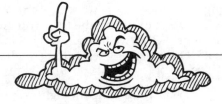

Funk-y Facts

Americans volunteer for one or more causes an average of 4.2 hours a week or 218.4 hours a year, according to a report issued by the Independent Sector, a private nonprofit organization. The major reason: They feel satisfaction when they reach out to others. Entitled "Giving and Volunteering in the United States," the report points out that teens and the elderly are the two groups that volunteer the most. The causes that attract the greatest number of volunteers include education, health, and human services.

The Top Three Relaxation Exercises

Meditation used to be something that just your hippie friends, college professor, and manicurist did to stay "centered." But now, nearly everybody does some form of relaxation exercise—Wall Street executives, computer geeks, and even your cleaning crew! The reason: It relieves stress, clears your mind, slows down your system, helps you feel rested and peaceful, and strengthens your immune system against stress-related illnesses.

The three most popular relaxation techniques include:

➤ Deep breathing

➤ Meditation

➤ Positive visualization

Select one of these techniques or find another relaxation approach you like better and then do it regularly. It will benefit you over time and keep you from becoming stressed out. At the first sign of the blues, RELAX with one of these techniques. These exercises will also boost your spirit when you're down so that you can better handle problems that come up. Let's take a closer look at each of these relaxation techniques.

Dr. Ellen Says

Deep breathing, meditation, and positive visualization exercises help reduce stress. To get immediate relief when you're stressed, also try getting a massage, taking a hot bath, listening to music, and doing something that makes you laugh.

Take a Deep Breath

We've been breathing since the minute we were born. You'd think we'd have it down by now. But guess what? Most of us breathe the wrong way. So add that to your list of things you have to change! When we inhale, we suck in our stomachs, and deflate our bellies when we exhale. Our breathing tends to be shallow because we are usually slumped over.

To breathe the right way, your shoulders need to be straight instead of sloped so the breathing can come from the lower abdomen. You know you're doing it right if your belly expands like a balloon being blown up when you inhale, and it contracts when you exhale.

Breathing the right way is important for the following reasons:

➤ It lets you feel and experience emotion more deeply and intensely.

➤ It helps you stay focused on the present instead of letting your mind wander off.

➤ It makes you feel peaceful.

Deep breathing is used by Olympic athletes to release tension before a competition. When you feel stressed out or uptight, try deep breathing. Here's how you do it: Take a very deep breath through your nose, hold it and count slowly to 10, then release forcefully and

Blues Flag

Do you get nervous giving a speech? Are you hot under the collar when someone is criticizing your work? Do you break out into a sweat when you think about asking someone out on a date? If you answer "Yes" to any of these questions, try sitting back and taking three deep breaths. This will slow down your heart rate, calm your nerves, and keep you focused on how to regain control over your emotions.

completely through your mouth. Do this three times and you'll notice a significant release of stress and increased ability to focus.

Meditate on Feeling Good

You don't have to be a Buddhist, Yogi, or New Age groupie to practice meditation. Anyone can do this relaxation exercise. According to the *Webster's New World College Dictionary*, to meditate means simply to "think deeply and continuously; reflect; muse." When you meditate, your muscles relax and you are breathing properly so you feel tranquil, restful. Your mind focuses on a mental activity—like counting breathes or repeating a *mantra*—so you aren't focused on your anxious or blue thoughts.

For meditation to work it must be done regularly for 15 to 20 minutes each time. Here's how to do it:

1. Find a spot at home where nobody will bug you and unplug the phone.

2. Wear loose, comfortable clothing.

3. Sit in a comfortable position and close your eyes.

4. Concentrate on slowly relaxing each part of your body, allowing tension to flow out of your arms, legs, neck, and back.

5. Begin to breathe deeply and rhythmically. Your chest and abdomen should both move together as you inhale and exhale.

6. Try to picture a peaceful image in your mind—a stream, a beach, a quiet landscape, or a word or sound.

7. Maintain your focus on your chosen image, sound, or mantra. Let your thoughts continue to flow but do not dwell an them, merely note them and return to your point of focus.

Think Positive with Visualization

Sometimes transporting yourself through your imagination to a tranquil place can renew your

Dr. Ellen Says

Do you typically stoop over with your head down and your shoulders round so you look like you're carrying the weight of the world on your back? Most people who are depressed have this posture. If you're feeling down and want a quick boost, try lifting your head up, pushing your shoulders back, lengthening your neck, and taking three deep breaths. Stand tall and walk with your head up high as if a helium balloon were lifting your head and shoulders toward the sky.

Terms of Encheerment

Mantras are sounds that have a flowing, meditative quality to them which are repeated out loud or inwardly by the person meditating to achieve a calm, peaceful, and relaxed state. While some people use mantras as a focal point, others zero in their thoughts on a picture, an object (candle flames or flowers), or a person. There is no "right" meditation technique for everybody—so just use the one that works for you.

75

energy and soothe you. Select your favorite scene in nature and record every detail in your mind using every one of your senses (think about how it looks, sounds, smells, and feels). Most of us have the skills to do visualization since we tend to recall every sordid detail of really awful incidents like your boss firing you, or your girlfriend giving you the kiss of death speech of "just wanting to be friends."

Now you can apply that skill for something that will help you!

You can use positive visualization when you are stuck in a line or in a traffic jam by envisioning yourself in Acapulco sipping a cool drink by the sparkling blue pool. While waiting to go in for your performance evaluation, envision yourself climbing a mountain, resting to take a drink from the green water jug you used to trek across Europe during college. Taste the cold water from the jug and drink in the beauty of the nature around you.

Here's how you do it:

1. Sit down, close your eyes, and breathe slowly and deeply.

2. Become aware of each breath and concentrate on how your body feels.

3. Visualize a beautiful scene from the beach, mountains, desert, or any other peaceful relaxed setting you love.

4. Make the visualization as real as possible to all your senses. If it's an ocean scene you visualize, smell the salt air, hear the gentle sound of the surf, touch the grains of sand, and feel the balmy air on your face. Use deep breathing techniques to derail anxiety.

5. If your mind wanders back to the problem creating the stress, make yourself return to the peaceful thought and stay there for a few minutes.

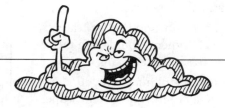

Funk-y Facts

Visualization can be a critical survival tool, as was shown by the released American hostages who survived years of isolation by mentally transporting themselves to a more comforting place. They realized that the only thing their captors couldn't control was their minds. Exercising this type of mind control kept them from going crazy and losing hope. And when they were set free, they readjusted to society more quickly because they had developed wonderful mind control techniques and were stronger mentally than many of those around them.

Put Your Finger on Your Emotional Pulse: Keep a Journal

Writing down your thoughts and feelings about an upsetting event, a stressful day, or other things that bother you will help you sort out what's going on in your mind. Through writing, you can more freely explore your thoughts and regain control because you aren't worried about what others think.

When you first start writing, you'll probably just pour out your most immediate, less profound thoughts. So don't blush or panic if you find yourself writing: "I have to do laundry," or "I wish I didn't have to go to this stupid reception." Once you've downloaded all the chitchat from your brain on to the screen or written it out on a page, you'll get to some deeper thoughts about how you are feeling and what is bothering you. Writing about your feelings will give you more control over difficult emotions and make you better able to solve your problems.

Journals are romantic, but the computer makes the writing process more immediate and convenient for many of us. Whenever you feel stressed, call up your file and write about your experience in a few words or sentences. Don't worry about how it reads or sounds. You are not writing the great American novel. In fact, you don't even have to write a grammatically correct sentence. You just have to get your thoughts on paper.

Consider how the following two people used an electronic journal as a problem-solving technique:

➤ A high school teacher who was overwhelmed with demands at school and home used her lunch break to write a letter to herself outlining all the pressures she felt. She then listed all the possible solutions to the challenges she faced. This system worked much better than what she used to do, which was simply brood or complain to her girlfriends about her problems.

➤ A writer who had little income, failed love affairs, and no motivation went away to the beach by himself and started writing his feelings in a journal. He asked himself questions a therapist would ask him and found that part of his unhappiness stemmed from him trying to live up to his mother's expectations—an impossible task. So he started to explore what he wanted from life instead of trying to live the life his mother had envisioned for him.

Blues Flag

When you start writing, you may hear a little gnawing voice inside you say, "It's not nice to have such ugly thoughts!" Ignore it! Many of us feel uncomfortable dealing with such angry feelings so directly. To break the barriers, commit to being less judgmental and more accepting of yourself so you can be honest with your feelings. Remember, anything goes as long as it's symbolic and you don't do it in the real world.

Writing in a journal—electronic or otherwise—in the morning or evening can save you pain, depression, and therapy expenses because it's one of our most effective forms of self-therapy.

Before you begin this self-therapy, remember these six key points:

➤ Write down your feelings as you experience them. If you feel like a victim in a relationship, write down how you feel about the other person and what you are going to do about it.

➤ Don't analyze your emotions or edit entries. Just get them down. If you're stuck, try drawing something to express how you feel. You don't need to be Picasso. A stick figure or a scribble is fine and often loosens up your feelings so you can return to writing as a way to further express them.

➤ Entries can be a few words, a few sentences, or a few paragraphs, whatever feels good to you. With each entry, note the time, place, and situation. This information is valuable because over time it will reveal the pattern and context of feelings and the times you may be more vulnerable to certain kinds of bad feelings.

➤ Keep everything you write safely hidden or in a locked drawer so your spouse, parent, or maid won't be able to read it over coffee while you're away from home. For your feelings to flow freely, you must feel that your writing is yours alone.

➤ If you want to share a journal entry with someone, wait at least several hours so you can reflect on what you've written. If your piece communicates anger, don't send it to the person because you may regret it later.

➤ Review your work periodically so that you appreciate the progress you've made and are empowered to make more deeper discoveries. Reviewing journal entries on your birthday, at the beginning of every new year, or on the anniversary of your marriage (unless you'd prefer to watch the wedding video) gives you an opportunity to learn new insights.

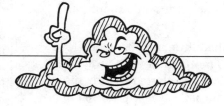

Funk-y Facts

"Think of your journal as a record of a conversation with yourself," says George Sheehan, medical editor of *Runner's World* and author of *Personal Best* (Rodale Press, 1992). "A life without a journal of some kind, whether biography or letters...is a life gone unexamined. It is as if a sailor had set out without charts or sextant and had no idea where he was..." Life, he adds, is full of wonderful experiences but "I will never know why unless I write it down."

Plan to keep a daily journal for a month. By then you'll find the process so valuable it will become a habit!

The Least You Need to Know

➤ When you're blue, identify what's triggered your bad mood if you can do so right away, otherwise put that off until you feel better.

➤ The Action = Energy = Power formula says that every action you take creates energy, and as your energy builds so does your power and potential to meet your goals.

➤ Identify a goal a day to keep you focused and help you feel productive.

➤ To perk up when you're feeling low, take a 10-minute walk instead of grabbing a candy bar or drinking a double espresso.

➤ Helping others makes you feel capable, kind, and giving—all feelings that will enhance your self-esteem.

➤ Deep breathing, meditation, and positive visualization techniques transport you to a calm, relaxed, and blissful state.

➤ Keeping a journal is an effective form of self-therapy and helps you sort out your thoughts.

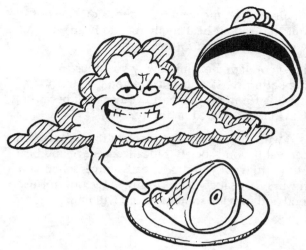

Chapter 7

The Moody Food Blues: Caving in to Cravings

In This Chapter

➤ The connection between food and blues

➤ When the brain commands, the stomach salutes

➤ Why men and women have different cravings

➤ Take the 4–12–minute test

➤ Triumph over the trigger foods

➤ Get more for less by eating five small meals a day

There it is—the chocolate chip cookie you've been coveting! You've made it through the whole day without nibbling on it, knowing that eating one bite could bring your diet crumbling down in no time, along with part of your confidence, self-esteem, and self-respect. First, you'd polish off the cookie, then because it tasted so good, you'd need to graze through the kitchen picking at crackers, muffins, chocolate kisses, and other goodies that seem to automatically slide down your throat and land on your hips.

When you're down in the dumps over what's going into your gut and you can't get a grip over your grub, you've got the Moody Food Blues. Boy, do I know what that's like! Like many of you, I tried to lose weight by going on every new diet, envisioning that my life would be wonderful if only I could shed those 20 extra pounds. It took several decades to realize that this attitude was a recipe for failure—no matter what I did, what fad diet I tried, I always failed. What finally helped me keep the pounds off was not any get-thin-quick scheme, but a new attitude about healthy living and healthful eating, along with a food and exercise plan tailored just for me.

Feeling bad about gaining weight can be good if you examine why you abuse food—and take active control over your eating patterns. Ask yourself: Do you give in to cravings because your body is really starving for nutrients, or do you overeat because you find food comforting when you feel lonely or bored or empty?

I know how hard it is to not be obsessed with your weight in a society that grades your worth by how thin you are. But you can get beyond society's idealized image and beat the Moody Food Blues by learning to listen to what your body really craves when you think you are hungry, feed yourself in ways that satisfy, and simply move on. In this chapter, we'll look at why we abuse food and provide some tips that will help you feed your body and soul.

What We Love to Eat When We're Blue

Our cravings are based on a mixture of psychological and physical factors. To get a grip on our love handles, we need to understand why we have cravings in the first place. A craving is an obsessive desire for a specific type of food that we think we must have because it will taste so good and make us feel so fine.

Studies show that the more times we are exposed to food that makes us feel good, the more we prefer it in the future. The foods we crave are usually rooted in childhood experiences, and we may have been born with a preference for certain foods over others.

If your mother gave you doughnuts as a reward for eating your vegetables, you're likely to reward or console yourself with the same type of food as an adult. When we are sad, lonely, or anxious we may reach for foods we enjoyed eating as kids at birthday parties, family gatherings, and other celebrations.

These are psychological explanations for our cravings—what we call emotional eating because we feel hungry for something other than food, but use food as a pacifier to numb our feelings and stuff our needs deep into our gut so we don't have to confront the fears associated with taking charge of our lives.

Whenever we let our emotions control our taste buds, we tend to abuse food and overeat (or in a few cases, undereat). So next time you reach for food to fill the void when you get bored, tired, anxious, or lonely, don't be surprised if you're experiencing the *Moody Food Blues*—the bad feelings you get when you eat to cover

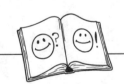

Terms of Encheerment

Moody Food Blues are the frustrated, anxious, and angry feelings we get when our food/mood connection is unhealthy and we turn to food to lift our bad mood instead of facing our problems. While it temporarily anesthetizes our bad feelings, in the long run moody food causes only deeper depression and unwanted pounds because it makes us feel more helpless, hopeless, and out of control.

up or erase your emotions. I call them the Moody Food Blues because you'll always end up feeling blue when you use food to try to feel better. You'll hate yourself more and more as the unwanted pounds and problems pile on because you've been using food to avoid dealing with those problems.

But the desire to eat is not just all in your head. There is a biological component to overeating as well—a physical drive inside us that compels us to reach for foods that will make us feel better, at least while we are eating them.

My Brain Told Me to Eat It

When we are under stress, tired, or dieting excessively, the *serotonin* levels in our brains—those chemicals that control our moods—drop and our bodies crave certain foods to bring the level of this neurotransmitter back up. This is our body's way of helping us feel better (thank goodness somebody is keeping an eye on us when we're in a funk!). Your brain must produce serotonin on a daily basis because you can't save it from one day to another, and all the production takes place at night. When our lives are balanced, when we are eating well and getting lots of sleep, our brain is producing enough serotonin to make us feel content. But if we are too stressed out, we aren't sleeping enough, or we're constantly on crash diets, our brain doesn't produce enough serotonin.

When our serotonin levels are low we usually crave sweets or carbohydrates. Antidepressants like Prozac or natural therapies like St. John's Wort will raise the level of serotonin in our brain and restore calmness. But so will eating certain foods. The only way to stop craving these foods is to eat small amounts of them. But that's not what those of us schooled in crash diets do. We are trained to think that giving in to cravings is bad and that we must deny ourselves the foods we love in order to lose weight.

But when we deny our cravings, they just get more intense. They build up a force and intensity of a tidal wave of enormous need. When the built-up wave crashes, we and all our intentions to diet drown under the force.

Terms of Encheerment

Serotonin is a chemical in your brain that is related to good and bad moods. If you don't have enough in your brain, you'll feel bad, even suicidal. If you have enough serotonin, you'll feel pretty good. You lose serotonin under prolonged stress, but raise the level of serotonin after eating carbohydrates.

Dr. Ellen Says

Research shows that chewing on crunchy foods like pretzels and apples release tension because of the sound and muscular action of chewing. If you'd prefer a more sedating effect, try eating creamy foods that are low in fat but may remind you of your childhood, like low-fat chocolate pudding or mashed potatoes with skim milk.

So of course, when we finally take a bite of the food we've been craving, we cave in with a vengeance by eating too much of it. This is why most diets don't work. In 95 percent of the cases, we gain back the weight 12 to 18 months later. The reason most of us gain back the weight is not because we lack the willpower, but because we don't know how our bodies work, we don't know how to create a healthy food/mood connection, and we don't know how to control our eating so we can feel healthy.

Real Women Chew Chocolate, Real Men Chomp on Steak

Our bodies may also be craving nutrients that we should be getting but we aren't. In *Why Women Need Chocolate* (Hyperion, 1995), nutritionist Debra Waterhouse says that women need starch, sugar, and fat to feel and look good because they have more estrogen and more body fat—and that's why many crave chocolate. A small piece of this yummy forbidden sweet, she said, is all they need to kill the craving.

Waterhouse eloquently explains (and her pearls of wisdom are quoted by chocolate lovers) that the forces which dictate female food needs are "biologically ingrained" and that's why cravings can't be controlled by willpower. The same biological force compels men to eat not chocolate, but meat. Men are more likely to crave steaks, eggs, hot dogs, and other protein sources because they have more testosterone and greater muscle mass.

The reason why men crave proteins and women carve out chocolate is based on evolution. Back in the days of the cavemen, men needed protein so they could beef up and be fit to hunt for prey. Women, on the other hand, needed extra serotonin boosters so they could improve their mood and be better fit to nurture children, according to Waterhouse.

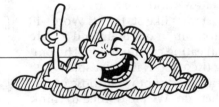

Funk-y Facts

According to Debra Waterhouse, author of *Why Women Need Chocolate*, women's cravings have cultural underpinnings dating back to the feast and famine cycles. In order to survive under harsh conditions, women had to find a way of storing food in their bodies when extra food was available, so they could keep going when the food ran out. Female food cravings, therefore, encourage women to eat higher calories, so that even in the midst of famine they will survive because they have the survival energy stored in fat.

You may be thinking, "Dr. Ellen is telling me it's okay to have my cake and eat it too, especially if it's chocolate!" But wait a minute! Don't rush to the refrigerator yet. You may feel better after eating that chocolate chip cookie only if you *really* need the food to fuel your serotonin levels—and, then, only if you eat just one, not a whole bag.

The problem is, though, that we often end up eating when we're bored or lonely—not necessarily when our bodies need the food—and we shove into our mouths too many of the foods we are addicted to.

If you're like me, you probably can't always tell whether your craving is based on biological or emotional needs. And most of the time, you couldn't care less since all you're thinking about is hunting down your prey. Why split hairs over motivation? Let's just eat!

Say, for instance, you figure out that the craving is biological. How do you ensure that you satisfy the craving (just a tad, thank you) without cramming too much down your throat? These are literally loaded questions, but they'll take a load off your tummy, thighs, and buttocks if you can figure out the answers.

And you will as you read on!

Women Are...	Men Are...
76% more likely to crave chocolate	78% more likely to crave meat
71% more likely to crave crackers	76% more likely to crave eggs
62% more likely to crave ice cream	69% more likely to crave hot dogs
62% more likely to crave candy	10% more likely to crave pizza
65% more likely to crave fruit	10% more likely to crave seafood
6 times more likely to "love" chocolate	5 times more likely to "dislike" chocolate
22 times more likely to eat chocolate to feel better	1½ times more likely to exercise to feel better
2 times more likely to feel good when they *fulfill* their food cravings	4 times more likely to feel good when they *deny* their food cravings
2 times more likely to binge on their craved foods	2 times more likely to follow a very low fat and sugar diet
2 times more likely to feel fatigued and depressed	2 times more likely to feel satisfied with artificial sweeteners and fake fats
Women Are Most Likely to Prefer	**Men Are Most Likely to Prefer**
#1: chocolate	#1: red meat
#2: bread	#2: pizza
#3: ice cream	#3: potatoes (65% of the men left this part of the survey blank!)

Men and women have different food cravings. Source: Why Women Need Chocolate *by Debra Waterhouse (Hyperion, 1995).*

Put the Timer Where Your Mouth Is: The 4–12 Test

To find out whether your body really needs the food you are craving or just wants it out of habit to cure boredom or calm anxiety, take the "4–12–minute test." Check your watch or the clock and try waiting 4 to 12 minutes to see if the craving passes. According to Dr. Stephen Gullo, author of *Thin Tastes Better* (Food Control Center, 1995), research shows that the average food craving tends to last a mere 4 to 12 minutes, even though it seems like an eternity when you're drooling over a Snickers bar.

When the 12 minutes are up and you still crave the food, your serotonin supply may be too low and need replenishing. Go ahead and eat part of the chocolate bar. You may be thinking, as many of my clients do: "What are you, crazy? Do you think I'd have this weight problem or the Moody Food Blues if I could just take two bites of a chocolate bar and throw the rest out?"

I understand your doubts only too well. Believe me, I'm no stranger to using food as my favorite source of stress reduction! When I'm exhausted at night and I still have hours of chores to do, I sometimes feel I can't continue if I don't have a comfort food to make me feel better and provide some much-needed energy. So if a chocolate bar is your favorite junk food, and you can't eat just one, then sneer at the Snickers and find an acceptable substitute. Pick out some other chocolate-based food that you don't feel addicted to so you won't eat too much but it will still make your brain happy.

Your brain knows what it needs, so learn to listen. It's not that picky about whether it gets a Snickers bar, a cookie, or a fat-free chocolate chip granola bar—so long as it's sweet and has some fat. You'll need to experiment with your substitutes to make sure they *aren't* addictive but *are* tension-reducing.

What unhealthy foods do you often crave, and what healthy food substitutes have worked for you in the past? List them here. We've listed a few to get you started.

Foods I Use as Unhealthy Drugs	*Foods I Use as Healthy Friends*
cookies	fat-free graham crackers
ice cream	fat-free frozen yogurt

Study your list and see where you can substitute the "drug" food for a "friendly" food. What new foods can you add to your list of potential healthy substitutes? What do your friends use? Try a new friendly food for a week until you have identified two or three favorite friendly but healthy foods you can turn to in times of stress or the blues.

Now I know this substitution process isn't easy, but it's not impossible either. We can probably agree that crunching on an energy bar is not the same as sinking your teeth into a warm, doughy, buttery sesame-seed bagel. But if bagels do you in and you've never been able to take just one bite—be it at your grandmother's brunch, a singles potluck event, or while just hanging out watching reruns of the *The X-Files*—then you can't afford to go near bagels! You must develop your friendly food substitutes or you'll never beat the Moody Food Blues. And you need to learn more about what your trigger foods are and why they are so deadly to your health, which is what we discuss next.

Pull the Trigger on Your Trigger Foods

Dr. Gullo suggests that you don't negotiate at all with *trigger foods*—those foods that prompt chain eating and that you can't stop munching on until the supply runs out. I'm sure you know which foods tickle your fancy—those high-fat, high-calorie snacks that we love to consume between meals.

The biggest lie of dieting, Dr. Gullo says, is the phrase that most people can't abide by: "I'll just have a little." The problem with this statement is that once you've tasted the food, you want more. So you have a little more today, then a little more than that tomorrow. A day after you may have more still, and eat it more often.

And voilà—before long, you've found the pounds you lost and you're addicted again!

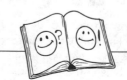

Terms of Encheerment

Trigger foods are the foods that you don't have any control over once you begin eating them—the bag of potato chips, for instance, which is empty before you know it. They are called *trigger* because they trigger an addictive process, much like a drug, where you have to have more and more of it to be satisfied. Typically, these foods tend to be high-fat, high-calorie snacks that most of us love to eat between meals while watching TV or just visiting with friends.

No Taste, No Waist

The fact is that you can't control trigger foods with logic because taste buds have a memory and power all of their own. Your physiological reaction when you eat is, "Get me more," not "Oh, thank you, but I just couldn't have another bite."

Dr. Gullo suggests that next time you are tempted to try "just a little" of one of your trigger foods—regardless of whether your body really needs it—tell yourself: "If I don't take the first little taste, I don't begin. I don't have any problems."

It may sound corny, but it works! I know because I tried it.

Some of my trigger foods are gum, candy, and butter on hot bread. Once I start, I can't stop. I used to buy huge cartons of gum at the store—and put the packets on my desk next to the computer or by my reading light at night. Two days later, the only evidence that the gum ever existed was the overwhelming smell of peppermint in the room and a trash can full of wrappers stuck together by wads of gum.

Y-u-u-u-k!

What foods do you go bonkers over?

You may be thinking: "Oh, that's just about everything I eat." But you might be surprised to learn that there are just a small number of specific foods that you go "goo goo gaga" over and can't control yourself when they're around.

There are certain times and places that you are likely to abuse your trigger food the most. Knowing which foods you are addicted to, when you abuse them, and how you feel just before you binge on them will help you control your eating patterns.

What are your trigger foods?

To find out, keep a record of your eating pattern over a period of a week. Divide a piece of paper into columns that list what you ate, where and at what time you ate it, and what triggered the desire to eat, like we show here.

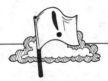

Blues Flag

You can avoid the Moody Food Blues by knowing what your trigger foods are and when you're most likely to binge on them. Your danger time zones may be when you first get home from work, in mid afternoon, or on weekend afternoons and evenings. Once you know your trigger foods and when you're likely to eat them, the easiest thing to do is to simply avoid them and then the struggle never begins.

Time	Place	Food	My Emotion/the Stressor
8 a.m.	home	cereal/milk	breakfast
9:30 a.m.	office	doughnut	boredom

Make sure you record everything you eat, including the corn bread that you inhaled while stooping over the kitchen sink, the leftover ice cream you sopped up from your son's bowl, the handful of sweetened cereal you grabbed on your way down to the den, and all the food samples you tasted at the supermarket.

After a week, take a look at your food log and ask yourself these questions:

➤ What foods did you have trouble limiting yourself to just one?

➤ How often did you eat these foods?

➤ When did you eat them? During meals or in between? At what times?

➤ Where are your food danger zones? Did you eat these foods at a restaurant, in your house standing in front of the refrigerator, or laying on the couch in front of the TV?

➤ Who was with you when you abused these foods? Were you alone in your room, having lunch with friends, or having dinner with the kids?

➤ What were you thinking or feeling right before you ate the food? Were you feeling lonely, sad, or hungry?

For instance, your log may indicate that you snack on bagels, cereals, and crackers after 8 p.m. on the three nights that you come straight home from work (the other nights, you are at classes). You plopped yourself in front of the TV and started noshing on these foods because "I was so tired, I couldn't think of what else to do," your log may state.

If this describes you, you're normal! Many people tend to consume more of their calories at night or in between meals than during meals, because they are bored, lonely, or exhausted. If you are sitting home with food as your only source of entertainment and company, and you feel a craving for a trigger food coming on, first take the 4–12 test and see if you can wait just 4 to 12 minutes so the craving can pass.

So now we have four action strategies for you to control trigger foods instead of having them control you: keeping a food/mood journal for a week; identifying your trigger foods; planning carefully for the dangerous times and places of the day when you're more vulnerable to eat a trigger food; and using the 4–12 test as often as possible to ride through the urge to self-destruct.

The other action strategy to master trigger foods is the "Just say NO!" approach. It helps enormously if you've made a deal with yourself that a particular food is simply not negotiable because it's too much trouble to keep trying to limit that food for the pleasure the food provides. I was amazed at how well this works.

Last summer, I was at the Golden Door Health Spa for a week giving talks to a group of female executives from YPO, the Young President's Organization. Toward the end of a glorious week of great company, exercise, and eating right, it dawned on me that I hadn't had any butter or candy for nearly seven days, and I was still alive! If I could do this for seven days, why couldn't I continue it when I got home? So I did. I made a deal with myself that I could no longer have butter and candy, and my life became instantly easier. I didn't have to fight with myself about how much, when, where, or what, and then feel bad when I always had too much of one of my trigger foods.

It's been almost a year now and I still have not had butter except in cooking. The only candy I had came from my kid's Halloween bag, and those chocolate bars suddenly didn't taste nearly as good as they had the year before. It has been so much easier simply to say "No" that I'm truly amazed at the effectiveness of this strategy. I love the calories I've saved and pounds I've avoided. Give it a try for yourself. Contract with yourself to avoid one of your trigger foods for at least a month and tell yourself that no matter what, you simply can't have it. After a month, you'll probably find the thrill is gone from the trigger food. You have more control, self-esteem, and health. Not a bad trade!

Don't Use Food to Beat the Boredom Blues

If your body is craving something other than food because you are bored or lonely, get away from the food. If you are at home, don't sit in the kitchen where you automatically grab a snack whether you're hungry or not. Instead, try the following:

➤ Call a friend or relative to chat.

➤ Talk to your spouse about your day.

➤ Toss a ball around outside with your kids.

➤ Brush your pet.

➤ Take a 10-minute walk.

➤ Read five pages of your favorite book.

➤ Learn a new computer program or surf the Internet.

➤ Take a warm bubble bath.

The key is to distract yourself until the craving eases and disappears. It helps to remember that the craving you feel is emotional, not physical. What you need is not food, but something interesting, fun, and stimulating to do or a person to connect with so you feel less lonely. Grabbing a bag of chips when you are in this state may feel good at first, but before long, you'll be thrown into the throes of the Moody Food Blues, and that sends you in only one direction: down.

Of Parties and Pig-Outs: Social Finger Foods

How many times have you gone into a party, happy hour, or other social setting and dashed to the refreshment table to avoid talking to people or search for something to drink that will reduce your social anxiety? I've done that and I'm an extrovert! Many of us get anxious when we enter a social setting, and it's natural to duck for cover around the food table or hang out at the bar.

But noshing on peanuts, cream dips, hummus, tortilla chips, and other finger foods—many of which are favorite trigger foods—when we're feeling shy or anxious can easily get out of control. And who feels like striking up a conversation when they're pigging out? It's hard to shake a new hand when it feels greasy from a trigger food splurge.

What can you do to stop? Don't go near the refreshment table or bar in the first place!

This suggestion will sound so logical that you'll wonder why you haven't thought of it yourself. Well, of course you've thought of it, but the fact is that physically leaving the food site is hard because you have to fend for yourself in the social swamps and risk rejection. Can you withstand the anxiety of talking to a guy whose eyes are roving around the room looking for a more interesting (or attractive) woman? Or get stuck with one of the most boring women at the party and not know how to move on?

I still have a hard time with rejection—I don't think we ever fully accept it, or grow to like it. But eating myself into oblivion so I don't have to confront my fears isn't worth it either. Dr. Gullo offers other useful tips on ways to tip the food scale in your favor during social gatherings:

Guiltless Pleasures

If you crave chocolate, your body may need the fat and sugar that the chocolate provides. So go ahead and eat SOME. The good news is that chocolate isn't high in caffeine or cholesterol. It's not as high in calories as other snack foods. So next time your friend gives you a box of Godivas, have a guiltless treat! Then put the box out of sight and reach for it again when your craving reappears.

➤ Don't go to a party on an empty stomach and tell yourself "I'll snack there and skip dinner." This is a mistake, because you'll probably consume a lot more calories—and still want dinner when you get home.

➤ Make eye contact when you talk to a person and stop scanning the room for baskets of chips. The process of craving begins when you see foods that look good to you. So avert your eyes and see no evil.

➤ When your host offers you a piece of cheesecake, don't tell her, "No thanks, I'm on a diet." There is bound to be a wise guy in the room who says, "Oh, diets are meant to be broken," or "You can always start tomorrow." Instead, blame it on the doc. Just say, "No thank you, my doctor says I have to watch my cholesterol."

Five Small Meals a Day Keep Your Pounds at Bay

Another way to take control of your eating is to eat less food more often. Most of us are hooked on three meals a day since everything in this world seems to be timed around when breakfast, lunch, and dinner take place. But who says that it has to be that way? The answer is, it shouldn't.

In fact, increasingly, experts suggest that you eat five small meals a day to keep your blood sugar levels stable throughout the day—a factor that will curb your hunger and cut down your cravings. Recent research has also shown that the five-a-day plan helps you burn up calories instead of gaining weight as you age. Over a long time, people who ate five small meals a day and exercised moderately did not gain the weight their contemporaries did who ate three large meals a day and did moderate exercise.

But these meals are not supposed to be in competition with the Last Supper. You can eat the same total number of calories, but just spread them over more meals. A meal, for instance, can be a snack of one of two of the food groups instead of covering all four.

Many of us still enjoy a nice big dinner after a long hard day. But while we are relaxing, the calories we just consumed are ready to turn in for the night, camping out in your fat cells. The calories we take in during the day are usually burned up, but the ones consumed at night stay in our nice, cozy, snugly bodies.

Many Americans sticking to the three-meals-a-day plan are now inverting the pyramid by eating their heaviest meal at breakfast and eating lighter during the day.

It's tough to believe that caving in to cravings is good for us if we can do it moderately and with foods that we won't abuse. But we've all been raised with crash and slash diets that have taught us to deny our cravings and deprive ourselves of foods our bodies are yearning for. We can take control of our food—and stop letting food control us—by learning to listen to our bodies and working with them to achieve our goals. When we learn to do that, we can beat the Moody Food Blues and use our food/mood connection to build health and strength, not weakness and inadequacy.

The Least You Need to Know

➤ Food cravings are based on a mixture of psychological and physical factors, and are usually rooted in childhood experiences.

➤ When the serotonin level in your brain drops, your body craves carbohydrates to raise the level back up—which restores a feeling of well-being.

➤ When you get a craving, wait 4 to 12 minutes to see if the hunger passes. If it does, then your craving may be psychologically based.

➤ It's best to say NO to trigger foods than to try to negotiate portions. To fulfill a biological craving, eat satisfying substitutes.

➤ If you want to eat because you're bored, distract and act: Call a friend, take a bath, or do something else to distract your attention away from eating.

➤ Eating five smaller meals a day instead of three big ones helps you control your eating and avoid gaining extra pounds.

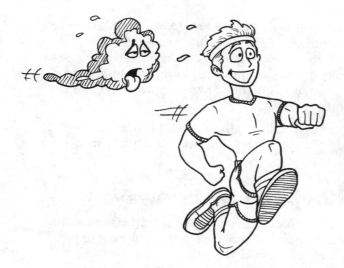

Chapter 8

Beating the Blues: Let's Get Physical

In This Chapter

➤ Exercise: the number one blues buster

➤ Working exercise into your daily routine

➤ What are endorphins and why are they good for you?

➤ The 20/20 formula: a win–win for your brain

➤ The terrific trio of aerobics, strength, and flexibility

More time! More effort! Even more sweat! Just the thought of it makes a busy grownup want to cry. We have so many reasons for not exercising, some wonderfully creative: "I don't have the time." "I'm allergic to spandex." "I get too depressed looking at those 'body beautifuls' at the gym." But the bottom line is this: *You will not beat the blues if you don't exercise!* Regular exercise is so essential to your mind/body health that there's no getting around it. You must figure out a way to put some type of exercise in your daily life because it's the only way you'll protect yourself from the blues, now and in the future.

Along with these excuses, however, there's a strong counter force in our society: the body perfect expectation. Most of us grow up facing pressure to look lean and muscled and to be able to climb to the top of Mt. Everest or successfully run the New York City Marathon. Some people are hard core about this kind of fitness, and I admire them. Most folks, however, are like me—a strung-out working person trying to squeeze in exercise before, after, or between office meetings, car pooling, and household chores.

In spite of these cultural pressures to achieve the perfect body, you don't have to be a maniac to be fit. You can begin to get in shape simply by increasing the amount of physical activity in your everyday routines—like taking the stairs instead of the elevator, walking to the bus stop instead of driving, or stretching during television commercials instead of going to the fridge for cookies and milk. Even simple chores like vacuuming or washing the car count as exercise!

In this chapter, we outline how and why you can fight funk with fitness—through both proven exercise strategies and a plan to increase physical activity as part of your daily routine.

Move and Groove to Keep the Blues Away

You roll out of bed, flip on the TV, and come across two very fit, tanned, and chirpy women in bright orange bikinis bouncing up and down a stepper to upbeat music, looking like they're having a blast getting in shape. The palm trees are swaying in the background, and you can almost smell the salt water, feel the warm wind brushing up against your skin, taste the piña coladas after the session...

And then you feel the extra fat flopping over your own belly!

I'd rather listen to pundits pontificate over political campaign reform than watch these bathing beauties perform. Who wouldn't want to switch the channel and tune out fitness? And talk about feeling blue before you even brush your teeth! So why bother trying?

If this is how you feel about exercise, then slide over to the other end of the couch to make room for most Americans. A recent Surgeon General's Report on Physical Activity and Health shows that more than 60 percent of American adults are not physically active regularly and at least 25 percent barely budge at all.

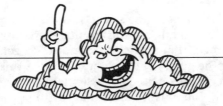

Funk-y Facts

The word "exercise" really turns off a lot of people because we've been pressured to do too much, too soon, too often. In fact, aversion to the "e" word is so extreme that many health professionals have changed their terminology to refer to exercise as "movement" or "physical activity." Even the U.S. Surgeon General's office has caught a whiff of the ill winds over use of the "e" word—and called its 1996 document "Report on Physical Activity and Health." So call it anything you want, but "Just Do It."

Yet, sitting idle for too long rots your body and your mind. When you don't engage in physical activity you are at significantly higher risk for the following:

➤ Heart disease

➤ Obesity

➤ High blood pressure

➤ Colon cancer

➤ Osteoporosis

➤ Depression

➤ Anxiety/stress

Exercise is the number one blues buster because when you are engaged in a physical activity you create energy, feel better about yourself, and get stronger mentally and physically. If you exercise for more than 30 or 40 minutes, your body releases feel-good chemicals called *endorphins*—a group of substances formed within the body that naturally relieve pain, regulate the body's response to stress, and determine mood. Exercise strengthens your immune system, bones, heart, and mind. So, if exercise is so good, why do we moan and groan so much about it?

How Did We Become Such a Motionless Mess?

As a civilization, we haven't always been so inert and weak. Our ancestors were constantly on the go, first hunting down prey for food and clothing (the mail catalogs were so slow back then), then working the fields picking crops. When the Industrial Age arrived, machines moved for us and took over much of what had been done manually. What did we do with the extra time? Why, watch TV, of course!

Blues Flag

Sitting idle for too long can be lethal! According to the American Heart Association, physical inactivity is a major risk factor for heart attacks and strokes—claiming the lives of 250,000 people every year. You can reduce the risk of contracting heart disease by filling your day with bursts of physical activity or slower prolonged activity, like walking 30 to 45 minutes a day.

Terms of Encheerment

Exercise simply means moving and getting your heart to pump stronger. It doesn't mean you have to become a marathon runner or mountain climber. It does mean walking at least 10 minutes a day, climbing stairs instead of using the elevator, carrying groceries home instead of driving, and playing catch or soccer with your child. Exercise means a life style, not a particular event.

The Information Age nipped the heels of the Industrial Age (not a minute too soon, since most of us were getting tired of watching reruns of *Green Acres* and *Gilligan's Island*) so many of us became computer nerds instead. Nearly all of our chores can now be done at the stroke of a keyboard without ever having to change out of our pajamas. And we wonder why obesity and depression are reaching epidemic proportions these days!

There is no doubt that we've progressed electronically beyond our wildest dreams—but we've regressed physically. Granted, few of us miss seeing those meticulously polite bank tellers, grumpy bureaucratic motor vehicle registration clerks, and the cranky cashiers at the supermarket. But efficiency has a price tag attached to it. And the cost of our physical lethargy is way beyond our health budget.

Haven't Got Time for the Pain

The number one reason most of us give for not exercising is: "I don't have time." If I had even a nickel every time I heard a client or friend say that, I'd be a rich woman today! All of us are time-starved no matter what we do for a living. But if Bill Clinton can find time to get out of the Oval Office and run a few laps around the White House, you should be able to sneak away from work to flex your muscles, go for a walk, or just stretch.

When people say to me, "I don't have time to exercise," what I'm really hearing is "I don't WANT to exercise." Who does, except those of us lucky enough to be born with "I just gotta move" genes? What finally made me get off my buns 15 years ago was the dawning knowledge that exercise was my only real life insurance. As we age, it's a pay now or pay later plan—and if you pay later, you pay a lot more, because you lose your ability to move.

It also became clear that exercise was the only route to preserve my mental and physical health and not die before my children became adults. I can't unnecessarily abandon my kids by getting really sick or dying, or deteriorate simply because it's easier for me to become fat and lazy. So I swing onto that exercise bike nearly every morning, no matter how much I hate it and don't want to do it. The equation is simple: The well-being of my children and their having a healthy mother is more important than my negative feelings about exercise. So I use the Nike slogan and "Just Do It" for them when I can't do it for myself.

But don't be fooled by the simplicity of the Nike message. There are many steps to achieving "Just Do It." To "Just Do It" even sometimes, I have to do a major league attitude adjustment, reorganize my time so that exercise is a business appointment with myself that cannot be easily moved, change a number of my life-style habits over a long period of time, educate myself with books, observation, and training about how, where, and when to exercise—and learn to find the inspiration within me and from others on the same exercise paths. Whew! No wonder this makes us sweat in more ways than one.

Body School Blues and Breakthroughs

I'm one of two staff psychologists at La Palestra Center for Preventative Medicine, a health-focused fitness center in New York City that trains people to become strong and healthy in body and mind. Working at La Palestra has been one of the best experiences I've ever had because I've learned so much from the staff and the curriculum that has changed my life. Pat Manocchia, owner and director of La Palestra, understands that true preventative medicine means integrating fitness as a way of life, and he's designed a program that teaches us to do that. One of the trainers, Mark Tenore, has taught me how to channel and release my aggression and depression into boxing, running, and other exercises, and even how to eat for fuel rather than for comfort.

From what I've learned over the years and particularly at La Palestra, I can honestly say that I'm stronger and healthier today than I've ever been in my life. I don't feel the effects of aging like many people my age report, and my energy increases, not decreases, with each passing year. I don't have those flaps of fat under my upper arms, and know I can protect myself if attacked. All this from someone who hates exercise and spent much of her life 30 pounds overweight and completely out of shape.

So how does such an exercise miracle happen? SLOWLY.

I'm certainly not someone with the discipline or passion to exercise consistently since birth. It has taken 12 years to get to this point and to move through the grades of Body School. I've flunked a grade or two and have been sent to the principal's office countless times for a bad exercise attitude, but along the way I learned some valuable lessons: It helps me a lot to exercise with someone else or in a group; it is very useful to work with a trainer sometimes, so I can learn how to use the machines or run properly or stretch without killing myself; and I feel so much better exercising regularly that I must do it for the rest of my life.

Motivation Matters

Many of our clients at La Palestra participate in some kind of athletic event as a way to focus and further their training. They train for and participate in marathons, mountain or rock climbing, bike races, or whatever event interests them. They come to someone like me for consultation on mental fitness, stress management, and exercise motivation.

The question I deal with all the time is this: "What do I do to feel or stay motivated to exercise?" These clients are committed to get and stay mentally psyched as well as physically fit—and they come because fears, inhibitions, or other bad feelings are preventing them from reaching their physical and mental fitness goals.

I tell them that motivation doesn't come naturally or magically. It's a learned skill, a mental muscle you build up, just like your biceps or leg muscles. If you feel good during and after a particular kind of exercise, chances are you'll try it again. Feeling and seeing the results is inspiring! For your fitness to become a lifelong habit, your motivation must come from within—and it must be for the right reasons.

To understand what works for real exercise motivation, we recently did a detailed research study of 40 people at La Palestra. Some were training to run the New York City Marathon, some dropped out of the training, and some were in a control group of people who work out but did not want to run the marathon. We studied changes in body image, weight, motivation, and mood before, during, and after the marathon.

The fascinating results were published in *SHAPE* magazine in June 1998 and in *Psychotherapy: Research, Theory and Practice*, a journal of the American Psychological Association. Results showed that those who stuck with the training and made it through the marathon felt deeply motivated by *internal* goals of increasing their strength and health. Their efforts focused on doing their personal best every day and working with a team of other members in training. They shared pain and pride, carbs and bandages. They became deeply connected to one another and their shared goals so that after they ran the marathon, their first question was: "Is everyone else okay?"

Those who didn't want to run the marathon or dropped out of the training, however, focused on competing and beating others, rather than doing their personal best, and they chose to train alone rather than work in a group or with a partner. They were motivated by external goals like losing weight, looking better, and claiming bragging rights at cocktail parties about having run the marathon. The research clearly showed that, if you want to participate in an event and feel good about it, the external goals of comparing and competing are not nearly as powerful as the internal goals of increasing health and strength.

So if your goal is to exercise so you can lose weight and please your husband or girlfriend, you aren't likely to remain motivated for very long. You'll have better luck at staying inspired if you strive to be healthy and fit so you can do whatever you want without tiring so easily. Picking an exercise you enjoy will also help you stick with the program for the long haul.

The Surgeon General recommends that you do at least 30 minutes of moderate physical activity every day if possible—and you don't have to do the activity all at once to get the cardiovascular benefits of exercising. You'd be surprised at how time flies when you are getting fit by walking up the stairs instead of taking the elevator, carrying your own groceries to your car, or washing your own car instead of taking it through the car wash.

The Terrific Trio for Health: Aerobics, Strength, and Flexibility

Any formal or informal physical activity plan must include three types of movements for you to build and achieve health:

➤ *Aerobics*. Activities that make your heart and lungs stronger so you don't run out of breath as much when you are running around doing chores.

➤ *Strength.* Activities that build up your bones and muscles so you can lift heavier things and feel stronger.

➤ *Flexibility.* Activities that help your joints and muscles stay flexible.

These movements can be incorporated into your everyday routines without ever going near a gym or watching a video narrated by an instructor who flashes a nice, clean, sweatless smile as she delves into her 98th jumping jack! Aerobics can be performed by riding a bike or walking; strength can be gained by lifting a three- or five-pound weight while talking on the phone; and stretching can be done on a desk chair or car seat or sitting on the carpet in front of the TV while watching *ER* or the *Today Show*.

Move Smart to Start

Those of you who would never set foot in a gym can become active by building physical activity into your own routines. The American Heart Association (AHA) suggests we make an effort to be move stronger and smarter. Here are some ways you can build exercise into your daily life:

➤ Walk two miles to work instead of driving or taking the bus.

➤ Walk into the school to pick up the children for carpool instead of pulling up at the pickup lane.

➤ Park in the farthest spot possible so you have to walk farther to get to the shopping mall.

➤ Throw a baseball to your kid for 10 minutes before dinner.

These are all physical activities that will make your heart happy. Other types of movement that will strengthen your muscles and keep your body flexible include the following:

➤ Squeeze a tennis ball to improve your grip and release hand tension while reading your e-mail.

➤ Get on the floor to do sit-ups or stretch while a coworker comes in to schmooze.

➤ Walk with your child while he tells you about his day at school.

➤ Do lunges as you vacuum, or stretch to touch your toes as you pick up fuzz off the rug.

➤ Do leg lifts while talking on the phone to your in-laws.

➤ Roll your head around slowly to stretch your neck and shoulder muscles while sitting in a traffic jam.

Climb a Mountain, Ford a Stream

Once you've mastered this informal physical activity plan, you can consider whether you want to go further and delve into a more formal exercise routine. Many people do want more structure after they jiggle and wiggle their bodies in these new ways because they begin to experience how much better they feel when they're active. The key to getting off on the right foot for a more formal exercise plan is to start off your program small, slow, and smart.

Be realistic about your abilities. Seeing a physician can be very helpful at this stage because as your health partner the physician can help you decide what you can and can't do to avoid injury. Doing too much too soon will do you in and turn you off to exercising! So be careful about your expectations. Statistics show that most people start and stop exercise programs five or six times before they begin doing something regularly.

Some people like to exercise at home—especially if they feel too intimidated to go to a gym. They keep treadmills or exercise bikes in their bedrooms, weights in their basements, or mats in their living rooms for stretching. If you chose this option, I suggest you get a personal trainer to come to your home for one session to help you assess your level of fitness and talk to you about fitting exercises into your life. You can find a trainer by asking friends who they know, visiting your local gym or YMCA, or calling your community recreation department.

Another tip for success is to ask a friend, spouse, or relative to be a coach for you, as you will be for that person on his exercise program. You're looking for a buddy who is as serious about working out as you are and can help keep you motivated. It's easier to bail out of exercising if nobody is looking or waiting for you.

Blues Flag

You need to talk to your doctor before starting any exercise program—especially if you're older, overweight, or have any health problems. It also helps to see a trainer even if it's for one session to help you determine the types of exercises you should be doing and at what levels. To find a trainer, go to your local YMCA or gym. Even if you're not a member, you can often use a guest pass to try out the place and work with a trainer for a session or two. Write down what the trainer says so you can try it at home and ask about exercises with free weights, not machines. You may also find it useful to consult with a nutritionist at the start up of an exercise program to ensure you are eating healthfully.

The same study of La Palestra members who were training to participate in the New York City Marathon showed that people running with "fitness buddies" and seeking the advice of a fitness trainer stuck with their program and successfully completed the race. By contrast, marathoners who dropped out tended to work out alone and didn't want to consult with any expert.

Aerobics on the Run: These Shoes Are Made for Moving

The word *aerobics* simply means "oxygen." Aerobic activities help you work your heart and lungs so you can take in oxygen better. The better your body uses oxygen, the more active you can be without getting tired.

Typically, aerobic activities use the large muscles in your legs, arms, and back. Familiar aerobic activities include:

➤ Walking

➤ Jogging

➤ Bicycling

➤ Dancing

➤ Swimming

You can do most of these activities at whatever levels of intensity you are comfortable with and you'll build more endurance as you go. You get the same benefits whether you walk briskly for a short time or leisurely for a longer time. You can race across the pool (trying to beat the guy in the next lane) or just take your time with long, slow, graceful strokes. The point is to find your aerobic range (the number of heart beats per minute necessary for your heart to build strength at your particular age) and stay in that range for 20 to 30 minutes minimum three to four times a week.

Choose Your Favorite Sport

If you've been totally inactive, select one activity that you like and do it three times a week for 10 minutes; or if you've been moving around some, do it for 15 to 20 minutes. Then build to 20 to 30 minutes three or four times a week.

Ideally, you should get to 45 minutes four to five days a week, because that's when the endorphins regularly start kicking in, and it becomes easier to begin exercising because you remember how good it can feel.

Dr. Ellen Says

If you are too uncomfortable going to a gym, buy or rent an exercise videotape. Look for tapes that cover aerobics, strength, and stretching activities and whose instructors are certified by the American Council on Exercise, American College of Sports Medicine, Aerobics and Fitness Association of America, or Cooper Institute for Aerobics Research. Stick with the more recent tapes because they incorporate the newest knowledge about physical and mental fitness—in this field, things change quickly.

Dr. Ellen Says

If you've been doing a lot of sitting, I suggest you start becoming more active by walking. This is a simple physical activity that you can do anywhere, at any time, without any special equipment. You don't even have to change clothes. That's why walking is the nation's most popular exercise. The pace at which you walk will give you different benefits, depending on how fast or slow you move.

The 20/20 Formula—A Win-Win Strategy

I used to do 20 minutes—and not a second more—on my exercise bike nearly every morning. I felt okay afterward, but always wondered whether all this "runner's high" stuff was just a bunch of hype, since I never felt it. It turns out the "exercise high"—that feeling of euphoria and well-being that comes with exercise—is not hype. I just wasn't exercising long enough to get the benefits of those endorphins, which typically kick in after 30 to 40 minutes of physical activity. During the first 20 minutes your body just burns calories, but in the next 20 it burns fat and usually produces endorphins. That's the 20/20 formula.

What keeps me inspired to get on that bicycle and spin away five or six days a week? Knowing how great I'll feel when I finish and that I'll feel really bad if I get fat! The 20/20 formula works so well that I'll often fit it in no matter how busy my day is! So I just get up a half an hour earlier each morning and get on the bike.

Bear the Weight and Spare Your Waist

The stronger your muscles are, the more you can lift, push, or hold. Having strong muscles also helps prevent injuries and reduces lower-back pain and gives you the stamina you need to do more physically rigorous activities without running out of breath so quickly. Sit-ups, push-ups, and leg lifts are all muscle-strengthening exercises—your body weight is used as the resistance on certain muscle groups. Lower-back pain is one of the symptoms of depression, so sit-ups and back-strengthening exercises can be another way to beat a potential symptom of the blues.

Many people use hand weights and weight machines to build strength into their arms, shoulders, and chest. You can start out with two-pound weights and build up to heavier ones. But you don't have to buy these if you don't want to. Just go to your pantry, grab a couple of cans of soup and start counting sets of 10.

I try to do weight training twice a week, once at La Palestra and once at home. We have a variety of weights of different shapes, sizes, and colors hanging against our bedroom wall. Sometimes I do the weights with the kids after school. Twelve-year-old boys who have begun to care about their bodies are great exercise partners. They push themselves and it's embarrassing not to keep up with them. Whether it's adults or kids, I encourage you to find a buddy to do these exercises with—you'll feel more motivated to push that weight instead of quitting to get some ice cream.

Guiltless Pleasures

Are you so stressed out that you are fit to be tied? Get away from it all by treating yourself to a health spa for a fantastic day or week of fun and fitness. Spas can be expensive, but the rewards are well worth it. You'll eat fine, healthful cuisine and work with top-notch trainers who are eager to teach you how to keep your mind and body in shape. Afterward, you'll feel refreshed, rejuvenated, and ready to roar once again!

Stretch Your Body and You'll Stretch Your Mind

We do stretching exercises all the time without even thinking about it. After sitting for hours at your desk, you get up and stretch your arms and back, moving your head from side to side to stretch your neck muscles. Afterward, you feel a little less tense, a little more relaxed.

Stretching before and after exercising is critical, although, unfortunately, stretching is the first thing we give up if we're short on time. Stretching helps keep your muscles from tightening up and makes you feel more flexible, which is especially important as you age because your muscles and joints become less limber and want to shrink. Without stretching, you feel stiff, can't move around as well, and are more at risk of being injured.

Stretching activities are easy to do and you don't need any equipment. To get some ideas on the types of stretching exercises you could do, buy a videotape on stretching or check one out from the library. Several books on stretching include pictures to show you how to do the exercise (a good one to check out is *The Complete Idiot's Guide to Healthy Stretching*, Alpha Books, 1998). You might also try an exercise class or a yoga session.

Try starting your day by sitting on the edge of your bed and stretching your back and spine by hanging over the side of the bed with your head and arms limp like a big rag doll almost falling over. You get two benefits from one movement: It stretches your back for the day and wakes up your brain for the morning.

Whether you stretch or grow heart, muscle, and brain through exercise, it all comes down to this: To beat the blues, you've got to do a certain amount of physical activity every day. You don't have to get all decked out in the latest aerobic fashions and join a gym to get a cardiovascular workout—and you don't even have to stick to traditional forms of exercising. You can start getting in shape by adding physical activity to your daily routine; then decide how you can move to a more regular exercise regimen.

Remember, it's better to sweat than to fret!

The Least You Need to Know

➤ Exercise is one of the best ways to fight the blues.

➤ When we engage in physical activity for more than 40 minutes, our brains produce chemicals called endorphins, giving us that "exercise high" that elevates our mood.

➤ A workout can take many forms: walking instead of riding, standing instead of sitting, carrying a child instead of pushing the stroller, vacuuming your living room instead of sitting in the dust balls.

➤ Studies show that sitting idle for too long is bad for your mental and physical health and only gets worse with age.

➤ All you need is 30 minutes of some physical activity at least three or four days a week to keep in acceptable shape.

➤ To be fit, you should include: aerobics, weight-bearing exercises, and stretching routines in your exercise program.

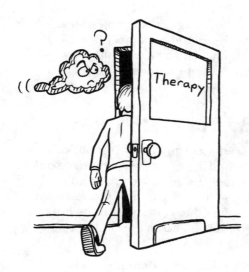

Chapter 9

When Self-Help Isn't Enough

In This Chapter

➤ Acknowledging when you need help

➤ Crossing the line from blues to depression

➤ The five types of depression

➤ The ABCs of therapy

➤ The top three therapy approaches: interpersonal, behavioral, and cognitive

➤ Three is a crowd—four or more is a support group

One of the hardest four-letter words many of us will ever say is: "Help!" It's tough to acknowledge that there are times when you can't do it yourself, whether it's fixing a broken marriage, drying up a drinking problem, or owning up to the fact that you have an illness like depression. Why? We *hate* to acknowledge vulnerability. None of us is supposed to have any vulnerabilities and weaknesses, yet every human being does.

But only by acknowledging that we need help can we begin to recover from depression and pave the way for a happier, healthier, and more meaningful life. Had I known that the depression I had was a curable illness, I would have sought therapy and medication sooner. I'd like to spare you the pain and confusion I went through—and that's really the reason I'm writing this book. In this chapter, I'll spell out the different types of depression and the various forms of therapy available to help people overcome this condition.

So if you fall into the category of "when self-help isn't enough," seek professional guidance. You owe it to yourself and those who love you! And remember that although "Help" can feel like a terrible four-letter word, when you finally say it and *mean it*, your real recovery has begun. You're no longer alone and it gets easier from that point forward.

When You Can't Get Over It By Yourself

When was the last time a miracle visited you? I haven't had any lately. Yet our culture zealously encourages our belief in miracles and the "quick fix" as the solutions to our problems. I can't tell you the number of times I've appeared as an expert on a TV talk show and been asked to give the "five tips" to solve some very complex problem that was just described in great, gory detail on the show. I used to comply with the host's request and quickly rattle off five tips to solve the problem, just as the closing credits started to roll and the show's theme song began. But I always felt bad.

As helpful as I thought this kind of advice could be, I was also promoting the idea of a quick fix and supporting our culture's denial that it's *not* hard work to solve these problems and somehow with luck they'll solve themselves. I became afraid that if people followed my advice they would fail and feel even worse. So I stopped doing those TV shows and began to explore what really does work when you're vulnerable. Here's what I've learned so far about how to achieve real solutions to your problems:

➤ *Acknowledge your vulnerability.* This can be such a relief but it's also scary, so you're brave to do this. But if you speak from your heart about your vulnerability and weakness, people have no choice but to listen and will usually want to help. Never forget that *all* of us have broken places inside and vulnerabilities because we are all human, even if some of us are better at hiding them than others. And sharing vulnerability is how true intimacy in a relationship grows.

➤ *You can't manage the big problems all alone.* No man or woman is an island and no true solution has ever been carried out without the help of others. I remind myself all the time that "it takes a village to raise an adult" and that it's a strength, not a weakness, to ask others to help you when you're vulnerable. It's important to your health to recognize others have something to give you that you can't give yourself.

➤ *See yourself as a problem solver, not a victim.* Don't give up—keep learning about the problem. Try new approaches to the problem and be open to feedback about what needs to change in your approach. Eventually you'll find a true solution that works for almost any problem.

These three steps to problem solving are especially important for you when self-help approaches are not enough to fix your blues or depression. To acknowledge your vulnerability, learn the difference between having the blues and experiencing real depression—read books like this one and talk to others. Then be honest with yourself about which description applies to you.

If your bad feelings go away before two weeks, chances are you've got the blues. But depression may be setting in if the symptoms last any longer than that. If you scored in the black on the "Are You Blue or Are You Depressed?" quiz in Chapter 2, don't be too hard on yourself! It's just a vulnerability rising to the surface, just like some people are more prone to heart disease or cancer. The fact that you're depressed is not your fault. Remember: Depression is curable. I'm living proof of that! After years of psychotherapy and experimenting with medication, I was finally able to join the ranks of the generally happy and usually empowered.

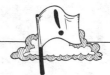

Blues Flag

Be careful, because the symptoms of depression and the blues appear similar on the surface; but the main difference is how *long* you've felt down and out.

Drawing the Line From Blue to Black

As we've seen in the previous chapters, there is a fine line between feeling blue and sliding into the pit of depression, and that's why taking the quiz in Chapter 2 is so important. I encourage you to take it if you haven't already done so, or take it again next time you feel particularly down. For most of us, falling into depression is a gradual process; it creeps up on us as we face a series of disappointments and failures in our personal and professional lives. Many of us teeter on the edge of depression for years before we just topple over and get sucked into the dark pit of this black mood.

You migrate from having the blues into experiencing depression if you:

➤ Have a good reason to be upset but then deny your bad feelings, or feel too emotionally stressed to cope with them, so you sweep them under the rug (where of course they continue to grow and eventually become so large they trip you).

➤ Have too much unresolved pain and loss from your past so you can't cope with normal, everyday problems that would make anyone upset.

➤ Are stuck in a pattern of negative thinking even if you've got good reasons to feel pessimistic.

➤ Have few relationships even though anyone in your shoes would have a tough time feeling close to people.

➤ Are vulnerable to inheriting depression.

The insidious nature of depression is that once you experience it, you're likely to get stuck in it—which is why you need professional treatment to get out of it. Self-help techniques won't be adequate if you're trapped in a real depression, so before you end up spinning your wheels and achieving few results, get professional help to guide you.

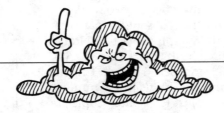

Funk-y Facts

In 1990 and 1991, the American Psychological Association National Task Force on Women and Depression concluded that in 80 to 90 percent of all cases, symptoms of depression can be significantly reduced in 12 to 14 weeks with the right kind of treatment. Unfortunately, only one out of five people with depression will ever get help. The rest continue to suffer silently, afraid that people will ridicule them if they knew they were depressed, or resigned that nothing can be done to lift their dark moods. Or, even worse, they have depression and don't know it. These sad folks think it's normal and natural to feel so bad for so long.

The first step in overcoming depression is accepting that *it most likely won't go away* if you just ignore it. Or, if it does go away, it will come back, usually stronger than ever! Biological, economic, cultural, family, and psychological stresses typically trigger vulnerability to depression and so it must be treated by examining your relationship with your family, your feelings about yourself, your view of the world, your behavior, your biology, your economic strengths and weaknesses, and other factors that make you who you are today.

The second step to breaking free from depression is to get an in-depth evaluation by a psychologist or psychiatrist who specializes in treating depression. If you are afflicted with depression, you need to find answers to the following questions: What kind of depression do you suffer from? How severe is the depression? What treatment approach would be most effective?

Be warned that these questions are deceptively simple. First, it's hard to find specialists you like and trust; second, some health professionals say they treat depression but they're not real experts; and, third, depression is a complex disorder that is often overlooked or misdiagnosed. But there are also many good therapists out there.

When I was president of the Division of Psychotherapy of the American Psychological Association, I represented a group of about 6,000 Ph.D. psychologist psychotherapists nationally and some internationally. I can say without a doubt that many of these psychologists were skilled healers and some of them were the most decent, caring people you'll ever meet. Try to find a therapist like that. With effort, you will.

The first place to start is by asking people you know and respect if they can recommend a therapist they like. You can also call your state's psychological association (usually located in large cities or state capitals) for lists of therapists in that area. To get the phone number of the association in your area, call APA (American Psychological Association) Practice Directorate at (800) 374-2723. Medical schools also have departments of psychology or psychiatry with therapists who are experts on depression on staff. Interview several therapists if you can, even if it's through a brief phone consultation, to see who you like as well as who's qualified.

Interview several candidates on the phone to see who "fits and feels" the best to you, and ask them questions like, "How would you go about deciding which treatment is right for me?" What they answer is important, but the way they answer is even more crucial. If they seem annoyed by your queries, that's a red flag! Before you are ready to make your decision, check the person's credentials. But remember: All the credentials in the world won't help you if you don't have a good feeling about the therapist. So trust your gut!

The Depression Diagnosis: "Doctor, What's Wrong with Me?"

The best way to guard against getting the wrong diagnosis is to arm yourself with as much information as you can about depression, and work with your mental health practitioner to find the proper treatment. There are five major types of depression, as discussed in the following sections.

Dysthymic Depression

This type of depression, also known as "neurotic depression," is the most common type of depression and twice as common in women than in men. It's characterized by a sense of helplessness, inability to get what you need, a feeling of being deprived, a defeatist attitude about your past, present, and future, and a constant state of sadness or anger over real or imagined loss. This depression can be caused by our inability to communicate effectively with people and from living in a culture that makes us feel inadequate about our appearance and accomplishments. People afflicted with this form of depression can still function, but they perpetually feel bad about themselves or those around them. They often think pessimistically and have little faith in the goodness of the future or their own value and worth.

Atypical Depression

This type of depression—also more common in women than in men—is camouflaged by other disorders such as bulimia, anorexia nervosa, compulsive overeating, oversleeping, and excessive irritability. People experiencing these disorders don't know that the depression is underlying their feelings about themselves. People who find themselves craving too much sleep (hypersomnia), experiencing huge appetites (hyperphagia), or increased sexual drive over a period of at least two weeks may be suffering from atypical depression.

Dr. Ellen Says

People have a genetic vulnerability to major depression if they have close relatives who were depressed. Biochemical changes in the brain either cause this depression or occur because of the depression. This is the reason why people afflicted with major depression often need medication to help balance their brain chemistry so they can benefit from psychotherapy.

Major Depression

People with major depression usually can't function in one or more areas of their lives for more than two weeks and may be feeling suicidal. Although slightly more women than men suffer from this form of depression, gender differences are not as pronounced because major depression seems to be the type most related to biological and genetic causes. This kind of depression is hard to identify and treat because it's often a recurrent, progressive illness. Depression is a mood cancer and like a physical cancer, it can go into remission, but it's likely to come back more quickly and with more intensity if it isn't treated.

Bipolar Disorder

People suffering from bipolar disorder, also known as manic depression, experience periods of deep depression followed by elation and hyperactivity. While feeling manic, people believe they are invincible and all-powerful. They get little sleep, spend money they don't have, and make unrealistic plans for their future. But after days or weeks of feeling that they are invincible, they crash, and view their world as dark and dreary. Both women and men are equally susceptible to having a bipolar disorder, and some evidence suggests that creative people tend to have a higher degree of this type of depression. Like major depression, a bipolar disorder seems to be the result of a biochemical imbalance in the brain and can be treated with a combination of medication and therapy.

Seasonal Affective Disorder (SAD)

As we discussed in Chapter 5, symptoms of seasonal affective disorder typically peak during the fall and winter and disappear in the spring and summer, although a few people experience the opposite pattern with more problems in the summer. Most people go through some phase of the winter "blahs," a period of sluggishness when it's cold and gray; however, those who suffer from SAD are much more seriously affected by the lack of light. SAD is the most easily treated depression, but also the most commonly misdiagnosed. As a result, people who have SAD often end up in "talk" therapy sessions when what they need—literally—is more light in their lives. Those affected by SAD can find relief from their depression by sitting in front of light boxes for a half hour to an hour a day. These light boxes treat SAD very effectively, without resorting to other costly treatments. Your therapist or physician can give you more information on this type of therapy.

Finding the Right Professional for Body and Mind

Depression can be scary not only for the person experiencing it but for those around him as well. But the good news is the chances of successful treatment have never been better! And you can find a cure for this condition without spending the rest of your life on a therapist's couch or draining your entire bank account!

Because there are so many different types of therapy—and each one has a slightly different angle—I wanted to devote the rest of the chapter to this topic. First, though, I'd like to give you a brief overview of the goals of any therapy.

Can We Talk? The Benefits of Psychotherapy

Ever wonder why psychotherapy was dubbed "talk therapy"?

It's because *psychotherapy*—defined as a treatment for mental and emotional problems—relies on verbal and nonverbal communication between the therapist and the person seeking help. The founder of modern psychotherapy was Sigmund Freud (1856–1939), who started treating patients in late 19th-century Vienna with the early techniques of psychoanalysis. His techniques probed the patient's unconscious conflicts and motivations to explain the patient's behavior and bring about change.

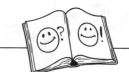

Since Freud's time, over 400 different therapy approaches have been developed and many have flourished, including interpersonal, behavioral, and cognitive therapies, which we'll discuss in just a moment. Most psychological treatments take place within a confidential relationship with the therapist, who supports, accepts, and gives hope to her client. The right kind of therapy can change your life profoundly—I know that it has done that for me. Without psychotherapy, I absolutely would not have learned the necessary life and relationship skills given my background of loss and poor education. Without therapy, I would not be able to function today, much less enjoy being a mother, wife, and professional.

Terms of Encheerment

Psychotherapy is a proven form of treatment that is based on resolving emotional and mental conflicts by talking about the problem and trying new behaviors to solve the problem. As I tell my kids, therapists are the "talk doctors." We identify problems and offer a lot of support, ideas, and skills about how to change, rather than give shots or medicine to help people feel better.

Three Good Reasons Doctors Prescribe Therapy

All forms of psychotherapy will give you a chance to see yourself in a new light and offer support to try new behaviors that might work better than the old ones. The self-growth and deepening self-knowledge that results from therapy is so attractive that many people who've got the blues—not just those who are depressed—pursue this form of treatment for their short- or long-term goals.

Most forms of psychotherapy have three goals:

1. To alleviate psychological pain and teach stress management so that you feel less distressed, upset, and anxious—and you can begin to deal with the problems that are preventing you from leading a happy, productive life.

2. To modify your behavior patterns and change aspects of your personality that have worked against you by preventing you from getting involved in healthy relationships or satisfying jobs, for example.

3. To increase self-awareness and insight so you can develop a better sense of judgment and become more flexible emotionally.

Psychotherapy can be conducted with individuals, groups of clients, couples, or families. You can be in therapy for the short term or long term, depending on when you and your therapist agree that your goals have been met.

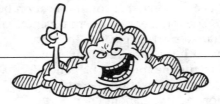

Funk-y Facts

Most people who are getting psychological or psychiatric help today are in individual therapy, a technique that focuses on the person's specific problems, coping mechanisms, defenses, and troubling behaviors, and what the person can do to solve the problems. Some psychotherapists give advice and are active participants in the treatment, while others sit back and let the patient explore and free-associate in order to get to the bottom of the depression. The latter is a more traditional, analytic approach that is typically not as effective in the initial stages of treating depression.

More active approaches are especially valuable to women because they emphasize action instead of just talking about problems. People who go to these therapy sessions learn to develop relationship skills that will allow them to enter into healthy alliances with other people. They also learn to change their behavior so that they become more independent-minded and think more positively, focusing on what they *can* do rather than what they can't.

The most effective approaches for the treatment of depression offered by trained mental-health professionals are:

➤ Interpersonal therapy

➤ Behavioral therapy

➤ Cognitive therapy

Let's take a closer look at each of these approaches.

Interpersonal Therapy (IPT): Can We Connect?

Interpersonal therapy is one of the newer short-term psychotherapies that focus mainly on relationship skills: assessing the quality and quantity of your relationships and teaching you better ways to achieve intimacy. It's based on the notion that symptoms of depression often evolve from problems in relationships. Because a woman's sense of self is primarily developed through her connections with people, IPT has proven to be particularly helpful to women; but men also benefit. IPT is based on a partnership model: The person seeking help is called a "client" instead of "patient" because he or she is not regarded as being sick or in need of a cure. The emphasis is on improving the client in his or her relationships at home and at work, focusing on the here and now.

The problem with IPT is that some clients need longer-term analytical technique, and IPT is short-term and aims to change behavior.

The first several sessions are spent exploring and defining current relationship problems and coming up with a goal for treatment. Then in weekly sessions over three to four months, clients and therapists work together on solving relationship problems that may be the cause of the depression. You might, for instance, feel depressed because a loved one died, or because you are constantly fighting with your partner. Throughout therapy you would learn about the importance of developing better communications skills so you could improve your relationships and feel better about yourself and your future.

Terms of Encheerment

Interpersonal therapy (IPT) is a short-term psychotherapy that focuses on developing and applying relationships skills. Through IPT, the therapist helps clients understand how critical positive relationships are to their well-being and then helps them assess the quality and quantity of their relationships.

Dr. Ellen Says

A major study conducted by the National Institute of Mental Health in 1989 on the treatment of depression found that 57 to 69 percent of clients who finished a 16-week course of IPT no longer had depressive symptoms. They were more effective at work, in leisure activities, and in the way they interacted with family members and others. More recent research reports even more promising results.

The focus of IPT is in the "here and now," and the client leaves each session with homework that he or she must do before the next session. The relationship with the therapist is very important and one of the ways the client learns relationship skills. In IPT, the therapist is very active and engaged with the client, serving as a coach, cheerleader, and janitor (to help mop up the mess created by the problems) all rolled into one. IPT is the primary focus of the therapy I do with depressed clients, although I use many other techniques as well. It is really fun and productive to do, and clients love it because it produces better results faster than many other approaches.

Behavioral Therapy: Positive Reinforcement at Work

Behavioral therapy focuses on changing a client's behavior. It is based on the idea that the depressed client isn't getting enough positive reinforcement in his or her life and needs to create more sources of rewards in order to trigger behavioral changes. The therapy emphasizes the connection between the behavior and what triggers it, not on childhood history or the deeper emotional processes underlying psychological conflicts. Analytical therapy is better suited to do that kind of in-depth exploration.

Many of the techniques used in behavioral therapy began with the discoveries of Russian physiologist Ivan Pavlov (1849–1936), who showed the principles of classic conditioning when he trained a dog to salivate at the sound of a bell. His experiments showed fundamental ways in which behavior is learned and how it can be changed.

You can change your behavior too—not by learning how to drool when you hear a bell ring like Pavlov's dog, but by charting your behavior. Once you realize that the behavior isn't serving you well, you can devise your own system of benefits and rewards for behavioral change.

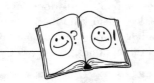

Terms of Encheerment

Behavioral therapy is a type of short-term psychological treatment that zeroes in on changing specific behaviors by using positive reinforcement, learning the antecedents and consequences of their behavior, and practicing life-management skills to behave more effectively.

Say, for instance, you're too terrified to drive on the highway because you are afraid of getting into a car accident—and this fear prevents you from doing many activities that require driving, like going to the mall or taking a job across town. To "unlearn" your fear, you could do relaxation exercises, so whenever you start feeling the anxiety about driving, you can take deep breaths, calm yourself, and get on that beltway ramp despite your fear. Once you've succeeded, you could give yourself positive reinforcement—take yourself out to dinner or buy yourself a new CD to listen to in the car when you drive on the beltway ramp again. You will then start associating the dreaded event—driving the car in the beltway—with a positive feeling and experience. The experience of driving will become more rewarding than punishing so your fear will lessen and your behavior will change accordingly and be more likely to stick.

Because behavioral therapy is very focused and problem-specific, your therapist will first conduct a careful assessment of which behaviors you want targeted and the consequences of each unwanted behavior. As in IPT, the therapist will train you in new life skills and give you homework so that you can start learning to exercise more control over your environment and give yourself more positive reinforcement to overcome certain fears, vulnerabilities, or self-defeating behaviors.

Cognitive Therapy: Get to Know Your Thoughts

Like behavioral therapy, *cognitive therapy* is a short-term treatment that targets specific symptoms, but it focuses on the person's thoughts rather than behaviors. Originally developed by Dr. Aaron Beck, cognitive therapy identifies logical errors in thinking which are common among depressed people. It's based on the assumption that the way people feel is the direct result of the way they think—and because people's thinking is often distorted, their feelings are based on thoughts that aren't true. So if you think that you can't get a better job, for example, you probably won't look for one or do well in an interview because you've already accepted defeat regardless of how qualified you may be. Such negative thinking leads to negative experiences.

Cognitive therapists will intervene in this thinking process by helping a client identify her thoughts, check their accuracy, and then correct these thoughts to more accurately reflect the person's reality. Cognitive therapy is very simply a technique to teach you how to convert your negative thinking into positive thoughts, and then harness the positive energy that's released into constructive change.

Cognitive therapy is an especially vital tool for depressed women, because it trains them to label and understand these typically self-sabotaging distortions and to realize when they are having them. It also appeals to men because it stresses productive thinking more than a demand for them to express feelings. Men often find intellectual,

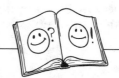

Terms of Encheerment

Cognitive therapy is short-term and seeks to change distorted thinking that often contributes to feeling depressed. Cognitive therapy works so well because the quickest way to change how you feel is to change how you think, and how we think is something we can all control.

Blues Flag

If for more than two weeks you've been drawing negative conclusions about yourself, taking blame for events that aren't your fault, or explaining situations in black-and-white terms (most situations fall in the gray area), there is a good chance that you are depressed and could benefit from cognitive therapy. Seeing a cognitive therapy specialist can change how you think!

action-oriented approaches easier than emotional exploration and they have been very successful improving the quality and quantity of their thoughts with cognitive therapy approaches.

Join the Crowd: Group Therapy

Group therapy is an increasingly popular form of treatment for depressed people because it's more efficient and economical than many other forms of therapy. All kinds of group experiences can be helpful for someone beating the blues or depression, including groups in clinics, churches, schools, and just about anyplace that has a group gathering for a specific purpose. If you have a depression, group therapy is helpful because it more specifically addresses the causes and cures for depression. In group therapy, a trained therapist leads the group and uses interactions of members to help participants improve their relationships and bring about behavioral change.

Group members become like a big family. You'll probably love some of them and hate some of them, but you'll need to learn how to resolve conflict with all of them. In group therapy, you work out your feelings and communicate your needs to a variety of people. Groups are like social laboratories where you can try out new behaviors in a safe place with a trained expert and symbolic brothers and sisters who can all help you evaluate what works, what doesn't, and why.

In group therapy you can also learn about the mistakes and triumphs other people have. A good group becomes an ongoing source of support and learning and is a huge help in resolving lonely and inadequate feelings. I've been a member of groups or lead them for over 30 years, and more than ever, I believe they are one of the most powerful healing tools we have for resolving depression.

Dr. Ellen Says

Check your newspaper's health section for listings of groups that deal with depression or related problems. Or call a local medical school or hospital and ask about what groups they offer. You can also try asking local therapists where groups are being held, even if you don't want to see the therapist for individual therapy. Therapists usually know who's leading a group, what the focus is, and whether there's room for new members; and most will be happy to help you find a group that fits your needs.

Group therapy offers many benefits:

➤ It costs less than individual psychotherapy, so it's more accessible to people with lower incomes or limited time.

➤ People end up demonstrating their relationship and communication problems by how they interact with other group members, rather than describing their problems as something that happens in the outside world. With the problem "in your face," there's more opportunity to fix it as it occurs.

➤ Groups provide a sense of community so people feel others are in the same boat—and many have overcome the same difficulties.

The result: People help each other work through their problems and come up with solutions to overcome depression quicker and more effectively than many other therapeutic approaches. In my private practice, I encourage clients to use the group as an extension of individual therapy after we have had a number of individual sessions. Eventually, they replace individual with group treatment. Many like the group experience so much that they choose to remain in the same group for several years.

Self-Help Groups: 12 Steps to Recovery

Groups who share a common need, stressful life experience, illness, or concern make up the most popular form of group support in the United States. These self-help groups offer encouragement, give spiritual direction, provide hope (especially for substance abuse recovery), and pave the way to personal growth so that group participants feel empowered to improve their life.

Look at the calendar in the health section of your newspaper and you'll see self-help or support groups for medical conditions you never knew existed. Call Alcoholics Anonymous (AA)—they're in the phone book—and they will provide you with a list of self-help groups in your community dealing with a wide range of topics, in addition to alcoholism. The popularity of these groups supports this notion: People appreciate the value of sharing their pain and feelings with others who understand what they're going through.

The most well-known self-help groups include Alcoholics Anonymous and Overeaters Anonymous, but there are dozens of other 12-step programs that address a vast array of addictions ranging from shopping to gambling. These programs help people who are depressed because their addiction gets in the way of healing, so if they can lick the addiction they've got a better shot at overcoming depression.

Self-help settings may be the only settings in which some people seek help. Many people who'd never be caught dead in a therapist's office would venture to an AA meeting, for instance. Such groups teach people that they are not responsible for their disease, but they are responsible for taking corrective action.

But these groups have limitations as well. While they give you a chance to express your feelings, they rarely offer feedback about what you can do to work through your problems. Most people who are depressed need a professional to guide them through various levels of growth until they feel better about themselves and can better cope with life's problems.

So when self-help isn't enough, either in these kinds of groups or from your own individual effort, then please push through your doubts and fears and say: "Help!" A trained professional will hear and help you in ways no one else can, until both of you find ways to beat the blues and depression too.

The Least You Need to Know

➤ There is a fine line between the blues and depression—and it's crucial for you to know the difference.

➤ The five major types of depression are: dysthymic, atypical, major, bipolar disorder, and seasonal affective disorder.

➤ Psychotherapy tries to alleviate your psychological pain, modify your behavior patterns, and increase your self-awareness.

➤ The most common types of psychotherapies for depression treatment include interpersonal therapy, behavioral therapy, and cognitive therapy.

➤ Group therapy costs less than individual therapy, and gives people multiple sources of support and problem solving and a sense of community so they don't feel so alone.

➤ Self-help groups established by people who share a common need, stressful life experience, or illness are the most popular form of group therapy in the United States today.

Part 3
Easy Clues for the Ordinary Blues

So, you're getting older, you don't think you look so hot, or your body doesn't seem to work as well—and you're so burned out most of the time that none of it matters anyhow. In other words, you aren't having any fun on this planet!

But don't beat up on yourself so much! You've got plenty of reasons to feel down. The fact is that nobody can fulfill the body-perfect standard society has set for us even though we all try like crazy to be trim and attractive. And it's tough to be upbeat about getting older when everything you hear about aging makes you want to dig your own hole before you hit 70. But you can beat these blues by challenging societal notions of beauty and age. These chapters tell you how to do just that so you can accept and feel good about who you are through all your ages and stages.

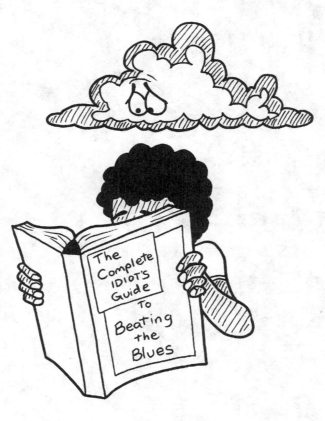

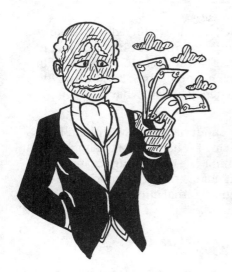

Chapter 10

"Can't Buy Me Love..." or Happiness, Either

> ### In This Chapter
>
> ➤ Debunking the myths: Wealth, attractiveness, and youth don't guarantee happiness
>
> ➤ How self-esteem and happiness go hand in hand
>
> ➤ What are the qualities of happy people?
>
> ➤ Quiz: How happy are you really?
>
> ➤ Replacing negative thoughts with positive ones
>
> ➤ The keys to happiness

I hate to admit it, but I've been unhappy more of my life than I've been happy. With the losses I had as a kid and the poor emotional management skills I had as an adult, it was almost guaranteed that unhappiness would be a frequent companion in my life. But the good news is that these unhappy experiences have made me more determined than ever to reverse the pattern. As I enter the second half of my life, I am fully committed to creating many more happy than sad days. And the best news is that now I can finally succeed because I know what works. The action strategies described in this chapter are the best tools my clients and I have found and used to create a happy life.

How about you? Have you been happy or unhappy most of today, this past week, or last month? Which feelings tend to run stronger in you: the blues or those sunny yellow ones? Asking yourself these kinds of questions is the first step to beating the blues. The second step is to learn what happiness truly is, not what we're told by the media it's supposed to be.

It's tempting to think that being rich, famous, attractive, and well-liked will make you happy. But you could be a millionaire, look like George Clooney or Sharon Stone, have a plaque in your room naming you the "best-liked" or "most likely to succeed" from high school and still be unhappy. Why? Because true happiness has little bearing on how much money you make, what title you have, where you live, what race you belong to, how old you are, or how you look.

In this chapter, I'll debunk some of the basic myths about happiness with hard facts. Then I'll show you how you can create your own recipe for happiness: enhancing your self-esteem, taking more control over your life, banning negative thoughts and learning to think positively, and making other important changes so you can join the ranks of the satisfied and genuinely happy, regardless of the external circumstances in your life.

"If I Were a Rich Man (or Woman)..."

MYTH: "If I had more money, I could move out of this dump, eat at fancy restaurants, quit my lousy job...and be really happy."

FACT: There is little correlation between well-being and being well-off, according to David G. Myers, author of *The Pursuit of Happiness*. Studies show that once you've got enough money to take care of your basic needs—food, drink, and shelter—you get the same shot at happiness whether you live in a dump or with Donald Trump.

I'm not saying that buying a large-screen TV to put in the larger home you just purchased isn't fun. But it's a quick thrill and then comes the chill. Before long, that big screen looks boring as you get used to everything looking bigger. And you're reminded, once again, that bigger is not necessarily better as you plot and scheme for your next expensive toy.

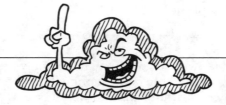

Funk-y Facts

According to David G. Myers, author of *The Pursuit of Happiness*, the good news is that our buying power has doubled since the 1950s; the bad news is that we are not any happier for it! In 1990, as in 1957, only one in three Americans told the University of Chicago National Opinion Research Center that they were "very happy." Darn, it just goes to show that what the Beatles said back in the 1960s is still true: "Money can't buy me love"—or happiness, either.

But buying is cool, you might be thinking. Not as cool as love or feeling proud of yourself. The character Tevye from *Fiddler On The Roof* may indeed have been a happier man if he knew that he already possessed all the wealth a man could have—food on the table, a loving family, and a roof over his head, shaky as it was. So, before you buy, don't lie. Ask yourself, will this purchase bring me real happiness? Then listen closely to yourself for the answer.

Ahhhh...to Be Young Again!

MYTH: "If only I had my youth, I'd be so happy."

FACT: People who say they'd be happier if they were young again probably forgot what it was like to be young. According to Myers, studies show that happiness doesn't align itself with any particular age. And recent research has shown that in fact our younger people are more unhappy than those age 30 and above. Over the past 20 years, those middle aged and above have a declining suicide rate while suicide for teens has sky-rocketed by almost 300 percent.

And for older folks, national surveys confirm that the empty nest is generally a happy place once those moody young adults have moved on. The kids have flown the coop, and the parents finally have a chance to focus on themselves and each other. But for kids, growing up is increasingly difficult, dangerous, and sometimes, just the pits. So don't think if you were younger you'd be happier. Instead, count your blessings along with those wrinkles.

Happiness Is in the Details

Happiness often comes from embracing the details of life. It's a feeling of contentment that runs like an undercurrent in our lives, a sense that at this point in your life, you feel good about yourself, your relationships, and the way you live.

Happiness pops out from small, little, seemingly insignificant things. You love your mutt Milly so you don't mind carrying a pooper-scooper and a plastic bag when you take her for walks. You look forward to eating your cereal and reading the box again for the tenth time. You can't wait to put together the data base at work even though you know nobody in the office will appreciate it but you.

That doesn't mean that people who are happy lead hunky-dory lives all the time. Even the happiest cheerleader falls, fails, and frets at times. But these changes in our emotional weather are quite useful to us. They keep us from becoming bored, teach us to appreciate the sunny days even more, and help us create deeper connections with others when we share our sad and bad feelings and discover we're not alone.

The Secret to Happiness

Happy people cope better with stress and anxiety, and they don't beat themselves up when they do something wrong or when somebody does something awful to them. Let's take a look at the qualities of genuinely happy people:

➤ Happy people are flexible, loving, and tolerant.

➤ They like themselves and accept that they will make mistakes. They believe there is always more to learn to become better people.

➤ They are confident, eager to try new experiences, and work hard.

➤ They don't believe anybody owes them anything and they take responsibility for their own happiness and their own lives. They are not blamers.

➤ They are optimistic about their future and willing to help others make their future better too.

➤ They feel in control of their lives and are able to say "No" if they are too busy.

➤ They have a strong network of support from friends and family.

➤ When they are wrong, they feel bad at first, but collect themselves, correct the problem, learn from it, and move on.

Dr. Ellen Says

The ingredients in the recipe for happiness are positive self-esteem, an optimistic outlook about the future, control over your life, connections with a close group of people, helping others, a strong commitment to something good outside yourself, and the courage to face your fears. Mix these ingredients and bake for one hour. You'll have enough servings of happiness to feed not only yourself but an entire tribe!

Boy, do they have their act together! Such maturity! Sometimes, I'm totally jealous. No wonder unhappy people love to hate them! But remember, nobody is happy all of the time. And everybody has the capacity to be happy because happiness is a life skill that needs to be learned and practiced by all of us. Let's look at how you can develop better happiness skills for your own life.

Are We Happy Yet?

To become a gourmet cook of the good life, it helps to see where you fit on the Happiness Scale. It's easy to confuse having happy moments in your life with being happy—that is, being content with your life as a whole despite its difficulties. So roll up your sleeves, get yourself a cup of coffee or tea, and dive into your inner spirit with your eyes open. Are you really happy?

(Hint: After answering the questions for yourself, you might take the quiz again about someone you love to understand their happiness equation and how you can better support them to be happier.)

Happiness Scale: How Happy Are You Really?

Please mark (T) for true and (F) for false. Answer as honestly as you can, because the only person who will see this is you!

1. I'm not sure I know what true happiness is (or I did know and I forgot). ____

2. To be honest, I don't enjoy my work but I need the money. ____

3. I usually don't have a good time without drinking or smoking or eating too much. ____

4. I can't get by unless I have a "little help from my friends." ____

5. Those who know me would probably say I'm often an unhappy person. ____

6. I often feel lonely and unsupported. ____

7. I don't think I have much control over my life. ____

8. Deep down, I think there is something wrong with me. ____

9. I tend to feel like I don't get enough love or have enough material possessions. ____

10. I feel helpless or overwhelmed more than I feel like a problem solver. ____

To see how you did, count up the number of statements you answered "True." Here are the scoring ranges:

0–3 True statements: Congratulations! You're in the normal happiness range. You've learned how to live a happy life. Keep it up and spread the wealth.

4–6 True statements: Beware! You're in the gray zone, between black and blue. You have normal blues and doubts, but too often and too many. These blues can easily turn to depression, so focus on building your happiness back to normal levels and removing your unhappiness blocks.

7–8 True statements: Uh-oh! You're in the black zone, which means real trouble. Your world is unnecessarily black and unhappy. Get support from friends and family and/or see a mental health professional to find out what's wrong and learn better happiness skills.

9–10 True statements: Emergency! With this level of unhappiness your body will get sick, if it hasn't already, and your mind is in the grip of a clinical depression, so get to a mental health specialist in depression management right away.

Many of us score in the 4–6 range—meaning life is okay but we periodically get the blues from overworking or trying too hard to meet unrealistic expectations or societal standards. Let's look at what it takes to have more inner peace and the feeling that you can handle whatever curve balls life throws in your direction.

Self-Esteem: "Is That All There Is?"

Liking who you are and feeling good about yourself, your family, job, and friendships is crucial to being happy. Easier said than done, right? Some days my self-esteem feels like Swiss cheese, with enough holes in it to allow the wind to whistle through!

Dr. Ellen Says

Self-esteem is not an end goal—it's an ongoing, lifelong process of learning to like yourself. To feel good about who you are, you must learn self-care skills for each age and stage of your development, such as resolving your negative feelings about aging or taking good care of yourself the first time you live away from home. Practicing self-esteem is a psychological workout. To keep that esteem muscle strong and toned, use it or lose it!

What self-esteem means, technically, is "esteeming yourselves," loving and respecting who you are, making your own needs a priority. When you love yourself, you take care of yourself—make yourself a cup of tea when you feel sick, treat yourself to a hot fudge sundae or a new shirt to celebrate some achievement, or look for another job if your current boss is a slave driver.

In other words, you're nice to yourself because you've learned to like who you are!

But most of us don't know how to make nice to ourselves. We are not raised to love ourselves. We've been trained to believe other people's needs are more important than ours, to worry about what others think of us, and to try to please people whose love or influence we want. Our self-worth may depend on something outside ourselves, such as:

➤ A job that pays us a lot of money

➤ A good-looking spouse

➤ Living in a fancy house

➤ Friendships with the rich and famous

But what happens when we get fired from our jobs, our partners dump us, our house is destroyed in a fire, and the famous person we thought was our friend doesn't remember our name? We feel awful. Horrible. Terrible. For a long, long time. We feel we deserve these misfortunes and that we are really worthless after all. The fact is, we are always at risk for unhappiness when we let someone else or something else outside ourselves define us.

The truest test of self-esteem was described in the Bible with the Job approach: Lose everything you have and still like yourself—feel you are worth loving by God and yourself. I don't suggest you try this unless you love plagues and boils! But there are many reasons why people suffer from low self-esteem. Here are some common ones:

➤ You were raised by parents who were unable to show their love and support or who were abusive physically or emotionally.

➤ You experienced failures or losses early in life that you never overcame.

➤ You had teachers or peers who told you that you wouldn't amount to anything.

➤ You had a physical or learning disability or were prone to anxiety or depression and kept feeling like something was wrong with you.

But even if you had a lousy upbringing and a sad past you can still conquer the blues by taking on new challenges, improving your outlook, and raising your self-esteem.

The most important thing to remember is that at any age, you can build your self-esteem by practicing some of the following esteem boosters:

➤ *Do something you like every day.* Make a list of 10 things you love to do—reading, taking a hot bath, walking around the block, visiting a friend, writing in your journal. Every day try to do at least one activity for at least 15 minutes.

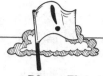

Blues Flag

A 1991 American Association of University Women study found that girls and boys start school with similar levels of self-esteem, but girls lose much of it by the time they reach adolescence. That's also when many girls shy away from pursuing math and science, and their IQ scores decrease unnecessarily, because they learn it's not as "cool" to be smart as it is to look good in our society.

➤ *Write down something good you've done every day for one week.* Before your head hits the pillow, grab a pen and paper and write down three good things you've done that day—gone shopping for the family, done car pool, helped a colleague at work—so you can see that you are much more valuable than you think. In a week, you'll have at least 21 reminders of why you need to like yourself.

➤ *Make a self-esteem treasure chest.* (This strategy is also effective to teach kids self-esteem.) Collect things that make you feel good about yourself and put them in the treasure chest: a touching thank-you card for something you did; a favorite photo with those you love; a great paper or report you wrote with glowing feedback; medals, ribbons, or certificates of winning performances; an affirming e-mail or a tape where you collect all the wonderful messages left on your answering machine that make you feel good about yourself. You can even take this idea to work—create a "smile file" to keep in your desk or office. Look at your treasures (or in your smile file) whenever you feel low to get an instant boost of self-esteem.

➤ *Do more of what you do well.* Make a list of what you do well, then write down different ways of expanding that activity. For example, if you're a good skier, make a point of skiing more often, go to different ski areas, or join a ski club.

➤ *Do what you've always wanted to do.* Set up one goal of something you've always wanted to do. Then, to accomplish your goal, break down what you need to do into little realistic steps. Ask someone to coach you if you're not sure how to set up your action plan to succeed at your goal. You'd like to be more active in your child's school? Join the PTA, volunteer to help at school functions like plays and dances, ask the teacher how to become a room mother (the person in the classroom who is the liaison between the teacher and the parent), volunteer to serve school lunches.

➤ *Remember what's good about you.* Make a list of the best things about you on an index card. Come on, don't give me that look! Everyone has at least 10 wonderful qualities and one special talent and I want yours, front and center! If you just can't come up with 10, ask your family and friends to list your best qualities. Make several copies of your list and keep it in your face for at least a week—posted on the refrigerator, on the dashboard of your car, or taped to your bathroom mirror. Check your list several times a day until you know it by heart and can recite it to yourself from memory the next time you're feeling bad about yourself.

Happiness Means...Learning to Think Differently

People with low self-esteem tend to be pessimists. They live in a dark cloud that follows them wherever they go and makes their world look gray, grim, and gruesome.

They don't want to try new foods because "I probably won't like it anyway." They don't want to learn to play Pictionary "because I'm no good at games, I always lose." They have trouble making up their minds about what movie to see ("whatever") or what clothes to buy ("I can't tell which one looks better"), or even what food to serve for dinner because they fear making the "wrong decision."

What causes them to be so negative? Generally, unhappy people have nasty messages running through their minds spewing statements like "You can't make any good decisions," "No way you'll ever succeed," "What are you, stupid?" Most of these messages were recorded in childhood by, guess who? That's right—mommy, daddy, and anyone else who had any say in our upbringing.

This negative noise in our brains has been on automatic replay for so long we don't even hear it. Yet, these messages impact us every minute of our lives (even in our dreams). To improve your self-esteem, you must get rid of the old tapes and record new, positive ones. Sometimes this task requires short- or long-term therapy with a mental health professional, but often you can teach yourself ways to change your self-image if you practice often.

Record a Kinder, Gentler Message

When you hear a voice inside you say, "You are so dumb," say instead "STOP!," turn it off, and slip in a new cassette that has a more soothing and positive message. For example, say you've just written an important letter and made 500 copies when you notice you've spelled "pubic" instead of "public"—one of the most dreaded typos (unrecognized by spell check) haunting every proofreader from an English-speaking country.

You may think: "Oh, God, I'm s-o-o-o-o stupid! I can never do anything right, and now I'll probably lose my job. This is so typical!" This self-deprecating thought will make you feel a host of emotions—anger, fear, self-hatred. STOP THE TAPE, and ask yourself:

➤ Do I really do everything wrong? What about the praise I got last week for the two reports I wrote?

➤ Would I really lose my job when my job performance record was so good?

➤ Is this an understandable error? What can I learn from it to prevent it from happening again?

➤ I'm only human, right?

You'll probably realize that you exaggerated the consequences of your error, and that nothing bad is going to happen. So you erase the old message and record a new one that says: "Yes, this was a silly mistake. I'll be more careful next time. But otherwise my job is going well."

Once you change the way you think about a situation, you change the way you feel about yourself. This happens because our thoughts determine our feelings. But our thoughts are so automatic (you are thinking all the time, even when you're telling yourself, "You are not thinking!"), that we often don't realize when the negative messages are playing. All we know is that we're feeling lousy and we don't know why.

A Different Take on the ABCs

You can train yourself to track down the negative thoughts and change them. In *What You Can Change and What You Can't* (Fawcett Books, 1995), Martin Seligman suggests that people pay attention to their feelings for a day or two and record five negative thoughts in a daily log. They should then check to see if these thoughts are factually correct, and, if not, dispute them.

Dr. Seligman suggests that people use a model developed by pioneering psychologist Dr. Albert Ellis to "identify ABC." Here is how Ellis explains it: When we are faced with any *Adversity* we react by thinking about it. These thoughts turn into *Beliefs*, which have *Consequences*—they become part of what we know about ourselves. The thoughts determine what we feel and do next.

Dr. Seligman then suggests that these thoughts be challenged. In the following excerpt from *What You Can Change and What You Can't*, he gives an example of a middle-aged woman, Judy, who had returned to school and was in a state of despair over her test scores—and how she changed those feelings into hope and a course of action after going through the ABC process:

> *Adversity:* I recently started taking night classes after work for a master's degree. I got my first set of exams back and I didn't do nearly as well as I wanted.

Belief: What awful grades, Judy. I no doubt did the worst in the class. I'm just stupid. That's all. I might as well face facts. I'm also just too old to be competing with these kids. Even if I stick with it, who is going to hire a 40-year-old woman when they can hire a 23-year-old instead? What was I thinking when I enrolled? It's just too late for me.

Consequences: I felt totally defective and useless. I was embarrassed I even gave it a try, and decided I should withdraw from my courses and be satisfied with the job I have.

Disputation: I'm blowing things out of proportion. I hoped to get all As, but I got a B, a B+, and a B–. Those aren't awful grades. I may not have done the best in the class, but I didn't do the worst in the class either. I checked. The guy next to me had two Cs and a D+. The reason I didn't do as well as I hoped isn't because of my age… One reason…is because I have a lot of other things going on in my life that take time away from my studies…

Outcome: I felt much better about myself and my exams. I'm not going to withdraw from my courses, and I am not going to let my age stand in the way of getting what I want. I'm still concerned that my age may be a disadvantage, but I will cross that bridge if and when I come to it.

Using this format, record five of your own negative thoughts and follow the ABC process, then dispute your thoughts and write down how you feel afterward. This exercise will help you learn to stop the negative thoughts from bombarding you and give you a chance to record your own positive messages.

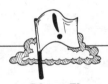

Blues Flag

To maintain self-esteem, don't just "hang." Structure your time, whether you're retired, unemployed, on school vacation, between jobs, an at-home parent, or addicted to TV. Never start the day without plans and a goal, and make sure you have at least one meaningful contact with someone per day. A lack of contact with others and no structure or goals means you'll lose time, focus, and energy and end up unnecessarily damaging your self-esteem.

Happiness Means…Getting a Grip

People who are happy feel they have some degree of control over their lives. The more choices you have, the better you feel about making them. Progressive employers give employees choices over where and what hours to work because they know that such freedom makes their employees better workers. According to a 1997 Families and Work Institute Study, 45 percent of employees can now choose when they begin and end their workdays, which means nearly one out of two workers has an easier shot at increased self-esteem.

One of the key secrets to increasing self-esteem is to take charge of your time and manage it effectively. In Chapter 13, "Battling the Burnout Blues," I'll give you some tips on how to be the master of your own clock. Beat the clock and you'll beat the blues—and feel great about yourself, too!

Happiness Means...Friendship and Good Cheer

Human beings are social animals. To be healthy, we need to be touched, loved, and held. Ever wonder why society's worst punishment is solitary confinement? Without human contact we simply can't flourish. People feel better about themselves if they have friends who support them and encourage them to pursue their goals. When we don't share our feelings with people, we become lonely—and looney. We feel like nobody cares about us, like we are in our own version of solitary confinement, and we become enraged and/or more withdrawn.

I know, some people are better at sharing their feelings than others. But, again, opening up to others is a skill that can be learned. Chapter 14, "The Bedroom Blues: What Happened to Marital Bliss?" will address how you can be intimate with others and what riches you'll gain when you share your feelings, secrets, and histories with people.

The Least You Need to Know

➤ Wealth, attractiveness, and youth do not guarantee happiness.

➤ Happy people are flexible, optimistic, outgoing, in control, and confident.

➤ Many of us have low self-esteem because we don't know what we want or how to take care of our needs.

➤ To build your self-esteem, do something you like, something you've always wanted to do, and learn how to truly take care of yourself.

➤ Remember what's good about you.

➤ Learn to think differently—erase negative thoughts and replace them with positive affirmations.

➤ Happy people feel in control of their lives and enjoy the support of friends.

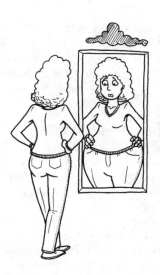

Chapter 11

Body-Blues News: You Can Learn to Love Your Looks!

> **In This Chapter**
>
> ➤ No one can meet the body-perfect standard
>
> ➤ The biggest sources of body blues for women
>
> ➤ Men: the newest recruits to the body blues
>
> ➤ Fat acceptance—the growing issue about shrinking
>
> ➤ Quiz: How do you feel about your body?
>
> ➤ Reject the body blues

Most of us are trained to judge people based on how they look—at least at first. It's hard not to when a great appearance is so highly valued in our society. Images of attractive people are everywhere we turn, on billboards, in magazine ads, and on television. And our nation's major industries promise us we could look like them if we buy this diet drink, join that exercise program, wear those clothes, or surgically remove a little here and add a little there.

The problem is, though, that even after a complete physical rehaul, most of us still don't look like the supermodels or superjocks we hoped to become. Our bodies just aren't made that way. A guy can't get taller no matter how many stretches he does, and most women aren't built or programmed to fit into a size 6 dress. But we still yearn to meet the cultural ideals. It's no wonder how many of us experience the Body-Image Blues!

But you can beat the blues by challenging the mainstream notion of traditional beauty and by learning to accept your own body shape and size. In this chapter, we'll look at the toll such unrealistic standards of beauty have taken on women and men and what we can do to liberate ourselves from these cultural stereotypes, and accept and appreciate our bodies as they are—imperfections and all.

Mission Impossible: Fulfilling the Body-Perfect Standard

Are you tired of waking up early to put on make-up and do your hair to pretend you look more like Cindy Crawford than a hassled working mother with an outgrown haircut and bags under your eyes?

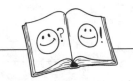

Terms of Encheerment

The *Body-Image Blues* are the negative feelings of shame, contempt, and disappointment in our bodies that most women and many men experience as they try to meet the unrealistic cultural standards of physical perfection, beauty, sex appeal, youth, and fashion.

Are you fed up with pumping iron at the gym so you can flatten that tummy, broaden those shoulders, and bulk up those forearms so you can look like Arnold Schwarzenegger or a superhero?

Are you angry that the one ad in the personals that sounded halfway decent was from a guy who was seeking someone preferably "thin" and "tall" and "youthful"?

If so, then join the rest of Americans—men and women—who try their damnedest to look the way they think they are supposed to look but always fall short (literally and figuratively) of meeting society's ideal standards for physical beauty. Feeling bad about the way you look is so common that I've labeled this emotion the *Body-Image Blues*.

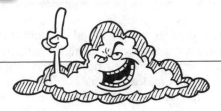

Funk-y Facts

The average American woman is a little under 5 feet 4 inches tall, weighs 146 pounds, and wears a size 12/14. Less than 25 percent of American women are both tall and thin. Yet, in the early 1990s, 95 percent of fashion was directed at this tall, slim, "model" customer. Today, over 100 specialty stores cater to larger women, and department stores are adding large-size clothing divisions to accommodate the fastest-growing market in women's retail.

When you've got the Body-Image Blues, you feel that something is wrong with the way you look. If you're a woman, you probably feel that your tummy is not flat enough, your breasts are too small, your hips too big, and you have no discernable waist. Or you may not be able to point to anything in particular that's wrong, but feel plagued instead by a general sense that your body just isn't right.

If you're a guy, you've got other problems. You may feel your shoulders and chest aren't developed enough, you're too short, and you've got stubby legs. You may gasp at your receding hairline, even though you're only in your 30s. Or it may be that your penis needs fertilizer.

Mirror, Mirror on the Wall...Uh-Oh!

Women are particularly susceptible to getting Body-Image Blues because for centuries society has taught them that how they look is more important that who they are. Even women who've always pursued intellectual subjects with confidence—like your high-school valedictorian or the infectious-disease doctor who lives down the hall—have not totally escaped this cultural trap. The level of insecurity women have about their bodies varies depending on the woman and her history.

But health officials estimate that at least one in four women suffer from some sort of an *eating disorder*, be it bulimia, anorexia, or compulsive eating. Few of us escape the body blues and its destructiveness.

Most women don't have eating disorders, but their weight occupies much of their thinking—and almost always, such thinking turns negative and leads to feeling the everyday blues. Corporations are cashing in on their insecurities by offering women all types of solutions so they can look better—which convinces women that there is, indeed, something wrong with the way they look naturally. Making women feel bad about their bodies is really good for big business.

Consider the five biggest sources of body blues for women:

1. Diet industry: $33 billion
2. Cosmetic and toiletries industry: $18.5 billion
3. Fashion apparel industry: $181 billion
4. Cosmetic surgery industry: $300 billion
5. Media: too big a number to count

No wonder it's become "mission impossible" for us to escape the Body-Image Blues!

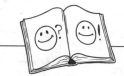

Terms of Encheerment

Eating disorders include anorexia, bulimia, and compulsive eating. Victims of anorexia will starve and exercise excessively to get well below their recommended weight. They look like sticks but still think they're marshmallows. Those with bulimia alternatively binge on food and purge through vomiting or taking laxatives. Compulsive eaters stuff themselves with food even when they are not hungry to distract themselves from and alleviate emotional pain.

Dr. Ellen Says

If you want to feel better about your body, *don't* try quick diet fixes! They just don't work. Nearly 98 percent of people who follow rigid diet programs regain their original weight within a couple of years. Why? Because diets don't address the reasons people overeat in the first place, and dieting slows down their metabolism, actually making it *harder* to lose weight. Also, scientists are discovering that obesity is often hereditary and requires different treatments.

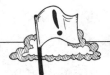

Blues Flag

Men who are obsessed with the size of their bodies may develop eating disorders and plunge into depression unless they learn to like and accept their bodies. Male athletes in particular might use steroids to achieve low body fat or muscle definition, but studies show a number of negative physical and psychological consequences associated with using anabolic steroids and other substances to bulk up or slim down.

Men: The Newest Recruits to the Body Blues

In the past, a guy could 4look like a schlump and get away with it. Who cared if he wore polyester suits, his beard was scraggly, or his buttons were bursting, revealing a dirty undershirt? So long as he brought home the paycheck, he looked good enough to his spouse!

And the more rich or powerful the guy was, the less it mattered how he looked.

But those days are gone. Although men still have more leeway in what they can wear and how they can look than women because society cuts them more slack, the social pressures of making good impressions are bearing down on them too. In today's corporate world, everybody must fit the image of being fit, young, and polished. It's good PR. It's good marketing. It's good business. We live in the information age, where image and data manipulation is everything. In short, most men can't afford to be slobs, unless they work at home and are seen only by family, friends, and the mail carriers—and even then it's increasingly risky.

Look at the huge success of Rogaine, a product that regrows hair. It's been used by over five million men since it was introduced in 1988. Losing hair is losing power, according to the body-perfect standard. So, a bunch of guys have become "Rogaine Ambassadors," whose job is to get out there among men heralding the coming of the new era when bald men can regain their masculinity (and power) growing a new crop on their top.

Another sign that men are becoming worried about their looks is the increase in eating disorders as men—like women—become obsessed with having a perfect body and either starve themselves until they get really sick or engage in the same eating/bingeing cycle that has ruined so many women's lives. Recent estimates show that nearly 5 to 10 percent of all anorexics are men—and men are one of the fastest-growing groups with eating disorders. These men, like women, increasingly end up in treatment where they need to figure out what drove them to such behavior as part of the recovery process.

Fat Acceptance Is Growing by Leaps and Pounds

But many men and women are tired of fighting the battle of the bulge. They are fighting for the first time against such unreasonable cultural body types. Celebrities are weighing in with their punches. Actress Delta Burke, who has battled with her weight for years and was dropped from her series *Designing Women* because of it, has made peace with her curves. She urges women to accept themselves as they are and stop killing themselves with diets to reach the thin ideal. "Eve wasn't a size 6 and neither am I," she says on the cover of her new book, *Delta Style* (St. Martin's Press, 1998). She's also introduced her own line of large-size clothing for women.

Nearly every department store and every major fashion designer are making clothes for larger-size women. Some large-size companies are even renumbering the sizes on all their merchandise, changing real sizes 14 to 24 into 1 to 6—a change that makes women feel better because they can brag about fitting into size 2 pants.

New magazines devoted to large women are also now appearing on the stands, like *Mode*, whose credo is "Style beyond size."

Many organizations have also popped up to battle societal prejudices against over-weight people. The National Association for the Advancement of Fat Acceptance (NAAFA), for instance, works to eliminate discrimination based on body size and offers educational seminars on such weighty issues. NAAFA sponsors the Million Pound March and celebrates International No Diet Day when they spread the truth about the dangers of dieting and publicize size acceptance.

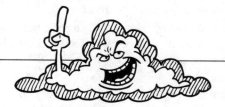

Funk-y Facts

Just being fat doesn't necessarily mean you are in poor health, says the National Association for the Advancement of Fat Acceptance. Research shows that health risks once associated with weight may instead be attributable to yo-yo dieting. Because obesity is so often caused by heredity and dieting history and because 95 to 98 percent of all diets fail over three years, it's apparent that remaining at a high but stable weight and focusing on personal fitness rather than thinness may be the healthiest way to deal with the propensity of being fat.

How Many Body Blues Do You Have?

Despite the efforts being made on the front lines to change views on size acceptance, most of us still live in the dark ages of starting new diets and breaking old ones—and of feeling blue about our weight or appearance. But you can fight the Body-Image Blues by challenging your own beliefs about size and learning how to accept your body. Before you plunge into the exercises in this chapter, figure out just how bothered you are by the Body-Image Blues. This quiz has been updated from my earlier book, *When Feeling Bad Is Good* (Henry Holt, 1992).

How Do You Feel About Your Body?

Answer "Yes" or "No" to the following questions.

1. Do you worry or obsess about the shape, condition, and/or size of your body every day? ___

2. Do you stand in front of a mirror and study your body for several minutes? Do you wish your body looked a lot different? If you can't even face yourself in the mirror, then skip the rest of the quiz, pass GO, and get to the action strategies, quick! ___

3. Do you feel fat no matter how much weight you lose or how much positive feedback you receive about your appearance? ___

4. Do you often feel intimidated by women or men you judge as thinner, stronger, better dressed, or more attractive? ___

5. Have you ever vomited or used laxatives to discharge food, or become so thin or heavy that your health has been affected (irregular or interrupted menstrual periods for women, impotence for men) because you were so unhappy with your body? ___

6. Do you feel frustrated that you "have nothing to wear" because you don't feel anything looks good on you, even though your closet is full of clothes? Do you feel clueless about fashion because you don't look like anyone on the cover of *GQ* magazine, even though your wife tells you which tie to wear? ___

7. Do you either dread the idea of shopping and trying on clothes or feel inadequate unless you're well dressed? ___

8. Have you ever seriously considered having a facelift, breast augmentation, penis enlargement, or any other elective cosmetic surgery because it would make you feel better about yourself? ___

9. Do you find that a new wrinkle, gray hair, or a few new pounds can wreck your day or morning? ___

10. Do you ever attempt to hide your body from your intimate partner or hide from yourself by avoiding looking in the mirror? ___

Total number of questions answered "Yes": ___

Do you have the Body-Image Blues? Let's see how you scored:

A score of 0–2: Congratulations! You've learned to love your appearance! If you scored within this range, go ahead and skip the rest of this chapter. You like the way you look and the way your body feels, even though you know it's far from perfect and you've somehow managed to duck the social pressures to look like an anorexic model or body builder extraordinaire. The down side is that your friends probably wonder what's wrong with you, since you don't hate the way you look like all of them do.

A score of 3–5: Warning! You're prone to getting the Body-Image Blues and may not realize when you're negative about your appearance. You get down on yourself because of the way you look more often than not. Do the exercises coming up in this chapter and you'll have a better understanding of why you are more likely to get the blues and be more able to keep them at bay.

A score of 6–7: Beware! You've probably got the Body-Image Blues. You don't like how you look and go out of your way to do whatever you can to make up for what you think are your flaws or shortcomings. The body-perfect standard has really gotten to you, bashing you over the head with its unrealistic expectations, and you must face up to your feelings or you'll feel worse and could develop a clinical depression or significant eating problems.

A score of 8–10: You're depressed! You haven't been able to escape the media and cultural image of how a woman or man should look and have taken to heart any bad things people have said to you about how you look. You may not even know how much you hate your body. But you do: BIG TIME! You could benefit greatly from professional help so your behavior can turn from self-destruction to self-satisfaction. It may seem impossible, but you can learn to love your body regardless of age, stage, shape, or size.

If you answered "Yes" to two or more questions, you have some level of the body blues—but you don't have to have ANY of them. Just remember: You can reclaim your body from the crazy body-perfect standard of our culture. Just read on!

Get Real: Rejecting the Body Blues

The best way to beat the body blues is to understand and challenge the notions on which you base your self-worth.

But how do you challenge something so basic? How do you learn to like the way you look when you've been programmed to hate your appearance? The exercises we discuss in the following sections will help you do just that. Many of these exercises are geared toward both men and women. Women will probably benefit from them most since Body-Image Blues are more ingrained in their heritage. But men will also learn a lot from them because they may be experiencing the Body-Image Blues for the first time.

Back to the Future

If you don't like the way your body looks now, think back to a time when you did like the way you looked or when you liked what your body could do. Was it when you were playing soccer in third grade and you loved the way it felt when you kicked the ball into the goal? When you went swimming at your neighborhood pool during the summer when you were 10 years old? Did you like the way the new dress your mother gave you felt around your legs when you were 11? Or your first men's-size tie at 12?

Once you identify the positive feeling or experience, find a picture (a childhood photo, a picture in a magazine, an image from greeting card) or make one that represents that experience. Think about or write down words or phrases that this image conjures up for you—impressive, cute, strong, capable, athletic. Then, close your eyes for several minutes and go back to that time in your life, to the good feelings. Really connect again to that feeling, fleeting as it may have been, of liking your body.

Dr. Ellen Says

Most of us don't feel the pressure to be physically perfect until we reach adolescence. So if you're rummaging through your thoughts about childhood and you can't find any good memories after age 10 or 11, don't panic. That's normal. But think about it and more memories will come to you, or switch to adult time and remember a time you really appreciated your body.

One woman pulled out a picture of herself dancing on the balcony of her apartment when she was six. Next to the picture, she wrote: "Cute, free, creative, sweet, lovable, festive, self-contained, self-confident, not caring what others think. Cute body that flows nicely." She told me: "I can't remember the last time I felt like that. Maybe I should put on some rap tonight and get down again. See if I can feel the spirit of that little girl again."

Wouldn't it be nice to find your spirit again? Mount this picture or image on construction paper, attaching a list of good associations, and put it somewhere you'll see it often. Let the image inspire you to reclaim your grace and dignity.

Happy Days No More: The Teenage Body Wars

When we become teenagers we often start warring with our bodies as much as we war with our parents. We are more critical of our bodies at this stage than any other time in our lives. Hormones spurt and surge, we grow too fast or slow, and we never, ever look as good as think we should. The slightest critical comment can shatter our egos into a thousand pieces on the floor of our souls. Body blues sprout as quickly as pimples in adolescence.

So what can you do? Buy several teen/adult magazines such as *Seventeen*, *Jump*, or *YM* for girls and *Teen GQ* or body-building magazines for boys. Look carefully at the pictures to see evidence of the body-perfect standard. Do this with a teen and discuss what you see, if you can. How did the perfection standard work in your adolescence? How much do you still carry today?

"If you get too thin, you'll get sick," were the words murmured by a competitive mother who was really feeling her age in contrast to her daughter's blooming youth. Mom's words and attitude are the seeds for an extra 20 pounds on the girl as an adult which she can't seem to lose. Why? Losing weight means getting sick. She's no fool. Mom said so!

A second exercise is to write the five sources of body blues we mentioned earlier in this chapter—diets, cosmetics, fashion, cosmetic surgery and the media—as you look at the magazines. Think back on how each of these related to you and write your thoughts on a sheet under each category. One woman wrote down under media: "I always thought that tall men had more fun and won the women." Under diets, another woman wrote: "I started starving myself one day and bingeing on 5th Avenue candy bars the next day. Didn't my mother ever notice how many candy bars were gone?"

Understanding how attitudes you adopted as a teen were a direct result of your cultural conditioning will help free you from those chains today.

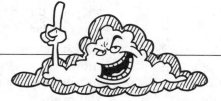

Funk-y Facts

No matter how thin women are, many think they could be thinner. A 1990 study in *Time* magazine indicated that 58 percent of the young women polled thought they were overweight, though only 17 percent actually were. A 1992 study from the Centers for Disease Control found that in a sample of nearly 12,000 high school students, more than one-third of the girls thought they were overweight, compared with only 15 percent of the boys. Forty-three percent of the girls, even those who thought they were the right weight, were dieting.

My Mother, Myself

Most of us have a tape recorder going on inside our minds that keeps playing negative messages—"Who do you think you are?" "You look so stupid in that." The worst comments usually come from our childhood (does anything come from anyplace else?), made to us by our mothers, fathers, brothers, and others. And even if they were inaccurate, we bought them and believed them.

Make a list of all the negative phrases you heard about your appearance growing up, noting who said it and how often. You might write how they made you feel.

Remember, you may feel temporarily lousy doing this exercise. But you are going back to see what messages were recorded, so you can erase them and tape new ones that will be more empowering and realistic.

Guiltless Pleasures

When you feel bad, be especially good to your body. A foot massage will make you feel warm and sensuous. Start by soaking your feet in warm water, then rub one foot (including the toes) with a soapy sponge. Turn on the water in the bath full blast (slightly hot) and put one foot under it, wiggling your toes. Once you're done, trim your toenails, and lather your foot with a creamy lotion. To add ambiance, use a candle in the bathroom instead of the lights, and listen to New-Age or classical music.

After making the list, note which vulnerabilities you grew up with, which ones came from the general culture, and which ones came from your family. Now become your own good mother and father and write down alternative positive statements next to the negative ones you grew up hearing. It's a good way to put negative feedback from your past into perspective.

Some examples:

➤ "That dress looks terrible on you. It makes you look fat." Say instead: "That dress is nice. There may be other styles you could try that would give you a different look and you can decide what you like best."

➤ "Why don't you work out more? You're so skinny. No one will pick you for the team and the girls won't be interested in you." Say instead: "You're growing so fast, you can be very proud of yourself!"

Read the positive statements over and over again whenever the old messages play back. Learning to nurture yourself will help you ward off the blues!

The Cinderella Complex

Most women were raised on fairy tales. We looked in the mirror for affirmation that we are beautiful, that we are the fairest of them all. We expect to look perfect, but the reflection in the mirror is less than perfect. Well, there is one way to solve this problem. Ditch the mirror that reflects cultural perfection and replace it with one that reflects the beauty within you.

Many of my clients liked doing this exercise using two mirrors. First, use your Ugly Duckling Mirror to appraise yourself. Study your body and note what you see in the mirror. Do you feel comfortable with your body? Satisfied? Do you like your body or does it disgust you? How does it differ from the body you wish you had?

Then, make a decision that you've got to stop hating your body—that you won't let cultural mores rule the way you feel about yourself.

Afterward, pick up your second mirror, Cinderella's, and make a list of five things you like about your body and appearance: your smile, your height, your strong, muscular legs. If you can't find anything you like about yourself, list things that you like that your body can do. Then put that list on your mirror. Focus on one thing you like and use it as much as possible for that day. It can be as simple as smiling at more people, or treating graceful hands to a manicure during lunch.

Reminding yourself of what you like about your body will help wipe away negative associations.

What Does Your Role Model's Body Look Like?

Role models are people we admire, with qualities we ourselves would like to possess. These people inspire us and drive us to improve ourselves and strive toward higher goals. Most everyone has a role model—perhaps a teacher, parent, actress, or politician. (Many of my clients chose Mother Teresa, Jodie Foster, or Barbara Bush.) Men favor sports heroes like Michael Jordan or titans of business or politics.

Take five minutes and make a list of women or men you admire. Then choose the top three contenders, and write a sentence or two about why you chose them.

People who do this exercise almost always find that what they admire about people they've chosen is not how they look but who they are—how they live and what they've accomplished. These role models refused to be defined by cultural standards and focused on what they could give, not on how they looked doing it. Consider these role models:

➤ Katharine Hepburn, the famed movie actress, was presented a Lifetime Achievement Award by the Council of Fashion Designers for "not giving a damn about clothes" and having enough self-confidence to turn her back on the arbiters of fashion.

➤ Frida Kahlo, a famous Mexican painter, was stricken by polio as a child and grew up with people making fun of her because she had a withered leg. She was left severely crippled after a major streetcar accident, lived through 32 operations, and had her leg amputated. But she enjoyed a rich life.

➤ Franklin D. Roosevelt and John F. Kennedy were two of the most effective presidents we've had, although both had great difficulty moving due to physical ailments.

➤ Christopher Reeve, the movie actor, is an outstanding example of the real Superman, defined by what's inside, his spirit and courage, and not what's on the outside, a broken body.

Changing our attitudes about how we look won't happen overnight. Most of us have grown up thinking we are defective in some way and that we aren't lovable the way we are. Accepting your body is priceless to your mental and physical health. Regular exercise is also one of the best body-blues blasters, so get thinking and get moving!

The Least You Need to Know

➤ The average American woman is under 5 feet 4 inches tall, weighs 146 pounds, and wears a size 12/14—a far cry from the size 6 cultural ideal that few women can or should meet.

➤ Millions of corporate dollars go into convincing men and women there is something wrong with them and that they need to diet, have cosmetic surgery, buy different clothes, and use more gym memberships.

➤ Men are having as much difficulty finding perfection as women, as evidenced by the huge popularity of Rogaine, the rising numbers of men reported to have eating disorders, and the use of steroids to build muscle.

➤ Recalling a time in childhood when you liked your body can remind you that it's possible to accept yourself.

➤ Reading biographies of role models can inspire you to want to change and overcome the Body-Image Blues.

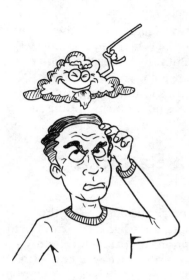

Chapter 12

Resolving the Age-Rage Blues

In This Chapter

➤ Why the golden years often seem blue, not golden

➤ How the media unfairly portrays older people

➤ Shattering the myths associated with aging

➤ Strategies for improving the quality of life as you get older

➤ The importance of cultivating a "family of choice"

➤ Male menopause: special considerations for men

➤ Good sex and intimacy can and should last a lifetime

Aging is one thing—but aging *successfully* is quite another. At some point in our lives, birthdays and holidays may become less bright, dimmed by the realization that we have one less year to live and the depressing thought that we may not be using our remaining time wisely or well. To begin to beat the aging blues we must accept one reality: Successful aging is a career, and with each passing year, we must devote more time and energy into better managing our minds and bodies. Aging well takes focus, effort, planning, positive thinking, and a good support team, but the results can be spectacular!

Margie is a recently widowed 67-year-old woman who told me that she couldn't wait until her 70th birthday. "What?!" I thought. "Is she nuts?" But years of clinical training suggested that might not be the best response, so instead I casually asked her:

"Oh...Why?" Margie cheerfully announced she would then qualify to join the Seventy Plus Ski Club, and get lift tickets for free or at reduced rates. "When Ted was alive we could never go skiing. He hated the cold and the snow. But now I have the chance and I can't wait!" Then she confided in a soft voice: "You know, many of the members have had bypass surgery or cancer and it's not easy." Then, she added brightly: "But the oldest skier is over 100. He can't find his hat but he has no problem finding his way down the hill!"

Say It Ain't So: Older People Get a Bad Rap in the Media

Practically everything we read about growing older, the magazine ads we see, the products sold on the market—all portray old people in a negative light. You can't help but feel sorry for old men and women who wait by the phone desperate for their children to call, or sit on park benches with blank stares on their faces, watching the world stream past them. Older people in the movies seem to typically be suffering from Alzheimer's, cancer, or heart disease, their bodies and minds broken, and their lives bleak, hopeless, and lonely.

Getting older gets such a bad rap in our culture that companies—eager to make a profit from our fears—are putting out products right and left to help us keep our age under cover: everything from wrinkle creams to hair dyes. Denial is big business! You can get a facelift to tighten up sags and liposuction to help you regain that sleek physique. Just imagine, dip into the fountain of youth, take a little here, add a little there, move a little here—and voilà, you won't even look like yourself but you'll have the illusion that you look younger!

With this image of the golden years, is it any wonder we feel blue instead of golden about the future?

I call these unhappy feelings the *Age-Rage Blues*, because it's natural to feel mad and sad at the way society devalues us with each passing year. We are taught to equate aging with a loss of independence, attractiveness, and influence.

But the truth is, these views on aging are based on wrong, outdated information. There is lots of research showing that most of us stay healthy for a long time if we keep fit, mentally and physically, and that we experience more value and true freedom later in life than ever before. We trade youth for wit, wisdom, and a greater capacity to love and be loved. Not a bad trade, if you really think about it! The point is we need to think about the *value* of aging instead of just feeling bad about the passing years.

Terms of Encheerment

Age-Rage Blues are the feelings of sadness and anger that men and women experience as they grow older in a society that values youth. Our culture teaches us that, as we grow older, we lose practically everything—our good looks, worth, mental acuity, and physical ability— and that we have fewer friends, less money, and little happiness. It's just not true! No wonder we rage as we age!

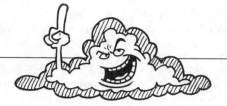

Funk-y Facts

How do popular magazines portray older women? That's one of the factors that author and feminist Betty Friedan set out to answer in her groundbreaking book, *The Fountain of Age* (Simon & Schuster, 1993). Her findings: The faces of older women rarely appear in magazines and when they do they're in a negative context. Their images are blacked out. In 290 ads appearing in *Vogue* magazine, for example, only one woman was shown who might have been over 60. That was for a me-and-granny shot. Great! We know what happens to grannies in the fairy tales: Their only real value is to serve as wolfburgers for the characters who really count!

In reality, however, older women are often adventurous and vital. In her book, Friedan counters the popular notion of aging only as "decline" and shows how ordinary women and men in their 50s, 60s, and 70s are discovering extraordinary new possibilities of intimacy, friendship, and work.

Update Aging Myths to Downplay Aging Blues

Our cultures' favorite images about aging are based on myths that older people are often sick, cranky, and inactive. Where do these myths come from? Until recently, aging was always looked at in terms of disease: We studied mostly what made people sick, not what helped them stay well. The *Baltimore Longitudinal Study of Aging*—known as the "original myth-buster"—uncovered answers to basic questions about what constitutes normal human aging.

The study, conducted by the National Institute of Health (NIH), was begun in 1958 and is still going on today. These findings can help all of us put aging into better perspective. Here are some of the findings:

➤ It was once thought that the health of the heart invariably declined with age. Not so. When older hearts are free of disease, the study found, they work just as well as those of younger people.

➤ The personality of older people does not changes over time. People who get old don't become nasty just because they're older. Those who were pessimists when they were younger remain negative throughout their lives, and those who were optimists remain positive.

➤ While it's true that older people are more susceptible to getting sick, they can prevent or control many diseases through diet, exercise, and up-to-date medical care.

➤ While some abilities decline, many remain stable, and some abilities can actually grow, like our capacity to love and connect with others. The declining changes occur very gradually. Any unusual change is much more likely to be due to disease than to aging.

➤ Only 5 percent of people over 65 are in nursing homes and not more than 10 percent will ever be—a figure so low it even surprised gerontologists.

Other studies confirm the *Baltimore Study* findings. For example, the National Center for Health Statistics, Illness and Disability recently found that for Americans over 65, only one person out of 10 has a health problem big enough to keep him or her from living an active life. In other studies, it's consistently reported that men become more caring and connected in midlife, not plunged into crisis because they don't have a red sports car anymore.

Long Live the Boomers!

If you really think about these findings, you can feel much more hopeful and positive about your future. So get your camping gear from your basement, take out your tennis racket from storage, and go for that class in philosophy! People today are living longer and healthier lives than ever. These statistics can not only cheer you up, but inspire and energize you to GO FOR IT, regardless of your age:

➤ Women who turn 50 and don't have cancer or heart disease will probably celebrate their 92nd birthday.

➤ Men who make it to 65 in relatively good health can plan to stick around and blow out 81 candles on their birthday cakes.

We also know a lot more than our parents did about how to use this extra time we've been given. Health-conscious *baby boomers* are revolutionary about aging just like so many other rebellions they have created.

With each age and stage, they chose to reinvent themselves instead of letting themselves deteriorate. *Every single model of successful aging added creativity to his or her life, if it wasn't there already.* They learned that creativity is one of the best companions we have as we age because it gives us a rich relationship with ourselves and the opportunity to discover and make new things. If others aren't around, we can always turn to our creative activity to make us feel alive and excited.

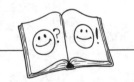

Terms of Encheerment

Baby boomers is a label used to identify the nearly 76 million Americans who were born between 1946 and 1964—the most fertile period in U.S. history. Baby boomers are known for their ambition, drive, and enthusiasm—and for redefining our cultural standards, life-long expectations, and aspirations.

At 60, Gloria Steinem is practicing to be a comic and is very funny; Jane Fonda traded her leotards for the role of the traditional wife and is flourishing; Burt Reynolds grew up and tried mature movie roles; and Warren Beatty recently directed and starred in a successful movie called *Bullworth*—a political satire that is fundamentally different from any other movie he has made and which was the biggest risk of his career. What's going on here?

According to Gail Sheehy, best-selling author of *New Passages* (Random House, 1995) and pioneer in the study of aging, these days real adulthood doesn't start until people turn 30. The first adulthood, she says, takes place between the ages of 30 to 45, the time we spend brown-nosing people we have to please (bosses, teachers, lovers) so we can accomplish what we need to do. But when we turn 45 we are ready to move on to the second adulthood phase of life and the independence it brings.

The decisions we make between the ages of 45 to 55, Sheehy explains, are crucial because they will affect what we do and how we live for the next 30 years or so. I'm now beginning my second adulthood, and I can honestly say that this is one of the most exciting periods in my life. I enjoy trying to apply and share all that I have learned so far, pursuing personal goals, finding new challenges, and still having the pleasure of raising my two sons who are only 9 and 12, because I was a late bloomer in the child production department.

Dr. Ellen Says

If you are a woman age 45 years or older, get ready for the best time of your life! Studies show that most older women tend to be happier and less stressed at this stage of their lives than at any other time.

But to make the best of the rest of my life, I've learned that I need to lay the groundwork for my future now. To help get you thinking about your second adulthood, answer the following questions:

➤ What do you really want to do in your next adulthood?

➤ Who do you want to be with in terms of friends, family, and coworkers?

➤ What new things do you need to try that you've been avoiding?

➤ How can you begin to give back to others? (If you just focus on yourself, you'll decline.)

➤ What changes in lifestyle (exercise, eating, doctors) do you need to make to take charge of the coming years?

➤ How long—and more important, how *well*—do you want to live?

Plan Ahead or You'll Stay Behind

The following strategies of "quality aging" are important to follow during any time of life—but especially as you look toward your older years. These are the top eight:

➤ Think about your finances and plan ahead so you can stay in control of your life in the future.

➤ Stay healthy by eating a low-fat, high-fiber diet and keeping abreast of the latest nutritional information.

➤ Just like you need air to breathe, you need exercise to stay fit and enjoy life. Develop a personal exercise program that combines aerobics and weight work, and/or a brisk walk. Don't skimp out on this. Just remember: Pay now, or pay later, and later it will cost you a lot more because you'll lose your mobility. The worst thing about aging is we lose our ability to move because we become too weak. Don't believe me? Thinking "Yeah, yeah"? Then consider this: By 65, the average woman has lost half her muscle and doubled her fat. By 75, she can't even lift 10 pounds! But the good news is that it's never too late to start a walking and free-weights program, which can reverse or prevent these losses.

➤ Don't smoke. Period. It's not negotiable and if you can't stop, put yourself in a stop-smoking program to help you gain control over your addiction.

➤ Build and maintain quality relationships. The more connected you are, the healthier you are, and this is especially true as we age.

➤ Plan each day with meaningful activities. Don't go into a day without structure. Plan things to stay active. My father-in-law is 90 and survived his quadruple bypass surgery 10 years longer than he was supposed to because every day he goes to the store he founded in Staten Island, Wexler's, and continues successfully to sell mattresses and furniture.

➤ Give back to the community. Despair is fed by staying self-focused and self-absorbed in your aches and pains and losses. Distract yourself by contributing to others and you'll have a daily dose of self-esteem and meaning in your life.

➤ Find and follow a creative activity. It can be anything as long as it involves two things: It must be challenging and meaningful, and it must

Dr. Ellen Says

In one study reported in the *New England Journal of Medicine* in 1994, frail older women and men increased their weight-lifting capacity by 118 percent in just 10 weeks of weight training.

Guiltless Pleasures

Just celebrated your 50th birthday? Congratulations! For your birthday present to yourself, sign up for an acting workshop, take a literature class, or take up a hobby you've been too shy, anxious, or busy to try. Then take your partner or a friend to dinner to celebrate your rebirth! Margaret Mead did her best work after she turned 50, as do many of the women ages 40 to 75 and even older who discover who they really are and aren't afraid anymore to show it.

involve learning something new. Build a garden, learn to bake, write an autobiography or family history, or learn to play bridge. Creativity will see you through some of the dark times because it's so rewarding and fulfilling for your spirit and renews your hope.

Get Real About Losses—and Their Gains

Most of us are terrified about getting older because we think of our body slowly deteriorating and our mental functions giving out. We do experience some losses as we age, and that's a scary experience for everyone, but there are many ways to compensate for the normal wear and tear of our bodies so that we can still lead satisfying lives.

Finding ways to cope with these losses can help us beat the Age-Rage Blues because we'll feel we have more control over our lives. It's true, for instance, that our vision decreases; but keeping our lens prescriptions up to date and getting surgery for glaucoma—by now a common procedure—will do wonders for people with severe vision impairments. Let's look at some other conditions that we may face as we age and then examine what we can do to alleviate the problem.

Loss: Our mental functions are slower with age.

Coping: An older mind functions as well, just not as quickly. It just takes a little longer to process and remember things. We don't lose our knowledge or our abilities to learn. In fact, our capacity for learning increases as we get older faster than our memory fades.

Loss: We're more vulnerable to illness.

Coping: Better nutrition, regular exercise, and stress management make all the difference in strengthening your immune system to scare off germs and bugs.

Loss: We are more sensitive to heat and cold.

Coping: Wear appropriate clothing when going outside, avoid extremes by staying inside when the weather is very cold or very hot, or consider living in a temperate climate.

Loss: Skin loses elasticity and becomes wrinkled, baggy, and dry.

Coping: Stay out of the sun, use sunscreen, and learn to appreciate wrinkles as badges of courage and life experience.

Write down your own list of losses and right next to each loss add ways of coping with it. If you don't know how to counteract certain losses, ask a friend, your physician, or do some research at the library. The important thing is to face your fears directly (writing them down helps) and know that there's a great deal you can do to reassert control over the aging process.

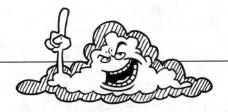

Funk-y Facts

When we are older we are better able to handle setbacks without becoming a victim, flying into a rage, or escaping into fantasy, as people between ages 20 to 49 tend to do, according to a study published in the New Haven: Yale University Press in 1989 entitled "The Middle Years: New Psychoanalytical Perspectives." After age 50, most women are well aware that adopting a defeatist attitude is a waste of time and energy. Most of us also lose our fear of death after middle age—when we begin to see death as a long sleep rather than a terrifying event.

Build New Friendships and Bolster the Old Ones

Your mother probably told you that blood is thicker than water. But it's not necessarily *better* than water. Many friends are more helpful, kind, and generous than family—and you need to connect to them. Even when you've got a wonderful family, or one that hasn't been fraught with divorce, abuse, or indifference, the great gains you get from creating a *family of choice*—a close circle of friends—decreases your chances of getting the blues. We treat our circle of friends like good brothers, sisters, fathers, or mothers; they are there for us when our own family is unavailable because of geography or unwillingness to help.

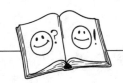

Terms of Encheerment

A *family of choice* is a core group of friends who function like members of a healthy family. They support and encourage you and are around when you need them in times of emotional, physical, or financial crisis. They don't criticize you, and they keep in touch with you, even if it's through a phone call once in a while. You support and invest time and energy in them as much as they do in you.

For women, keeping in touch with friends is particularly important several years after their spouses die—the time they are most vulnerable to depression. Men need a strong support network right after their partners pass away, but many of them are not likely to reach out to friends since they simply don't know how and for many years their wife was their only confidant. It's important that men develop those relationship skills as early as possible in their lives so that they can feel comfortable picking up the phone to call a buddy when they feel lonely.

Will any friend do?

No, don't just close your eyes and pick one. Align yourself with people who are loyal, trusting, capable of long-term commitment, and similar to you in personal growth and maturity. They need to be able to get close and be open about their desire to give and take more. There are different kinds of families of choice. Some women prefer a support group of female friends who all get together once a month to talk about their lives. Some men may want to just bond by going to the movies once a month. But with all family of choice members, we must feel safe, accepted, able to be ourselves, and be willing to give and get support.

Let's Get Physical

Can you imagine grandpa and grandma romping around between the sheets in the very same house your parents grew up in? Are you blushing now even thinking about it? If you are, you're in the majority who thinks that once you get old, sex goes out the window. Well, guess what? People over 50 have sex and love it! Sex doesn't have to diminish with age. Once women are beyond childbearing age, society assumes that they don't want to have sex because they are done with reproduction. But older women often enjoy it more than younger women, because they've shed their inhibitions with the years.

Dr. Ellen Says

A woman's sexual response changes little with age. Arousal and performance doesn't decrease by much—and any changes resulting from reduced estrogen after menopause can often be reversed with medication. Your male doctors may not talk about sex with you because they may be too embarrassed. But plenty of information about women's sexuality is available through women's health groups (see Appendix B, "Resources," for listings) and simply talking to other women. Don't be shy, girlfriend, too much is at stake!

Men: A Menopause of Their Own

Yes, men go through what Gail Sheehy calls "male menopause," too—they just don't talk about it.

This menopause usually hits men after they turn 40, and manifests itself in increased episodes of impotence. Sheehy reports that the largest study of impotence done since the Kinsey Report recently found that about half of American men over 40 have experienced middle-life impotence to varying degrees. But this condition is partly psychological, since adjusting to middle-life crisis, changing professions, and making other major life changes affects sexual function. It's partly physical too, because with age, the hormone most associated with male sexual functioning, testosterone, declines significantly.

That's why sexual function for men does ebb with age, but decline is gradual and men without major physical problems have enough sex hormones to keep going strong well into their 70s—if not longer! Men can overcome the menopause malaise by dealing with their feelings and talking to their partners about their problems. All of us—both men and women—should make a commitment that we won't allow our sexuality to evaporate because we're divorced, single, or widowed. The most powerful sexual tool for aging men isn't some technique or new position. It's intimacy. And if we add a healthy dose of Viagra, a drug that helps men achieve erections, older men may find a degree of sexual satisfaction they've never experienced before.

Here are some ideas for both men and women on creating and nurturing a sexual relationship as they get older:

➤ *Masturbate*. Don't be shy. Buy a back massager at a drug or department store and use it as a vibrator if you're too embarrassed to go to the adult sex shops, which tend to have lots of erotic paraphernalia—far more sophisticated stuff than ice cubes made in the shape of breasts.

➤ *Fantasize*. You ever get the hots for the technician who comes into your office to fix the machines? Or the cashier at the local supermarket who has a sexy voice? Think about them—what they may be like in bed, how they'd look in certain positions, what they'd say. You don't have to confess to your priest, rabbi, or partner that you are lusting in your heart. Just enjoy your fantasies!

➤ *Read nonpornographic, sexually oriented novels*. These books can be found in most major bookstores under "anonymous," or in the more respectable sounding "human sexuality" section of New-Age bookstores, near the crystals and sweet sounds of Kitaro.

➤ *Flirt with men or women of all ages*. Join a social club or go to dances. Whatever you do, try to keep emotionally connected and in touch with your sexual side.

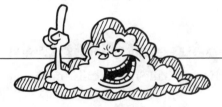

Funk-y Facts

Viagra is a prescription drug approved by FDA in March 1998 that is used to treat impotence in men. The drug, which research has shown increases the body's ability to achieve and maintain an erection during sexual stimulation, is viewed as being generally well tolerated. Side effects, like headaches, upset stomachs, stuffy nose, urinary tract infections, or others, tend to be mild and temporary. For it to work well, experts say, Viagra should be taken anywhere from 30 minutes to four hours before sexual activity. But before you take it, you should have a complete medical history and exam to figure out why you are impotent. Also, be careful because other medication that you are ingesting may have a bad interaction with Viagra, so be sure you tell your doctor what else you are taking.

Learning to age well is a challenge all of us face and if we fail, we will get the blues for sure. I can't say that it's been easy. Most of us feel a pang of sadness as we see wrinkles forming around our eyes and compare ourselves to the young beauty queens or jocks that jump out at us from nearly every magazine cover. But what really helps overcome the Age-Rage Blues is realizing that growing older brings on many more opportunities than limitations if we open up our minds to new possibilities.

Since writing on this topic, I've recommitted to taking control of my life and my aging. I reviewed my life insurance plan, updated my physical exams, and restarted a tired exercise program that will help minimize future problems caused by the normal process of aging. It's possible to feel very excited about your future, regardless of your age, and I hope you feel inspired to fulfill your potential as fully as you possibly can. After all, we've only got one life to live—and we get better at it as we age.

The Least You Need to Know

➤ Many people are challenging the stereotype that as you grow older you automatically become ill, get more irritable, and lose interest in living.

➤ Women who turn 50 and don't have cancer or heart disease can often live another 40 years; men who make it to 65 in good health can often expect to blow out the candles on their birthday cake when they turn 81.

➤ Boomers have put off growing old. The first adulthood takes place between ages 30 to 45; and the second adulthood extends from ages 45 to 65.

➤ The decisions we make between the ages of 45 to 55 are crucial because they will affect what we do for the rest of our lives.

➤ To beat the Age-Rage Blues, we should plan ahead, exercise and eat healthy, establish a support network, be realistic about our abilities, and maintain an active sex life.

➤ Male menopause usually hits men after they turn 40 and manifests itself in increased episodes of impotence.

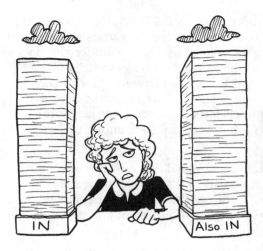

Chapter 13

Battling the Burnout Blues

In This Chapter

➤ Technology: for better or for worse?

➤ Why we push ourselves so hard

➤ Burnout Blues: Equal Opportunity Stressor

➤ Quiz: Are you burned out?

➤ It's true: You need to take time to make time

➤ Other strategies to beat the Burnout Blues: Get plenty of sleep, take a break, think positive, exercise

"Things have just been crazy lately. I've been so busy!" exclaimed a friend of mine who was "multi-tasking." That's the fancy new word for munching on a hot dog while doing a conference call on a cell phone while watching our kids' soccer game while trying to carry on a conversation with me and the other parents. You know how we give these important names to the foolish things we do so we don't have to stop doing them? Well, it wasn't "multi-tasking" we were seeing. It was the birth of the blues!

The Burnout Blues are the most common of all the blues because most of us are trying to cram in 48 hours' worth of work and activities into 24. In the process, we're feeling exhausted, overextended, overworked, and overwrought so we snap at our kids, growl at our spouse, and groan to our friends. We wake up the next morning vowing: Today will be different. But by two in the afternoon, the same burned-out, burned-up feelings have set in, and by 5 p.m. we're ready to incinerate any car, person, or pet who gets in our way.

It's no surprise that so many of us get the Burnout Blues. A 1995 survey conducted by *U.S. News and World Report* showed that 30% of the workers feel very stressed every day, 40% feel daily moderate stress, and 43% had visible physical or emotional problems from burnout. Whether we are married or single, whether we have children or not, whether we are housewives or CEOs, male or female, our days are filled to the brim. And when we can't do everything we feel we "should," we harp on ourselves for not "accomplishing" enough. The Burnout Blues begin to simmer, we make more mistakes and are more critical of ourselves, and the negativity feeds another blues growth spurt.

But the Burnout Blues can also be very productive as a signal that our lives are out of balance and we need to make a course correction. I know it's hard to brake when you're racing over the speed limit, but braking is the only way to have the time to think so you can take control of your time, determine your priorities, and restore balance to your life.

In this chapter, I'll show you how to slow down and focus on what's most important in your life, using the same principles I've used in working with my clients. Let's get started!

Keep Your On Switch "On" to Win the Burnout Blues!

Technology was supposed to make life easier for us as we struggle to juggle work and family in a frenetic world where traditional roles no longer define who does what. And, in some ways, it has. It's great to get cash 24 hours a day, surf the Internet, pop a CD-ROM in my computer to avoid a time-consuming trip to the library, or push a button to instantly fax or e-mail the latest joke to one of my friends.

But what gets me is that, although we are better informed, technology hasn't helped us become more patient, smarter, or happier. Have you ever noticed that our faxes and modems always seem too slow and that access to all this information doesn't give us wisdom or answers to the tough questions in our lives?

Instead of helping, technology often places a huge burden on us: With all these tools available to us, we are expected to be more competitive, successful, brilliant, and on the top of whatever pile is before us. Our society tells us that we must "accomplish" in every area of our lives—work, home, sex, fitness, appearance, parenting, income, spiritual—in short, everything. No wonder we're so tired!

So instead of taking a breather with the extra minutes we shaved off by not having to wait in line at the bank, we use that time to "accomplish things"—work harder on that proposal, squeeze in a load of laundry between bedtime stories, drag ourselves to yet another singles event to feel we are "doing something" to find Mr. or Ms. Right, push to do an extra repetition with the weights at the gym.

Why We Overdo It

What drives us to push ourselves to or over the edge?

Granted, there is a lot we have to do to take care of ourselves and our families. But most of us can alleviate some of the tension related to everyday living by asking friends to give us a hand, hiring a cleaning person to keep our house tidy, or accepting that it's okay to eat frozen dinners or a pizza when we're too busy to whip up a meal.

But we want to do it all—and do it all perfectly. Why? In the following pages we'll take a closer look at what drives us to push ourselves so hard.

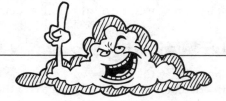

Funk-y Facts

In the Judeo-Christian tradition, work was ordered at the creation. "Six days shalt thou labor." A provision existed for taking a rest on the seventh day, but idleness was generally seen as wrong. "If a man will not work, he shall not eat," the Bible states. All work, regardless of how monotonous, was viewed as valuable for the individual, the family, and the community. This ancient tradition continues to strongly influence us to this day. But maybe we've gone too far. Modern technology does not have a day of rest. Instead, it provides 24-hour, seven-day-a-week access to our work and finances, so we may feel that unless we're working, we're not really living.

Blame It on the Pilgrims

All of us have been raised in a culture that judges our worth based on what we achieve and control. This is part of the Puritan ethic that our parents were raised under as well: A man is rewarded because of what he has done, not because he is just a nice guy. (How many "just a nice guy" awards do you see handed out? I think they would make better additions to someone's trophy collection than much of what is already there.)

Consider the following statements we grew up hearing:

➤ "She works very hard," a manager gloats about his employee, "she always takes work home."

➤ "Don't just stand there," your mother yelped when you just stared out your bedroom window, "get something done."

➤ "Actions speak louder than words."

➤ "He who would accomplish little must sacrifice little; he who would achieve much must sacrifice much," —James Allen.

The message here is clear as crystal: Doing is good. Not doing is bad.

The result: an anxious generation of people who are doing too much, not taking care of themselves, and not paying enough attention to their relationships. In fact, in a 1995 survey conducted by *U.S. News and World Report,* the only two places where people said they were really unhappy in their lives were not having enough leisure time and not having enough money. And here's the tricky part: Doing even more is not the answer, for if we keep up this hyper-level of activity and stress, our blues are bound to grow and, in some cases, turn into clinical depression or physical sickness.

Burnout Blues: Warning Signs

The *Burnout Blues* are those awful feelings we get when we are overworked, overwhelmed, and overloaded because we are trying to do too much and trying to do it perfectly.

People who have the Burnout Blues don't look bright-eyed and bushy-tailed; but they also don't have to look disheveled, scraggly, or wiped out. If you listen carefully to what they say and how they act, though, you'll see the burnout symptoms. You may recognize the following types (some of them may be living in your home—I know they live in mine!):

Here are the seven most common burnout types:

➤ *Overdoers* are constantly rushing from one place to another, "touching base" with subordinates and kids (checking up on them, really) via cell phones and beepers while zipping in and out of public places.

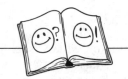

Terms of Encheerment

The *Burnout Blues* are the bad feelings we experience from being constantly tired, overwhelmed, stressed, and drained by the increasing demands and role conflicts confronting men and women today.

➤ *Shortcutters* are always in a frenzy and always trying to take shortcuts to shave a few seconds while driving to work. But if they get stuck behind a slow driver they blame themselves for "being impatient" and call themselves "stupid" for needing to take the shortcut in the first place.

➤ *Time optimists* overschedule and then cancel appointments. They are always coming into meetings late or leaving early. They chronically underestimate how much time a task will take so they maintain the illusion they can get it all done, then they're surprised and upset when they find out they can't.

➤ *Hyperdrivers* can't relax or sit still even when there is nothing pressing to do because they don't want to feel like they are "wasting time." Their foot is always on the gas pedal, never on the brake. Of course, they often have trouble sleeping, either falling asleep or staying asleep through the night.

➤ *Deniers* are swamped with things to do and won't take the time to eat right, get exercise, or see their doctors and dentists for annual checkups. They deny they have any physical or emotional vulnerability.

➤ *Speed parents* are in a constant frenzy and often resent having to spend time with family because they have so much to do and family time feels, well, slow. When they do get dragged to the zoo despite their protests, they spend their energy trying to find ways to cut the trip short.

➤ *Gotta be mes* are women and men who do too much and complain that nobody helps them do the chores or office work, but when someone asks what they can do to help, they can't seem to let go and delegate tasks.

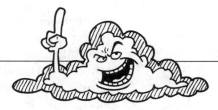

Funk-y Facts

In *The Time Bind: When Work Becomes Home and Home Becomes Work* (Metropolitan, 1997) author Arlie Russell Hochschild has found something quite interesting: Many of us actually prefer work over home because work is more comfortable and offers clearer rewards for our labor than home does. American homes are messy, pressured places these days where stress is high and "atta boys" are few and far between. No wonder an increasing number of us unnecessarily stretch out the hours of our workdays longer than they need to be to avoid the laundry and discipline demands awaiting us at home.

To Each His/Her Own Stress

Everybody who feels burned out wants to believe that they are much busier than whoever they're talking to. I've had the experience of being cut off by people who minimize my concerns with a "You think you've got it bad" comment. We seem to be competing for who has the worst pressures. The one who has the most burnout is assumed to have done the most and is therefore, a better human being than you and me.

Everybody's got their version of the big, bad Burnout Blues:

➤ If you're a married, full-time working mom, you're bound to be burned out just from the thought of all the responsibilities that face you each day.

➤ If you're married, work full time but have no kids, you try to "accomplish" a lot more in your spare time so your life feels busy and productive without children in the picture.

➤ If you're a full-time working single guy, you're burned out from working too much (everyone expects you to stay later since you have no family) and from going on too many of those blind dates or those awful, dreaded singles events just in case the "right" woman is there.

➤ If you're a married housewife with children, you feel stressed from doing all the household chores, shuttling your own kids (and the kids of mothers who work) to activities and feeding everyone—never feeling appreciated since you have the job society takes for granted.

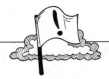

Blues Flag

Women are more vulnerable to getting the Burnout Blues than men because most work at least two jobs (at the office and at home), make less money than men, and have to put up with mistreatment from society. Most women do half to a third more than men in housework and childcare. And the men just don't get it, which makes the women feel even more burdened and frustrated.

➤ If you are a married man with kids who works full time, you worry about losing your job, you feel guilty that your wife has to work because you don't make enough money to support your family, and you feel bad that the kids are home alone until you or your wife get off work.

➤ If you are a single mom who works full time you have all the concerns of a married mom plus you worry about finding a partner and you fear losing your job.

The permutations on stress are as varied as our personalities. But the common denominator is this: We are all time-starved, and unless we change the way we value ourselves and use our time, our relationships and our health will be ruined. But there's hope! I know because I'm one of those people who nearly crashed from trying to cram in so many things at once. Are you? Take the following quiz to find out.

Is Doing Too Much Doing You In?

There is a lot we can do to better manage the stress in our daily lives—notice I say *manage*, not eliminate, since anyone who breathes is bound to experience some level of stress. The exercises in this chapter will show you how to beat the Burnout Blues, or at least keep these bad feelings within reasonable bounds so you feel you have more control over your life.

Answer the following questions "Yes" or "No."

Are You Burned Out?

1. Do you feel like you have to throw cold water over your face (or take other drastic measures) at dinner or breakfast to keep awake because you're wiped out from getting less than six hours of sleep? ___

2. Do you have an older parent who needs your care, or do you have one or more teenagers or kids under six? ___

3. Do you often feel like somebody "up there" is playing a joke on you by adding more chores to your "to-do list" while you're sleeping so your tasks are never done? ___

4. When you're driving, do you punch your horn at the guy in front of you when the light turns green and he doesn't instantly move? Do you threaten to get the refrigerator delivery guy fired because he showed up 10 minutes late? When everyday things go wrong, is your usual response one of the four-letter words?

   ___

5. Do you want to convert to Judaism during Christmas, to Christianity during Rosh Hashana, give up your birthday, and avoid all other holidays and celebrations because they just mean more work for you? ___

6. Do you do the dreaded "multi-tasking": operate in more than two roles daily or often find yourself doing several things at once (not counting walking and chewing gum)? ___

7. Do you find yourself losing or forgetting important things like keys, money, appointments, directions, or even your own name and address because you're always racing the clock? ___

8. When you're pooped or just down and need a boost, do you often eat a bag of chips or other yummies that you'd hide in a brown paper bag if you saw your nutritionist coming? Or would you light up a cigarette (even in front of a militant anti-smoker) if you're really stressed or tired? ___

9. Are you in a significantly unhappy relationship at work and/or at home? ___

10. Are you the only minority in at least one group important to you (for example, are you an ethnic minority, a lesbian, the only woman in a group of men, the only guy at a showing of *The Bridges of Madison County*, the only person in the group who likes your boss, and so on)? ___

0–2 "Yes" answers: Congratulations! Your life is a good balancing act and you haven't succumbed to societal expectations that you must be everything to everybody. Whatever you're doing, it's working great. Keep doing it (don't overdo it!) and pass the secret around.

3–5 "Yes" answers: You're vulnerable! Your life may seem balanced, but the demands on your time are a problem. Think twice before committing yourself to anything new until life simmers down and you feel less overextended. Focus on priorities; build in daily relaxation.

6–7 "Yes" answers: You are significantly burned out! You could sink into a depression. You are pushing your physical and emotional limits, doing more and enjoying it less. Your chances of getting sick are high. Your relationships are probably not as great as you'd care to admit because you have no time to nurture them. If you don't make some changes and reduce your role overload, you'll end up in the black.

8–10 "Yes" answers: You're running on empty! Your demands on time are extreme and you could be heading toward a physical or an emotional breakdown. You are totally overextended and are teetering on the verge of depression. Look at why you are doing so much and why you feel the need to be all things to all people. Get counseling and learn how and when to say no. Then practice, practice, practice stress management.

In the following pages I'll share with you some of the action strategies I've found to be most effective in banishing the Burnout Blues.

Take Control of Your Time

How many times have you had to shuffle around looking for keys when you were in a hurry to leave the house? Or pour through piles of books to find a slip of paper that has an important person's phone numbers? What about all those late fees you've had to pay because you forgot to return the library books (the ones that weren't lost) when they were overdue? Or those extra trips you took to the supermarket because you didn't make a list and get what you needed the first time?

If you have the Burnout Blues, these experiences are likely to occur frequently because when we feel drained we can't keep it all together, no matter how hard we try. Under the best of circumstances, it's hard in this pressured culture to feel in control with so many competing demands on our time. When we're tired, forget it! No way will we have the focus or energy to drain the swamps of our brains and clean out the garbage dump that our closet has become. When you feel the Burnout Blues and someone has the nerve to suggest that you take time to make time, you probably think "Kill!" and snap back, "I don't have time!" To feel more in control of your time, accept this fact: It does take time to make time!

Select one area of your disorganized life to fix and write out a cleanup schedule. Make a contract with yourself that you agree to follow and then program in a big reward when you're through and you've succeeded. Do one of these contracts a month and in a year, you will have gained many more hours of time because you'll be significantly more organized.

Most of the books and classes on time organization require so much time that we're often exhausted before we even start. But don't give up! You don't have to resign yourself to suffocation from the clutter and demands! No matter how much you may be suffering from Burnout Blues, there are a number of small steps you can take that will produce big results over time. Here are four of the best tips I've found for you to gain control over your time and life:

➤ *The time log.* Keep a time log for a day to see where your time goes. Not where you think it goes, or where you would like it to go, but where it *really* goes. Log in each activity and how long it took from the beginning to the end of your day. People usually underestimate how much time they spent watching TV and gossiping with an office pal and overestimate how much time they spent on household chores and boring office work. You'll be surprised to see that you are not spending your time as you thought. Once you're clearer about what you're doing, you can plan what changes to make so you can do what you want to do.

➤ *The military strategy.* Plan your attack on clutter and disorganization as if you're a military strategist. Plan ahead to win, but pick one of the easiest targets first: buying a better appointment book with more room to write so you don't lose so many slips of paper with important information; donating to charity all the clothes you haven't worn in the past two years; buying a beautiful basket or bowl for your keys so you find them in the same place each time; buying an accordion file and labeling each section so as soon as you pay your bills they are placed in the proper file categories to save you hours of frustration at tax time.

➤ *Lose the Lone Ranger.* One of the biggest sources of Burnout Blues is spoiled children. As time-starved parents, we tend to overindulge our kids to replace the time we can't spend with them. And the last thing we want to do in the time we do have together is to fight about chores and who cleans the bathroom. So we tend to expect too little of our kids, take the extra burdens ourselves, and do it alone.

One cure to the Burnout Blues is three words: delegate, delegate, delegate. Make a list of what needs to be done, negotiate, compromise, and delegate to both your kids and your spouse. Then be willing to work through the resistance they'll naturally have about being asked to do more. And don't forget, it's essential that you check up and follow through to make sure everyone does their job. Just remember, the conflict is worth it because your family's help will keep you from getting the Burnout Blues. You're also teaching your children critical survival and relationship skills that will be invaluable to their future development.

➤ *A "No a day" keeps the Burnout Blues away.* One of the hardest things we must learn in life is how to say "No," because often our "No" disappoints those we love. A boundary is a limit, something you can't or won't do, a line in the sand that can't be crossed. Learning when and how to set boundaries—to be able to say "No can do" or "No want to"—is one of the most important skills you'll ever learn to banish the Burnout Blues. Setting a boundary is a learned skill, so no matter how wimpy or whiny you are today, you can build up this muscle by practice and by challenging yourself. Learning to set appropriate boundaries helps you respect yourself and your time, so that others will treat you with respect and be more careful in what they ask you to do.

Begin by saying a "No a day" to something small (okay, miniscule), and then when you're stronger, practice and rehearse and ask friends for coaching until you can say "No" to one of the big drains in your life. The stronger you build your boundaries, the weaker your Burnout Blues will be.

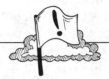

Blues Flag

Adults need about eight hours of sleep a night, but a study conducted by the National Sleep Foundation found that nearly one-third of the respondents got six hours of sleep at most during the work week. Sleep-deprived people also cause 1,500 vehicular deaths, 100,000 car crashes, and 71,000 injuries each year, according to the National Highway Traffic Safety Administration.

Dream a Little Dream for Me

It may seem like a waste of time because you are just laying there trying to get to sleep, but adequate sleep is crucial to your well-being. Yet, when we are overloaded, we get up earlier, go to bed later, or do both—and lose lots of sleep over it. In fact, in a recent Gallup Poll, 25 percent of adults think that if they want to be successful, they cannot have the "luxury" of getting adequate sleep. No wonder one in two adult Americans report having sleeping problems, usually saying that they're too worked up to get to sleep.

To keep the blues at bay you've got to catch your zzzzz—so would you try to dream a little extra dream for me? Here's how.

Learn the Art of Sleep Exchanges

Sleep exchanges are a bartering system in which you consciously trade something less valuable for the rest you need. To figure out what your bargaining chips are, make a list for a week of everything you do from 5 p.m. until your head hits the pillow every night. Then make a commitment to eliminate one or two activities from your list each night and turn off the light within the same half hour each evening. You let go of something less valuable (watching an old movie) for something more valuable (in the morning feeling like you're alert and strong and won't chop off someone's head at work).

One coaching client, for instance, did the sleep exchange exercise and could see that she was spending more than two hours a night on chatty phone calls to friends and colleagues. She decided to give up returning nonessential calls at night and found that calling friends back from work was more efficient because she could say, "I'm at work, I can't talk long," and she could get to the point more quickly.

Another client decided to limit himself to just one cable news show at night, instead of channel surfing every night all the while complaining that "There's nothing good on." He finished his TV surfing adventures each evening feeling empty and exhausted and would hate himself in the morning for being so tired and stupid. But channel surfing had become a strong habit because it was such a convenient way to avoid confronting his shyness and developing a more satisfying social life.

By doing this exercise, you should be able to go to bed 30 minutes earlier. Try the same tactic in the morning. You may, for instance, stop setting the alarm for 5:30, and then waking up every five minutes for the next half hour to turn off the snooze alarm, when you really don't intend to get up until 6:00 anyway. Just sleep the extra half hour and gain the energy from uninterrupted sleep.

Other suggestions: Establish a relaxing bedtime routine, drink warm milk before bed, use your bed only for sleep or sex, and invest in a white noise machine if sounds from outside keep you tense or awake. *The Complete Idiot's Guide to Getting a Good Night's Sleep* (Alpha Books, 1998) is a good resource.

Don't Be a Sap: Take a Power Nap!

Naps are for saps, you're thinking, right? Well, consider some of the power-nappers of our century: Thomas Edison; Lou Gerstner, Chairman of IBM; ex-president Ronald Reagan; an increasing number of women executives; and many of the people you know (only they won't admit it because they don't want to sound weak). Too bad, because instead of weak, they're smart. Science is beginning to recognize that between 2 p.m. and 5 p.m. the circadian alarm clock rings in most of our bodies and napping is our programmed biological response.

What happens if you listen to Mother Nature and grab a 15- to 20-minute nap? "You get a tremendous recovery of alertness—several hours' worth—out of a 15-minute nap," says scientist Dr. Claudio Stampi, who studies how to maximize sleep patterns for astronaut and pilot alertness at Boston's Institute of Circadian Physiology. And the National Aeronautics and Space Administration has shown that pilots who nap a half-hour during flight (don't even think about this one) perform significantly better at landing. So next time you're fighting afternoon fatigue and losing the battle, put your head down on your desk, sit in a restroom stall, go rest in your car in the parking lot, or lay down on the couch before the kids come home from school, and take your power nap. Power naps are one of the surefire ways to beat the Burnout Blues for that evening and—over time—for your life.

Take a Break to Brake

When you are barking at your employees, swearing at your computer, and just being a general grump, do yourself—and those around you—a favor. Take a time-out. This breather will help you recharge and refocus—and you'll be much more positive afterward.

167

Guiltless Pleasures

Take mini-breaks throughout your day to do things you like or to get organized. That's what the most successful women in America do, according to *The Female Advantage: Women's Ways of Leadership* (DoubleDay Currency, 1990), by Sally Helgesen. Some women take time during their lunch hour to sit and read a good book, while others set aside several minutes before important meetings to review what they want to accomplish.

Give yourself at least one 20-minute break a day, or two 10-minute breaks a day, and use that time to ask yourself a few questions:

➤ What do I need to get done? What activities will further my goals?

➤ Am I accomplishing my goals right now?

➤ Can I do this more efficiently? How can I work smarter, not harder?

Once you've had a time-out, you'll be able to see more objectively where you are, avoid making a bad situation worse, and correct your course to sail closer to your daily goals.

Get Rid of Negative Thoughts

What drives many of us to be workaholics and super-moms, and engage in other obsessive behaviors, is a deep-seated feeling that unless we accomplish everything or take care of everybody's needs, we just aren't good enough, smart enough—or worth loving. That's why we say things to ourselves like, "I can't do anything right" or "I'm totally incompetent" when we do something we think is wrong or fail to meet the impossible standards of perfection we set for ourselves.

Why might we have those thoughts? Somewhere in the recesses of our minds, we remember a parent, family friend, or teacher criticizing us when we were young because we made mistakes or failed to live up to their expectations. And we believed what they said about us. These critical comments still dictate the way we think about ourselves today. To beat the Burnout Blues, we need to challenge these negative thoughts, get rid of them, and replace them with positive affirmations.

If you've been working late every night and you haven't been able to find your shoes, watch, or Victoria's Secret catalogs because your house is such a pig sty, instead of saying, "I can't believe what a slob I am!" try saying: "It's okay that my house is a mess. This is a temporary situation. I'll make time to clean up this weekend, or, if I'm too pressed for time, hire a cleaning lady to do it for me."

For the next week, keep track of your negative thoughts by writing down critical statements you make to yourself. Next to it, write an affirmation. In this way, you'll be able to shift the way you think about yourself—and when you think good thoughts, you feel better.

Beat the Blues by Getting Physical

If writing down your thoughts or emotions on paper seems ridiculous or just one more demand, then I'll offer you an alternative. Here are some of my favorite physical outlets that will help you beat the Burnout Blues—and they won't hurt you or anyone else. When you're burned out, your body retains a lot of tense, built-up energy. To shake some of it loose, try one of these activities:

➤ Kick a soccer ball with some kids or colleagues or play football.

➤ Pick up some ice and smash it against the sidewalk, street, rocks, or the side of a brick wall.

➤ Hit a bucket of golf balls after work or stop at the batting cage and whack those balls.

➤ Take up boxing. It's one of my favorite physical outlets. I don't hit anyone because I don't have the stomach for that, but I wallop the punching bag and hit focus mitts with a trainer, or do a workout with the kids. This is a wonderful action strategy for releasing not only the Burnout Blues, but all the blues.

As hectic as our lives are, we've got to give ourselves a break and accept that we can't do it all or we'll lose it all. We lose what's most important to us—our relationships. I'm such a driven maniac charging through life trying not to miss the good stuff, that sometimes I forget the price my loved ones pay if I'm not available because I'm too tired or preoccupied. I had to learn too that it takes time to give ourselves time; but, if I learned to do it through making a million mistakes, maybe you can learn to do it by making just a thousand mistakes. So don't be hard on yourself, and try to take the breaks you need to refuel your energy. Just keep reminding yourself that you deserve it and so do those you love!

Dr. Ellen Says

Talking to a good buddy can help you beat the Burnout Blues—even *if* it's just a short phone conversation. Sharing your feelings and experiences provides an outlet for your pain and anger and helps you manage stress. Take what I call Five-Minute Intimacy Breaks when you feel burned out and you'll feel a stress load lifted off your back.

The Least You Need to Know

➤ Most of us try to cram 48 hours into 24, and as a result we always feel exhausted, burned out, overworked, and unfulfilled.

➤ We are driven to do too much because we live in a culture that judges our worth based on what we accomplish, not on who we are.

➤ Women especially get the Burnout Blues because they are expected to fulfill their traditional duties in addition to having a full-time job.

➤ Getting your office, closet, or some other area in your life organized will help you regain a sense of control and order over your life.

➤ Adults need eight to nine hours of sleep a night, but they generally only get about six.

➤ Being hard on yourself for not accomplishing everything you need to do is unfair and unhelpful. It's best to accept that you can't do it all, and let someone give you a hand.

Part 4
Beating the Blues in Relationships

When did your pillow talks with your spouse turn into pillow fights? Why do your parents still treat you like a two-year-old, and why do you feel like such as lousy parent to your own two-year-old? And why do you date so many losers all the time?

This section focuses on the various relationships we all have that become sources of the blues. We need them, we want them—but we don't quite know how to cope with them. Read the chapters in this section if you want to learn the best ways to find—and maintain—a relationship, get along better with your parents or children, or rekindle some sparks in your marriage or other relationship.

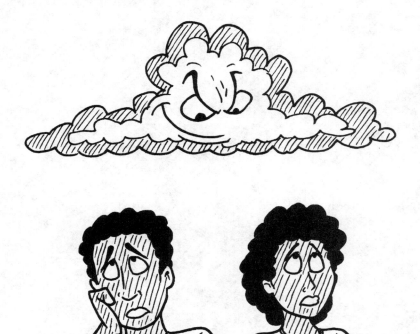

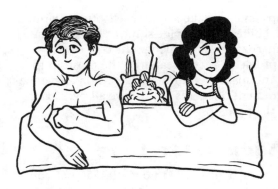

Chapter 14

The Bedroom Blues: What Happened to Marital Bliss?

In This Chapter

➤ Life in the relationship trenches

➤ Do you have the Bedroom Blues?

➤ Quiz: How solid is your marriage?

➤ Self-esteem builds up steam in marriages

➤ Can we talk? The caveman shutters up

➤ Make love, not war: tips to spice up your marriage

What is the #1 problem in relationships today? We can't live with them and we can't live without them! Go to any cocktail party in America, health club, supermarket, or restaurant, stand around the water cooler at any office, or wait in line at an ATM machine, and you're likely to hear people complaining about marriage—wanting it if they don't have it, not wanting it if they do.

Sound familiar? "I'm just not getting what I need out of my marriage," or "We never make love anymore." What about: "Things just aren't what they used to be" or "We never talk" or "I have to stay for the children." It always makes me sad to hear these comments. But given how common they are, it's amazing so many people still try for "and they lived happily ever after" after having their hopes dashed on the relationship rocks countless times.

It's even sadder to me that so many people accept that their marriage has lost its fizz and gone flat. They believe that being bored is inevitable—even stylish. It's "in" to be on the "outs" with your spouse. But it's normal for every marriage to go through a bad patch once in awhile, considering the stressful lives we all lead and how difficult it is for men and women to truly understand and accept each other.

Actually, feeling bad about your relationship can be good because it sets off an alarm that something needs your attention. Marital blues also provide some of our greatest opportunities for personal growth because marriage wars challenge the core of our being and test how well we can handle the problems that threaten us the most. In this chapter, we'll look at ways you can reignite the spark in your marriage. And believe me when I tell you it can be done—I've seen hundreds of clients fall in love all over again just when they thought love was a thing of the past!

Might as Well Face It, I'm Addicted to Love

Ever feel like your marriage is Vietnam, and you're constantly under attack? That you signed up for the army reserve and you didn't realize you'd be called to duty to serve your spouse? That no matter what you say it's the wrong thing and no matter what you do it's never good enough? Ever wonder if your marriage will end up like that popular movie *The War of the Roses*? Yet with all these doubts, you stay and hope for the best. Might as well face it, you're addicted to love.

If you are, you're not alone. All human beings are hard wired for love because without it, we can't survive. So we become addicted in our search for love and stay in unsatisfying relationships without knowing how to fix them. Our marriages roller-coaster through the dips and turns where we fight over our relationships, blame each other for feeling unfulfilled, feel disappointed over how things turned out with our mate, and wonder if the grass is any greener in the neighbor's bed. These doubts and feelings are normal because events happen in our lives that change us and we develop different needs at different times than our spouses. Negotiating these differences takes skill, time, and energy we often don't have, so most of us end up feeling the marital blues instead of marital bliss, and we become more addicted than ever in our quest for true love.

It's 10 O'Clock: Do You Know How Your Partner Feels?

Ten o'clock or any other time, you may not know what your partner is thinking or feeling because you're so busy juggling work and family matters that you don't bother to find out. As a result, you end up bickering over who takes Suzy to the birthday party, whose turn it is to do laundry, and why you never seem to have enough money no matter how hard you work.

You yell at your spouse for scheduling two play dates for Johnny at the same time—and for not planning anything else for the boy to do the rest of the three-day weekend. You reproach your husband for planning boys' night out on the same night that you have your stress-reduction workshop. You hate that your wife spends so much time talking on the phone to her girlfriends and so little time cleaning the house.

174

In the end, nobody gets to do what they want, everyone feels misunderstood and unappreciated, and you both go to bed tired, overwhelmed, and grumpy. Instead of whispering sweet nothings into each other's ears, you want to go after each other's throats. It's so uncomfortable, you don't want to look at what's really wrong because it will take too much time and energy to fix. So you rationalize your position. You convince yourself that loss of interest is inevitable, that your spouse is to blame, and that you're still doing better than anyone else you know.

You and your mate are probably just experiencing the *Bedroom Blues*, which are normal feelings most couples have for three main reasons: 1) the enormous pressures imposed by today's workplace on all of us; 2) the lack of communication skills most of us experience because we didn't learn how to talk about feelings when we grew up; and 3) the unrealistic expectations we all have that our marriage can fill us up and fix all of our problems.

If the spark was there at the beginning of your marriage, it's probably still there now, buried under layers of disappointments, dashed hopes, and unmet expectations—waiting to be rekindled. We all have the power to unleash the heat and fire of our passions. The key to opening up this emotional dam is intimacy. We feel intimate with our spouses when we create a safe, comforting environment in which we can both share our feelings and state our needs.

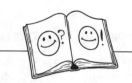

Terms of Encheerment

Bedroom Blues are the sad, mad, and bad feelings all of us have when we feel disappointed, frustrated, empty, or conflicted in our relationship with our partner. The Bedroom Blues are growing as a consequence of trying to maintain relationships in today's hectic, confusing, stressful, and nonsupportive world.

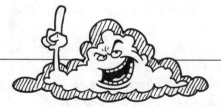

Funk-y Facts

Dr. John Gottman, a psychologist specializing in marriage research at the University of Washington, is considered the old man of marriage. He has studied over 2,000 married couples for over 20 years and can predict with 94 percent accuracy which marriages will succeed or fail. A successful marriage is less of a mystery than we would like to think. For example, Dr. Gottman has found that it takes five positive interactions to wipe out the effect of one negative interaction in a marriage. So watch your ratios on a daily basis and make sure your batting average is a least 5:1 positive to negative!

I know that it's much, much easier said than done. Maybe nobody ever taught you communication skills. Or perhaps your parents didn't know how to communicate their feelings so they couldn't teach you very much. And even those of us who majored in psychology and have studied emotions for years have a hard time in real life being intimate with our spouses (believe me, a Ph.D. is no guarantee of a golden tongue!). But speaking from my own experience and that of hundreds of clients, we can all learn these skills if we put our minds to it and create more fulfilling, meaningful, and exciting relationships.

Anyone Keeping Score in Your Bedroom?

Next time you are dusting your Marital bookshelves, take a look at your wedding picture or a photo of the two of you in the early days of your relationship. Do you wonder who that smiling couple is? Whatever happened to them? All of us feel we've changed a lot since the day we made our vows, but feeling estranged for too long could signal that the marriage is in trouble. Take the following quiz to find out where yours stands.

How Solid Is Your Marriage?

Answer the following questions (T) for true and (F) for false.

1. I haven't had sex with my partner since the last time I cleaned under my bed—at least a month to a year ago. ___

2. I remember all the bad things my partner has done in large-screen Technicolor, while the good deeds end up on the cutting-room floor. ___

3. Kissing my partner sounds like the most disgusting thing in the universe. ___

4. My partner is my best pal. ___

5. I can tell my partner that I feel gutless, slothful, and half-witted, and he or she won't alert the press or laugh at me. ___

6. We both want the same things out of life and share basic values. ___

7. My partner should have never become a parent. ___

8. My partner has a significant drinking or drug problem. ___

9. I put up with my partner's quirks, eccentricities, sense of humor, and other qualities I may not be crazy about because I love him/her. ___

10. Sign me up for the lifetime marriage plan. I'm sticking with my partner until the end! ___

How did you do? Count the number of true statements for items 4, 5, 6, 9, and 10 and count the number of false statements for items 1, 2, 3, 7, and 8. Then record the total of each:

___ True statements

___ False statements

Add these two scores together and see if your marriage is on solid footing!

A score of 7–10: Most excellent! Congratulations, the Bedroom Blues are not for you—you've got an excellent marriage! But are you sure you answered the questions based on how you feel and not on what you think the answer should be? Many of us like to see our marriage through rose-colored glasses—but this warped view does more harm than good because we may ignore the warning signs that our marriage is in trouble and don't try to fix it until it's too late.

A score of 3–6: Bedroom Blues time! Move over, you've got lots of company! Most people who fall into this category have resigned themselves to having an unsatisfying, boring relationship because they have no time, energy, or hope that they can reawaken their passion. Please don't settle for this dreary life. Beat the Bedroom Blues by doing the exercises in this chapter and reawaken the relationship flame that will warm and cheer your soul.

A score of 0–2: Divorce dangers! Your Bedroom Blues are destructive, and without help your relationship will continue to get worse and may end in divorce. You've probably never had a chance to learn the skills necessary to build and maintain a healthy relationship. This can threaten your happiness. Get help from a relationship expert, one specializing in building social and communication skills. Group therapy (see Chapter 9) may also be helpful because it provides a safe social laboratory to explore fears and failures and to learn about relationships as they unfold before your eyes in the group.

Dr. Ellen Says

Good news! You can have a good marriage even if you were raised in a dysfunctional family, according to research conducted by Judith Wallerstein, author of *The Good Marriage* (Houghton Mifflin, 1995). Of the 100 people she interviewed who considered themselves to be in happy marriages, only five said they grew up with good role models. The rest saw fighting, boredom, infidelity, and in some cases, abuse and abandonment. So what did they do? Taught themselves the basics of good relationships.

I'm Okay, I'm Okay (I Am Okay, Right?)

To have a good relationship with your partner, you need to feel good about yourself. Most of us tend to get lazy in our marriage and rely on our spouses to make us happy. When we are in a funk, we tend to blame our moods on our husbands or wives: *If only my partner was* (fill in the complaint du jour)...*then I'd be happy.*

We may feel this way because we were raised to think that once we find that special person, we'll be happy forever and we can stop taking responsibility for our own happiness. We don't have to continue hobbies, interests, and activities that filled our lives before we married. Our spouses will take care of us. While marriage will go a long way toward satisfying our hunger for love, the sad fact is, no marriage will make us feel happy or whole. Our well-being was, is, and will always be our own responsibility.

How do we become happy in a relationship? By learning to like ourselves. By knowing that we can rely on ourselves when the going gets tough. By believing that we deserve to be treated well and that we are worthy individuals even if we lose all our money, gain 50 pounds, get fired from our jobs, or get dumped by our lovers.

We'll never feel secure in a relationship unless we know we could leave it and be okay. If the thought of being alone is horrifying, our marriages just become parking spots for our growth, places where we go to get away from ourselves. And we are likely to stay in those marriages no matter how awful they are just so that we don't have to be alone and learn about who we really are.

Make Time for Yourself

One way to build your self-esteem is to do something slightly challenging by yourself every day. It doesn't have to be elaborate, just something that will make you focus on your strengths, resilience, and ability to take care of yourself. Some suggestions:

➤ Take a 10-minute walk after you come home from work before you start dinner or after dinner to think about what went right with the day, not what went wrong.

Guiltless Pleasures

Refresh your soul and take yourself on an adventure! I love to go to our childhood beach house on the Oregon coast to walk along the deserted beaches and read the diaries I kept as a teen. Many of us get married and stop exploring ourselves. It's not fair to ourselves or our partners for us to stop growing. Your break can be only a day or two, but the benefits can last a lifetime.

➤ Stop off at the library on your way from work and find a book or video about adventure. Picture yourself doing the activity as you read about or watch it.

➤ After the kids are in bed, take a drive to a diner or restaurant you've never gone to before and get some coffee or dessert.

➤ Take an overnight trip and stay at a bed-and-breakfast. Walk, nap when you feel like it, write in a journal, explore, think about your life and what needs to change. Develop goals and action strategies to solve problems.

➤ Go walking or jogging one morning before everyone wakes up, or while your partner fixes the kids' breakfast. Negotiate this exchange ahead of time and let your partner know what you're trying to do: Gain more inner strength and emotional independence so you'll be a better partner.

When you are alone, don't analyze why it's important to be alone or waste your time feeling bad or sad. Just do it and let your mind drift to other thoughts.

Among my fondest memories are the times when I visited Yosemite alone, hiking, carrying a canteen, an orange, and a note pad and pen to stop to write or draw whenever the mood struck me. Dozing in the sun on the warm rocks in the river or climbing, caked with sweat and exhaustion, to the top of the falls and plunging into the icy river became walks on the wild side of my self-esteem. They were "wild" things for me to do, especially alone, but the activities boosted my self-confidence in a way nothing else ever had before.

I still find these occasional trips or breaks alone to be essential—and believe me, it's not easy to get away when you've got two children and a husband who need you. But we can all squeeze in an overnight getaway at a country inn or city hotel or visit a friend's cabin in the mountains. This time alone can boost our self-esteem and remind us we can count on ourselves no matter what.

It all starts with you! With the foundation of increased self-esteem, your marriage is guaranteed to improve. It's an old therapy trick we use: Focus on helping you change *you* instead of your spouse. When you learn to control yourself, not your spouse, to count on yourself rather than be a dependent wimp, and to be fair but clear about what you need, your spouse *has to change* in response, and it's usually for the better. If it doesn't get better, then you'll have the strength to dump your partner. So, either way, increasing your self-esteem is a WIN/WIN strategy.

The Keys to Successful Communication

We often have trouble talking about *trouble*—those things that bother us, our vulnerabilities, intense needs, and vague desires. It's hard to tell people how we feel because many of us were raised to conceal our emotions and weaknesses. Plus, we often keep our feelings to ourselves because we're afraid that saying what's on our minds may hurt, anger, or upset someone else. But if we don't tell people what's bothering us, we become victims to their needs and we resent them, or we give up, withdraw, and give in to the blues.

Lashing out at your spouse (one manifestation of resentment or unmet need) is not an effective way to communicate, although we often resort to it because it temporarily feels good and often it's the ONLY way we know. It's much better if you can explain to your spouse why you feel hurt or upset by using a variety of communication techniques. One of my favorite action strategies is described by Dr. Robert Cooper in his book, *The Performance Edge* (Nightingale-Conant, 1991). He suggests the following structure for effective communications, especially when intense feelings are involved.

> "*When* you X, *I feel* Y, *because* Z." (You state what behavior bothers you, how it makes you feel, and why.)

Here's an example. Let's say you got home after leaving work early to do car pool, sign up a child for swimming class, and stop off at the market to pick up dinner. Your husband, who was reading the newspaper when you walked in, barks: "When I got home I wanted orange juice and there wasn't any. I hope you didn't forget to get it again."

You consider throwing the bag at him (sans orange juice), but you soon realize that you'd be cleaning up the mess. So instead, you chew him out: "You lazy bum, you're just sitting there relaxing while I'm rushing around like a maniac. You should be glad I go shopping at all! You need to help out around here, you live here too!"

You've got good reasons to be mad, for sure. But your response is likely to further escalate the fight and not solve what you feel is the major problem—that you're working too hard and shouldering too much of the household's responsibilities. Using Dr. Cooper's formula, here is a more productive response:

"When you yell at me for forgetting something at the market, I feel upset and resentful because I do all the food shopping and it doesn't seem fair. I'm so busy that I don't even have time to make a shopping list. How about if we shared the shopping and took turns going to the market or let's call in our order and have them deliver it? Let's make a list together so we don't have to make extra trips to the market because one of us forgets something we need."

What are the benefits of this approach versus just letting him have it for being such a jerk?

Your partner will be less defensive. He may not like what you're saying, but because you're not attacking him, he'll be more likely to listen. Defensive is bad because the person is spending his energy defending himself and planning his counter attack. Not listening. Not problem solving. Not respecting your legitimate needs. Hating you and your big mouth. Not good.

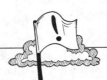

Blues Flag

Dr. John Gottman has found that men in troubled relationships become defensive and withdrawn, tending to "stonewall" their partners and shut down emotionally. They act this way to calm their minds and bodies because they are physically flooded by unpleasant stress chemicals when faced with conflict. That's why it's smart to let men have their "cave time" and try again to resolve the conflict when they've calmed down.

Put Yourself in the Other Person's Shoes

If you find yourself in an argument, you can also diffuse the anger by telling the other person you know how they feel. Women have been trained from birth to rely on intuition, to put themselves in another person's place so they could know how that person feels.

Before explaining your position, try starting with "I understand how you feel. It makes total sense to me," and then add some detail that shows you do understand and accept how the other person feels. "If I were in your place, I would feel the same way because...But it makes me crazy when I come home from work and none of the dishes are done."

Time Out! Chill on the Bench Before Returning to the Game

If these communication techniques don't work, and the argument continues to escalate, take a break from the action with a *time-out*. Sometimes the conflict can't be resolved because both of you are so emotional or mad that neither will listen to the other. Sometimes you're so hurt, you just want to hurt back. Taking a time-out gives you a chance to take a break so both of you can calm down and reassess your position so you can develop a more strategic approach to the problem.

Here are the rules for time-outs I use in the couples work I do:

➤ Either person can call a time-out and *both* must stop the negative interaction.

➤ Whoever calls the time-out asks for some time and suggests when to discuss the issue again; five minutes later or five hours, but not longer than one day later.

The point of the time-out is to separate from each other mentally and/or physically so each person can get back in control of him- or herself. Take a walk, a drive, a bath, or visit the local convenience store. The point is *not* to try to gain control of the other person. When you've regained control of *yourself*, come together and try again until you can resolve the argument.

Men and Women—Lost in Space

Couples would fight a whole lot less if they understood the differences between the way men and women handle stress. In *Men Are From Mars, Women Are From Venus* (HarperCollins, 1992), author John Gray says that when men get into a funk, they retreat to their caves where they go to solve their problems by themselves and then reemerge feeling better.

But most women don't realize that men want to be alone. When a guy comes home and hides behind the newspaper, she wants to know what's wrong. Typically, the guy will say, "Nothing's wrong, I'm okay," which, Gray says, is guy shorthand for: "I am okay because I can deal with this alone. I don't need any help. Please support me by not worrying about me."

But when women hear their men say "Nothing's wrong," they feel something is horribly wrong and that they're being rejected. Maybe they did something to upset their mate. So women pry further, egging their mates to "talk about it"—which is the last thing men want to do.

Dr. Ellen Says

When a man is upset and begins to withdraw, wise women back off for the moment and do something they enjoy to feel good about themselves. The last thing a troubled man wants to see is the worried look on his partner's face. During this period, women whose partners are down in the dumps should focus on doing some of the self-esteem—enhancing exercises suggested in this chapter.

A Few More Words Makes a World of Difference

There is an easy way to avoid the most classic communication breakdown between the sexes. All men have to do is say a few more words. Instead of just saying, "Nothing," for example, they could add: "I need some time alone to think about this, I'll be back." Just saying "I'll be back," Gray explains, makes a big difference because women feel reassured that they won't be abandoned or rejected.

Women, on the other hand, tend to deal with stress by talking about their feelings and free-associating until they stumble into some insight or good feeling. So, as women tell men all the possible reasons why they feel so terrible, men start to believe that the women are blaming them for it and they get defensive. Gray suggests that somewhere in their monologue women interject: "I really appreciate you listening, I'm sure glad we can talk about all this" or "I'm glad I can complain about all of this, it makes me feel so much better."

Replacing the Fizzle with Sizzle

When you find yourself trying to spice up your sex life, remember these three ingredients: surprise, warmth, and intimacy. If you sit back and wait for sexual passion to strike, you'll be waiting a long time. Just like writers must write to overcome their writer's block, couples must practice and make love to overcome their sexual inhibitions.

The more sexual contact you have, the easier it is to do it. Many of us have fallen out of the habit of making love, and the longer we go without it the more awkward and embarrassed we feel around our partners—and the less likely we are to initiate sexual contact.

Many of us don't have sex because we simply don't make the time and we get out of practice. The answer is really astoundingly simple: To regain your sexual intimacy, schedule an appointment, just like any other important activity. Stop thinking about it and just do it, small step by small step! A Saturday or Sunday morning is the favorite time of many of my hard-working clients because it's one of the few times in the week they don't feel too tired. They feel stupid at first setting up an appointment for intimacy, but they soon feel smart when it begins to work.

You don't have to go all the way! Any close physical contact—hugging, kissing, touching—counts as intimacy. Start with those steps until both of you are comfortable. Slowly graduate to the more intense activities until sex becomes one of the best expressions of your love.

The Fantasy Getaway

Some of my clients who are facing the Bedroom Blues make plans to go on a getaway to spend time together and break the routine. It can be one night at an inexpensive motel down the street or a three-day weekend at a five-star hotel far away. The key is that the getaway should cater to the whims and fantasies of your partner, even if it means you put your own needs temporarily on hold! The only rule is that no one can get hurt or be treated in an unsafe or disrespectful way.

One couple renewed their romance with a fantasy getaway. The woman made all the plans, telling her husband she had a surprise for him and to be ready to leave the office at 4 p.m. on a Friday. She told him that someone would call him with instructions on where to go. He arrived at the hotel lobby and saw his wife standing there in high heels and a trench coat (with nothing on underneath!). They spent the evening and the next day in the room, taking bubble baths, making love, ordering room service, and eating candy bars from a silver platter.

You may be thinking, "Oh, I'm not the type to do that," But neither was this woman! She hadn't worn heels in years, and had never walked outside with only a coat over her birthday suit! But she took the emotional risk of seeing herself differently, of doing something that she felt was not "me" but that would please him. It did more than please him. He was thrilled and she felt a new kind of power: the most female and sexual she had ever felt in her life because of her power to turn on and so deeply please her partner.

Many of us who feel sexually turned off often blame our spouses. They aren't exciting enough or sexy. But other people can't make us feel sexually excited, we have to be receptive to it first, and allow ourselves to be turned on. Taking your spouse on a getaway, doing something out of character, and breaking the routine in your life can go a long way toward helping you and your spouse rediscover your intimacy.

Here are some other ideas:

➤ Meet your spouse for lunch at a hotel, then surprise him or her by checking into a room.

➤ Buy your wife a dress that you'd like her to wear and take her out to dinner.

➤ Buy your husband a sexy pair of silk boxers and have him wear them to bed one night.

➤ Make love in the hammock at 2:00 in the morning.

Dr. Ellen Says

If the thought of a sexual fantasy experience turns you off, do something together you are more comfortable doing. The three main ingredients to feeling intimate are: *Focus, Fantasy,* and *Fun.* Focus your time and energy on creating intimate situations with your partner. Make your time fun, light, and playful. And be creative! Do something surprising and new so the two of you can become close by sharing an adventure.

The possibilities are limited only by your imagination. Your potential as a couple is limited only by the boundaries of your heart. Since love can grow and expand at an astonishing capacity, you're in for a rare treat if you put in the effort to trade marital blues for marital bliss.

The Least You Need to Know

➤ All marriages go through stages where couples fight and blame each other for the problems.

➤ Sexual intimacy can be revived in any marriage, unless it's abusive or the couple is totally incompatible.

➤ The key to feeling good about your marriage is to first feel good about yourself.

➤ Taking time off for yourself can enhance your self-esteem and help strengthen your marriage.

➤ Using techniques such as time-outs and putting yourself in your spouse's shoes can strengthen your communication with your spouse.

➤ Being aware of how men and women handle stress differently can avoid many fights.

➤ To rekindle romance and sexual intimacy, couples should get away by themselves, break the routine, and try new experiences together.

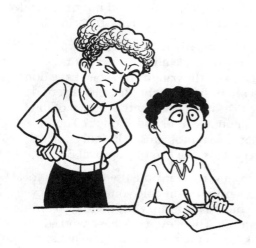

Chapter 15

Coping with the Parent Approval Blues

In This Chapter

➤ Coping with parents who are martyrs or dictators

➤ Desperately seeking parental approval

➤ Cutting the umbilical cord: better late than never

➤ Spot negative thoughts, then STOMP them out

➤ Empathic listening—one of your key survival skills

➤ Turn the tables: You set rules for time and talk

➤ When cutting the tie is the only way out

Like many people, I've spent much of my adult life still trying to please my mother and earn my father's respect. I needed their approval to feel good about myself. But my mother had a tough life, losing my brother and father in a car accident when I was 17. On top of other major losses and disappointments, there was nothing I could do or say that would relieve her pain or help her feel better about me because she was so overwhelmed herself.

My father was deeply damaged when his identical twin brother blew his brains out on the day I was born. Dealing with the details of his brother's messy suicide, Dad couldn't come to the hospital for my birth or the first three days of my life. When he did come to see us, he would not speak of his brother's suicide—not then and never again in his life. But I know that from that moment on, when he looked at me, he saw death as well as life. It deeply influenced how close he could be with me for the rest of his life. He always maintained a certain distance from me so he would not be reminded of the unspeakable tragedy that occurred for him at the time of my birth.

When parents experience this kind of pain and trauma, their energy is tied up in their own emotional and physical survival, not in meeting the emotional needs of their children. As long as the children are fed and clothed, the parents feel they have done their job and there's nothing left to give. And often they're right. But this lack of emotional support takes its toll on the children—leaving them with a legacy of low self-esteem, insecurity, and a constant nagging doubt: Am I good enough? These insecurities typically lead to failed relationships, social problems, self-doubts, neediness, and hunger for parental support: in other words, the Parent Approval Blues.

In this chapter, I'll share with you some tips on how to overcome the Parent Approval Blues. The exercises outlined here will help you examine the role your parents played in your self-image and how you can improve your relationship with them by learning to believe in yourself and taking charge of your life. These exercises have worked well for me, my clients, and friends. They can work for you too! Just don't give up, and keep trying. It took me more than 40 years to escape the Parent Approval Blues, so if you can do it in less time than that, my hat's off to you and a big congratulations!

Parental Approval: Want It, Got to Have It

I've had every aspect of the *Parent Approval Blues*. A first marriage that didn't last and too many relationship problems to count. I slowly but surely had to learn the relationship skills necessary to be effective and healthy in relationships.

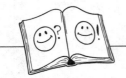

Terms of Encheerment

The *Parent Approval Blues* are the angry, frustrated, and hurt feelings we get when our parents dislike what we do, disapprove of how we feel, and criticize the way we think, or at least we think they disapprove. These blues can easily last a lifetime and screw up our lives from beginning to end.

And after years of therapy trying to fix these problems, I experienced the same truth shown so powerfully in the movie *Good Will Hunting*. In this film, Robin Williams, playing the role of a psychologist, is working with a cocky, brilliant, hostile young man who was and is burdened with severe abuse and abandonment from his childhood. The young man, Will, is taking his rage out on the world around him and in the process, trashing his life and potential for love.

When Will realizes why he's so angry and how devastating the abuse has been to him, he begins to sob and fall apart. The therapist grabs his shoulders and with great force and kindness says over and over: "WILL, IT'S NOT YOUR FAULT!" Will finally hears the therapist and for the first time in his life, begins to heal from the devastating pain of his childhood.

And so it went for me. I finally realized that my mother's unhappiness was not my fault and I stopped trying to change her. My father's pain was not my fault and I began to understand and accept what had happened to him and its impact on me. Instead of staying angry at them and trashing my life, I worked at understanding their experience and seeing it as being independent of me.

Slowly an answer emerged to the bottom-line question: Am I good enough? Yes! Not perfect, not even close, but *good enough*.

So my job was not to spend my emotional energy blaming them but to focus on improving my own life and learning how to acknowledge my own worth. What can I offer? What do I want to do? Who am I outside of their definition? How can I learn to treat others well? I needed to learn how to pick myself up when I was down, to stop being so hard on myself, and to think more positively. Not an easy job for a negativist like me.

My feelings about my mother changed too. I no longer felt threatened by her negativity, nor did I desperately seek her approval. I simply wanted to spend time with her and to get to know her through the eyes of the adult that I'd become. I hoped to connect her to her grandchildren so both could benefit. Our relationship is far from perfect; it's a lot of work for both of us, even in the best of times. We still have our moments of reverting to the past, when I feel overwhelmed by her negative feelings and diminished by my own powerlessness. She probably feels exactly the same about me. But these bad moments are increasingly rare and they're replaced by more and more good times.

Recently, my mother visited us in our home—it was the first time she has come to our house in 12 years. We leafed through family photo albums, talked about our past. I felt connected to her in a way I never had before and experienced joy in seeing her interacting with my two sons, who welcomed their grandmother with open arms. Her visit touched me, and I look forward to our future get-togethers.

At last, almost 40 years later, I've made peace with my mother.

But getting to this point was tough. You too can call a truce with your parents—it's never too late. But before you can get to that point, you'll find it helpful to understand the dynamics between parents and children.

Honor Thy Mother and Father? You've Got to Be Kidding!

You just slammed down the phone on your mother who told you that you're wasting your time being a writer because there's no future in it, even if you are talented. You hate her for not supporting you, but you also feel defeated, wondering if she's right. Maybe you should get a "real" job.

Your aging father complains you don't visit enough, even though you stop over at his apartment four times a week—often at the expense of going to your daughter's soccer game or working out at the gym. You resent his demands, but he is, after all, your father, who took care of you when you were a baby. So you keep going.

You are in a horrible marriage, but feel too insecure to leave it because you know your parents think divorce is a disgrace and dishonor. You resent their callousness, but you are too afraid to venture out on your own. So you stay with your spouse, dreading every single day.

Any of these scenarios sound familiar?

If they do (don't feel bad about confessing) then join the rest of us at the "kids at heart" club. You can't really tell us apart. We all look like adults on the outside—nicely dressed and well-spoken—but inside there's still a part of us who's a kid yearning for our parents' acceptance and depending on them for direction and support. "Daddy, Mommy, look at me!"

The fact is, no matter how old, successful, or well educated we are, many of us often do what we think our parents want us to do and accept their view of the world as our own, even though we're not aware that we are following *their* agenda and not our own. When we upset Mom and Dad by becoming a massage therapist instead of a cardiologist, by marrying someone who wants to transfer to Calcutta instead of moving into the house for sale next door, we feel as if we've failed them.

And disappointing our parents makes us feel guilty and bad about ourselves.

So we often put our parents' needs before our own, buying into the assumption that "good children" sacrifice their lives for their moms and dads, and accepting the fact that all of us eventually suffer from the Parent Approval Blues.

But these bad feelings we have about our relationship with our parents can be good because they serve as a warning that something is wrong with the way we think about ourselves and our families. And if we work out the problems, we can change our lives and have deeper, more meaningful relationships with them and ourselves.

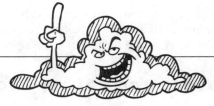

Funk-y Facts

Wonder why you feel so guilty for doing something that hurts your parents? Check out the ancient biblical teachings:

Exodus: "Honour thy father and thy mother; that their days may be long upon the land which the LORD thy God giveth thee." **Proverbs**: "Who so curseth his father or his mother, his lamp shall be put out in obscure darkness." **Proverbs**: "My son, hear the instruction of thy father, and forsake not the law of thy mother: For they shall be an ornament of grace unto thy head, and chains about thy neck."

I'm an Adult, So Why Do I Feel Like Such a Kid?

Imagine you are a successful professional in some field you love. People adore you, listen to you, respect you. You are wined and dined by VIPs, you own three summer homes, and get paid big bucks to tell large crowds what's on your mind. But when your mom asks you to do something you don't want to do, you stomp, whine, and throw tantrums. And then, with your tail stuck between your legs, you do what she wants anyhow because "I don't want my mommy to be mad at me." Why do we sometimes act like four-year-olds when we are with our parents?

The reason is simple: Many of us have never fully grown up—that is, never completely challenged our parents' beliefs and come to our own independent conclusions about the way we feel toward ourselves and the world. So we still rely on our parents to tell us where to go, what to do, and how to think.

They Say That Growing Up Is Hard to Do

It's hard to grow up because we have to take big risks and stand alone. Long after we leave our parents' house, we carry with us their beliefs, expectations, and opinions. If they say the world is square, then square it is and the hell with Columbus. If they tell us we are fat, then fat we are, even if the scale says otherwise.

How could we not believe our parents? After all, our relationship with them is the most important one in our lives. Its roots are so deep that they define and determine who we are and what we think more than anything else in the world. As infants, we depend on our parents to survive. They feed us, cloth us, protect us. We think they are Godlike, we watch their every move and imitate it. We listen to what they say and adopt their feelings, visions, and interpretations as our own. And we believe that what they say about us is true.

If our parents think we are wonderful, honest, and diligent, we are more likely to feel optimistic, self-confident, and decisive. We face the world on our own terms and try to do our best. But if our parents tell us we are stupid, unattractive, and clumsy, we grow up feeling insecure, worthless, and defenseless—and feel too vulnerable to go off on our own.

Most of us were raised by parents who were critical and judgmental because that was how they were raised by their parents and those were the parental norms of that generation. As a result of those parenting styles, our generations are more susceptible to experiencing the Parent Approval Blues.

The Umbilical Connection

To be happy, healthy adults, we all need to cut the umbilical cord. Otherwise, the cord wraps around our throats, and we end up choking ourselves with bad relationships, unsuitable jobs, extra weight, and unhappy lives. If you don't resolve your feelings about your parents, you could find yourself in a scenario such as the following:

➤ You may accept a job with an authoritarian boss who unconsciously reminds you of your father, and surprise yourself by getting into a screaming match with him that's reminiscent of your battles at home.

➤ You may be critical of and feel distanced from your spouse, the way your parents were with each other.

➤ You may withhold from your kids what was withheld from you, without even knowing that you are doing the same thing.

➤ You may see the world as a dangerous and cruel place where people take advantage of you, just like your parents viewed it.

The Bad Things Our Parents Tell Us and Why We Believe Them

Why do our parents say so many hurtful things to us? Even the most relaxed, confident parents have some trouble tolerating their kids' emerging independence and when the kids are strong, parents often feel weak in comparison. It's natural for all of us to want to keep the people we love close by and to feel competitive even with those we most love. But some parents can grapple with these feelings and still give their kids the freedom they need to explore the world.

Many parents, however, can't let go as easily. They may have grown up with authoritarian parents who ruled with an iron fist and assume that this is the best way to raise their own kids. Or they may feel insecure about their abilities, and project that on to their kids by making them feel bad about not being able to do well in school, sports, or other activities. For some parents, their kids are the repository of their unfulfilled dreams and the kid must pursue the dream of the parent, not their own dream, for all to go well.

Regardless of how we were raised, we can all take control of our lives by figuring out who we are and what we want. You can start changing your life by breaking old habits. You may think that this is easier said than done. And you're right! But if I could do it, after years of failure and feeling helpless and hopeless, so can you!

Guiltless Pleasures

Deep down inside, we love our parents even though we may feel they've done some pretty nasty things to us. After years of fighting with them, saying something nice to them will make you feel good—and can change the course of the relationship. So try focusing on the positive. Compliment your mom on how nice she looks, or tell your dad that you admire how organized he is. They may look at you suspiciously at first—but keep at it until it feels right to them and you!

Cut Off Parental Criticism at the Knee: Break Old Habits

If you've spent most of your life fighting to get out from under your parents' control, chances are you've felt pretty beaten down, discouraged, and dejected. Your parents probably told you that you were a bad person in some way and you probably bought into that opinion. It's time to learn how you can break those patterns and feel better about yourself.

Don't Play It Again, Sam

How many times have you said to yourself: "I can never do anything right!" or "There I go again, being stupid!" or "Nothing will ever work out right." These tapes still run through my mind once in a while. I call them "Insults For Ellen—The Top 10"—and these records have been on the charts for years!

And guess who recorded the messages? Probably your parents. These negative tapes have been on automatic replay since you were young, and by now you may be so used to them that you don't even hear the music.

To stop these negative thoughts from wreaking havoc on our self-esteem we need to be aware of when we have them, understand where they come from, and then *stomp them out*. Shatter those records and tapes into a thousand pieces and sweep them into the garbage. (And I'm not talking about the recycling bin, either.) Switch the focus from negative to positive about yourself. How?

Spot That Thought

Take a half an hour and write down on a piece of paper (or type at the computer) a list of negative things that you remember your parents telling you throughout your life.

Your list may look something like this:

➤ "You never do anything right!"

➤ "You'll never find a husband (or wife), you're too fat."

➤ "You don't look good in that."

➤ "Being a musician (or whatever) is a waste of time."

➤ "Why don't you understand anything? Are you stupid?"

There were many forces beyond your parents' control that influenced them to act a certain way—and understanding those forces may help you realize that how they treated you may have had more to do with what was going on in their lives than with anything you did or said.

The next step, then, is to try to figure out why your parents said negative things to you. Ask yourself: How do your parents feel about themselves? Are they proud of who they are? Are they happy with their jobs and their relationships? Do they seem content or anxious? What's their history? What were their parents like?

Parents who are unhappily married or divorced, for instance, may be critical of who-ever your bring home because deep down inside they don't think good marriages exist because they've never experienced one. A mom who tells you to ditch the arts and go for a Masters in Business may have had creative leanings when she was younger that were stifled by her own mom who said painting "wasn't practical." She was terrified to defy her own mother and equally terrified if you defy her, so in her world everyone loses the opportunity to find and follow their passions.

Be a Parent Detective

If you don't have a clue as to why your parents act the way they do, then get out your Sherlock Holmes cap, put on a trench coat, and become a parent detective:

➤ Talk to your own parents (if you feel comfortable doing that) or to relatives about doing a family history. Gather as much information as you can about the family to get a sense of how your parents fit in. Ask relatives what your parents were like when they were little kids. Were they popular? Happy? Sad? Rad?

➤ Look through old photo albums and watch home movies or videos (they won't seem as boring when you are actually looking for something) to see how your parents acted. Did they seem close to others in the pictures? How were they dressed? What image did they try to project—tough, cute, debonair? You'd be amazed how much you can learn about your parents when you're not busy trying to prove to them that you're right and they're wrong!

➤ Create a family tree. Relatives may be more willing to talk if they think it's for a good project for the family. As you plot people's positions on the tree, listen closely to the information provided and when you feel something important may be lurking behind the tree, ask gentle, respectful, leading questions like: "You're kidding! She drank every night until she was 94? What kind of person was she?" or "He had a hunting accident. How sad—it must have been such a loss for his family. How did they cope with it?"

STOMP on the Negative Parent Tapes and Throw Them Out!

Now that you've identified the voice and learned where it came from, the question becomes: How accurate is the negative message? We know your parents said it's true. But what do you think? Say, for instance, you've always assumed you were lazy, since that's what your parents called you ever since you could remember.

Are you lazy? Think about what you do with your time and when you are likely to see yourself as lazy. Is it justified? Chances are that you may have been lazy in your parents' eyes because you didn't do what they wanted you to do, but that your actual life is active and far from lazy.

If this parental statement is not true, *stomp on that tape and throw it out.*

The next time you put yourself down as being lazy, stop the thought by saying "NOT TRUE!" or just "NOT!" and turn your attention to an activity that will distract you and make you feel better—going jogging or dancing, reading a good book, calling a friend, or running an errand.

Eventually, the parent cassette recordings drilled into your memory will stop playing, and the music you'll hear instead will be a new CD containing the sweet melody of all the wonderful things about you. And technology is on your side. CDs hold a lot more memory than cassette tapes, so you can really pack in more good stuff about you in them!

You CAN Go Home Again (and Survive It)

Dr. Ellen Says

If the going gets real tough and you find you need outside help in communicating with your parents, consider going to family counseling. Through counseling—typically short-term—families can resolve current problems, learn to work together more cooperatively, and communicate more effectively. Counseling is particularly helpful when an older parent becomes ill and other family members have to pick up the slack and take on additional responsibilities or when a younger person is in crisis, such as with a drinking, drug, or school problem. Through counseling, family members frequently open up to each other—sometimes for the first time ever—and learn to understand and accept one another.

Even once you resolved some of the old bad feelings, going home for a visit can be hard because your parents may not have changed. I know only too well how it feels when you are determined not to let your parents get your goat, and then one comment throws you off and you're back to where you started—raiding the refrigerator to stuff your anger so you don't explode at them.

To avoid flying off the handle when your parents are pushing all your buttons, you need to be able to express your anger and needs more effectively.

Say, for instance, your parents are touting the benefits of a religious education right after you enrolled your child in public school. All you are hearing is them really saying: "See. You can't make any good decisions, and this is just another example. You're a lousy parent."

But you've given this subject much thought and chose public school. You may feel the impulse to convince your mom that times have changed, public schools are much better, multiculturalism is in vogue, and so on—*but don't fall into that trap!* Instead, you may want to practice "empathetic listening," a fancy term that really just means backing off and letting your mother talk, while you carefully listen without judgment. The way to listen is to put yourself in her place. *Be* her for a moment and really understand where she's coming from. You don't have to agree one bit with what she's saying, but you can benefit enormously by learning where she's coming from and why.

Dr. Ellen Says

Don't ask for your parents' advice if you don't think you're going to like what they say! This is a trap many of my clients fall into. If you know your parents don't like your girlfriend, asking them what they think of her is a sure way to start a fight. So unless you really want to hear an answer very different from how you feel, "Don't ask, don't tell."

So while your mom is pontificating, just nod and start your sentences with words like: "I understand why you'd feel that way..." or "I appreciate you saying that..." or "I know what you mean..." or "Let me think about that." If your mother begins insulting you, shift gears into a stronger approach by saying: "When you say that it hurts me because (reason). Could we instead..." (See Chapter 14, "The Bedroom Blues: What Happened to Marital Bliss?" for more communication tips.)

Once you let your parents talk without fighting with them and make an attempt to understand their position, they will be more likely to tolerate your position—even if it's different from theirs—without as much judgment and negativity. You might even learn to respect each other and tolerate each other's differences, which is a marker of real maturity.

Don't Step Into Those Guilt Traps Parents Lay So Well

Another crucial step in improving your relationship with your parents is setting guidelines for your visits. According to Harold H. Bloomfield, M.D., who wrote *Making Peace With Your Parents*, don't let your parents control your thoughts or actions.

In the following sections, I give you some guidelines to keep you from getting hot under the collar during those family visits.

Sorry, Got Places to Go to, People to See

Let everyone know ahead of time the length of your visit, otherwise you may spend the entire time figuring out how long you should stay and defending why you can't stay longer. And don't feel you have to spend every single second with your parents. Plan other things to do and let your parents know when you'll be going off to do other things, so that when you get there you won't get into a big fight about it.

If you aren't feeling great about your life and you know your parents will pounce on your when you're down, then consider putting off a visit or go and stay with a friend or at a hotel to minimize the tension. The more stressed you feel the more likely you are to fall into the Parent Approval Blues.

Don't Just Sit There Stuffing Your Face

Eat less and move more!

Many of us go home and fall back into old habits and old foods. If you're trying to lose weight, you may resent your mom for making your old time favorite meal—fried chicken with French fries—(even if she doesn't know you're on a diet) and blame her for your weight problem.

Eat lightly, sample a few pieces, say a warm "Thank you" and then get out of the house and go for a walk.

Build in Lots of Exercise During Your Visit

Exercise makes you feel stronger and more in control, and gives you a healthy break from your parents while relieving your tension. But just because you are exercising, don't try to get them to reform their lifestyle. If you do, get out the boxing gloves for another round—for old times' sake.

Prepare for the Worst

Think through ahead of time the worst possible case and what you'll do to cope with it.

If you know your parents will be rude to your girlfriend, let her know ahead of time what to expect and figure out a plan of action to take if the situation gets too hairy. Your parents don't have to love her, but they don't have the right to be rude to her either.

Cutting the Ties That Bind: The Last Resort

Blues Flag

If you and your parents can't agree on something, don't keep insisting they see things your way. Hang up the phone or leave their house and do something physical: Pound on a pillow, scream at the top of your lungs in a closed car, or kick your mattress. A punching bag is a gift to your mental health. Whatever you try, get physical, stay safe, don't destroy anthing valuable, and let it rip! The more you can let off steam, the less power your anger has to get you in trouble. Don't pretend your anger will go away if you ignore it, because that approach only makes your anger grow until it explodes uncontrollably and destructively.

When you finally change the way you behave and become true to yourself, you are testing how much your parents can handle. Many parents will be shocked with the new you; they may intimidate you or stop talking to you for a while. Most, though, will come back around, eventually saying "I've learned a lot from your changes." And the relationship will mature and grow deeper.

But unfortunately, some parents may never get used to the change.

Sometimes, we can deal with our parents' insensitivity by keeping our visits short, getting together with them only in large groups or public places, and making other arrangements to stay in touch while keeping our distance.

But if we have to deny all of our needs, if we can't share any aspects of our lives with them, and if seeing them becomes too painful or dangerous, we may have to consider breaking the tie. *But be careful*—this is a drastic step that should be considered only after all attempts at keeping contact have failed.

Before you take that step, answer the following questions:

➤ How long has it been since I started asserting myself?

➤ Have my parents shown any inclination toward accepting me more, even a small, tiny gesture or step?

➤ Have they spoken or acted any differently, given me more room, or tried to make things up to me?

➤ Are they still verbally or physically abusive to me after my efforts to get them to stop?

Blues Flag

If you absolutely need to sever ties with your parents because they are abusive or dangerous, seek professional counseling and make sure you are connected to a support network. This is a severe measure and it must be done carefully so you can integrate the change. I suggest you start by setting boundaries about what behavior is acceptable and what isn't. Visit less frequently (or not at all if they are abusive), stop calling as often, and take other gradual steps to exit from their lives.

Remember, it will take a while for your parents to change, so give them the benefit of the doubt. This is very important! Give the new relationship with them time to grow and mature. Be patient! It's worth it because every improvement you can make in your relationship with your parents provides significant improvements in your relationship with everyone else. That's how important our relationship with our parents is. It must be severed only when there's no other alternative and your health is at stake.

The only time to completely break ties with your parents is when they are abusive, destructive, and dangerous, and they will not change no matter what you do. Then breaking contact with them is clearly the best thing to do. But if you have to cut the ties, then I advise you to seek professional counseling and support about how and when to make the separation, because this is the most painful and important break you will ever make in your life, no matter how justified it is.

When we are little, we hold our parents responsible for our happiness and well-being. But as adults, the tables turn and we are responsible for nurturing ourselves and taking care of our needs and often their needs too. It's never too late to take charge of your life and learn to think independently. With courage, support, and inspiration, you can walk out of your parents' house and into a good home of your own. You can escape from the Parent Approval Blues by breaking their old disapproval tapes and replacing them with the music and beauty of your own spirit.

The Least You Need to Know

➤ Regardless of our age, level of education, or success, most of us still seek our parents' approval.

➤ We get the Parent Approval Blues when we let our parents continue defining who we are and determining what we think.

➤ To become healthy, happy adults we must challenge the rules we were raised with and learn to think and be on our own.

➤ Replacing negative self-defeating thoughts with positive, empowering statements about ourselves is a crucial step toward making peace with your parents.

➤ Your parents are more likely to accept you if you stop trying to convince them that you are always right and actually listen to what they have to say without judgment.

➤ When visiting family, set the boundaries about what you'll do at home, whom you'll spend time with, and when you plan to leave.

➤ Breaking all ties with your parents is an extreme measure that should be taken only if they are dangerous, destructive, or abusive and unable to change.

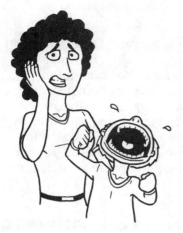

Chapter 16

The Pooped-Parent Blues: Calling the Shots When You Feel Shot

---

In This Chapter

➤ Who gets the Pooped-Parent Blues?

➤ Making the rules for your kids—and sticking to them

➤ Quiz: Are your kids making you blue?

➤ Using positive reinforcement to correct a child's behavior

➤ Understanding and dealing with your child's temperament

➤ Does your child have depression or a learning disability?

You've yelled at your eight-year-old to clean his room a million times and it's still a pigsty. You finally grounded your 16-year-old daughter for breaking her curfew after weeks of empty threats. And you know something is wrong—very wrong—with your 11-year-old who is way behind in school and may have a learning disability (maybe it's ADD on ADHD?). But you're too tired from working all day or caring for kids to face these problems, much less fix them.

I know how you feel. I often have these problems too. You really, *really* try to be calm when your kids misbehave or seem troubled. All the books tell you to, and so does your therapist, cardiologist, and next-door neighbor who sees you, well, losing it when you're with your kids. But after transgression #11, you lunge into your Mommie Dearest or Frankenstein routine, towering and hollering, threatening and nagging them. And afterward you feel guilty for being such a lousy, mean, and rotten mother or father (possibly like the one you had), and wonder how much damage you are doing to your kid.

If this scenario sounds familiar, you've got a case of the Pooped-Parent Blues—one of the most common blues known to any tired parent who loves her kids but can't seem to get them to listen, obey, and behave! But take my word for it: You can beat the Pooped-Parent Blues by keeping your cool and putting into practice effective discipline strategies, no matter what your level of exhaustion. These strategies actually give you more energy than they take to do. They have helped me and my clients significantly improve our relationships with our children and greatly increase our satisfaction in being parents. Rather than feel pooped most of the time, we feel pleased and passionate in our role as good parents. In this chapter we take a look at how these discipline strategies can help you cope.

Being a Parent Is the Toughest Job in the Universe

You hoped being a parent would be all about hugs and kisses, sharing hot fudge sundaes on warm summer nights and hot chocolate on frosty days, reading scary stories by flashlight in a tent, and having more Kodak moments than you could ever photograph or experience in one lifetime. At least that's what I thought when I first had kids.

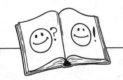

Terms of Encheerment

Pooped-Parent Blues are the sad, bad, frustrating, exhausted, and guilty feelings we get when we do what we think is right for our children but they don't react the way we expect them to and we don't know what to do about it. Most parents experience these blues because, with the increased demands on our time to make money and stay competitive in an increasingly complex world, it's hard to raise kids without good role models or support from society.

And like most of you, I do experience such snippets of time—moments when I feel nothing but sheer joy, love, and acceptance for my children. But I'll admit there are also times when I want to hurl household objects at them, use them for target practice, or drop them off at a friend's house and leave town without telling anyone.

Why? Because kids do things that drive us crazy!

They leave backpacks on the living room floor (that we trip on again and again) after we tell them NOT to a million times. They bop their siblings on the head after being warned to leave them alone. As teenagers, they're exquisitely adept at finding and pushing our hot buttons until we feel like a character in their newest violent video game. They refuse to eat what you cook, they don't study enough, and they whine, whimper, and wear you out just when you can't stand hearing their shrill voices another second!

Most of us try to get a grip on our kids' gripes by screaming, threatening, punishing, and bribing them, but that rarely works. Our kids know that many of our threats are empty ("If you don't eat your dinner, you'll never get dessert!"), and that if they nag at us long and hard enough we'll cave in to their demands.

Boy, do I know how terrible it feels when your kid has the upper hand and knows that you're a pushover! Do you know what I mean? That's why so many of us try to defend ourselves against our munchkins by turning into tyrants to regain control. But in the end, instead of feeling all-powerful we just feel all-pooped.

You have a case of the *Pooped-Parent Blues* if you feel you're doing a lousy job raising your kids, you don't know what to do about it, you fear your children will end up on skid row because you didn't do the right thing, and you're too tired to face or fix the problems.

Most of us feel insecure about our parenting abilities at some point. Let's face it: Raising children today is far more complicated, dangerous, and tiring than ever before. It's tough to give kids the attention they need when both parents may work long hours, reliable child care is often unavailable, and bosses often give only lip service to family-friendly policies.

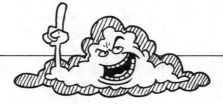

Funk-y Facts

Although single moms are the most susceptible to getting the Pooped–Parent Blues because they often raise their kids by themselves, single dads are following close behind. Today, nearly 28 percent of all households are headed by one parent, usually the mother. But the number of single fathers is on the rise, tripling since 1970 to nearly 1.3 million in 1990. Single moms and dads can better manage their parenting demands by being in a flexible and supportive work environment, having reliable day care with backup, scheduling time for themselves, getting connected to a network of singles in their communities, and seeking professional help when other coping strategies don't work so there's more support for the parent, not just for the kids.

And yet, our kids need us more than ever as the world they face is more difficult and dangerous than the world of our youth.

For example, our parents probably avoided us our entire teenage years or just gave us a book about the birds and the bees and left the rest to our imaginations. Parents today need to have heart-to-heart talks with their kids about sex, drugs, and AIDS...all before the kid is nine! The stakes rise dramatically when our children have emotional or learning disabilities and we are faced with so much contradictory information and medical insensitivity.

But feeling bad about our parenting skills can be good. It gives us the opportunity to evaluate how we deal with our children and improve our relationships with them by understanding more about our own childhood and the vulnerabilities we inherited as parents. Learning to accept our children for who they are, not who we want them to be, rewarding their good behavior, and letting them know they are loved are skills that can be learned and practiced. These parenting skills will make you feel good about being a parent—and give your kids the foundation they need to be happy, healthy, and responsible human beings.

The Parenting Blues Scale

Almost every client I have who has kids experiences the Pooped-Parent Blues to one degree or another. What most of us know about parenting comes from our own childhood, and the world has changed so much since we were kids that many of the lessons we learned back then no longer apply.

The definition of "good parenting" changes over time, as do suggestions on the best disciplining methods to use with children. Think about the "spare the rod, spoil the child" attitude so popular in the '60s and compare it to the current thinking that corporal punishment is not as effective as other disciplining techniques.

Do you know what philosophy to use in raising your child and do you feel confident about your parenting skills? Just where do you fall on the pooped-parent scale? Take the following quiz to find out.

Are Your Kids Making You Blue?

Answer the following questions (T) for true and (F) for false.

1. Some days I wish my kids had a one-way ticket to anywhere but here. ___
2. Other days I'd like to just sell them and at least make some money. ___
3. My kids can make me angrier than anyone I've ever known (or imagined). ___
4. When one of the kids start to whine again, the sound makes me want to explode! ___
5. There's nothing more terrible I can imagine than losing my kids. ___
6. Often I feel I'm just too tired to get it quite right as a parent. ___
7. No matter what I do, I never seem to have enough time with the kids. ___
8. Frequent quality time with our kids and both parents disappeared with *Father Knows Best*. ___
9. Our family resembles the Simpsons more than the Brady Bunch. ___
10. Children should be seen but not heard, and sometimes it's fine to skip seeing them too. ___

How did you do?

If you answered "True" to five or more of these questions, you've got the Pooped-Parent Blues! But don't worry, mom or dad, you've got lots of company and can get lots of help. Most of us are in the same boat—a dinghy, that is—and will be floating around for a while groping for our paddles since dealing with our children is a work in progress.

If you answered "true" to fewer than five questions, you're either a candidate for sainthood or you don't have any children!

Set Boundaries to Retain Your Sanity

Punishing your kids is one way to teach them to behave appropriately—and we all know how that works! You do time-outs. You take away TV and phone privileges and anything else your kids care about. This disciplining method occasionally works for my kids.

But I also found that they do a whole lot better when I pat them on the back for a job well done or when I give them a reward for good behavior.

Rules, Consistency, and Follow-Through

To practice good discipline we need to set rules, be consistent in carrying them out, and follow through with consequences when they are broken. Kids do better when they understand what type of behavior is acceptable, when they know how far they can go before they cross the line and get privileges taken away.

It's the parent's job to set limits—and stick to them. I know that this is easier said than done! After a long day at work, I'm so worn out by the time I get home that when my kids ask for the 20th time if they can play ball in the living room (which is against the rules at our house) I feel like saying "Go ahead" just to shut them up.

But I've learned how important it is to stick to the rules so our children know what we expect from them. The secret to getting your kids to follow the rules, though, is to explain the rules before you yell at the kids for breaking them. This way they will understand what the rules are and why they are in place so they can become active partners in helping the family. If, for instance, one of the house rules is that your son must clear the table at dinner, don't immediately shout: "You know you're supposed to clear the table, what's wrong with you?" Instead, sit down with him before dinner and calmly say the following:

> "Your mother and I have been thinking about how everyone can help out around dinner time. We'd like you to clear the table and bring the dishes to the kitchen. Try doing your best to remember that."

Be specific about what clear the table means. Put the dishes where? In the sink, the dishwasher? Does "clear" also entail cleaning the table with a sponge?

Kids are also encouraged in this way to do their best—and that's a reasonable expectation. Remember, your kid wants to please you more than upset you. And when he does achieve success, acknowledge his efforts by letting him know that you've noticed he is trying harder and you're proud of him.

To Each His Own Rules

Each family sets its own rules. For example, you could devise rules about how people should treat each other, what type of playing is (and isn't) allowed in the house, how long kids can watch TV, who gets to use the computer and when. You could also have a rule requiring people to tell each other how they feel—no name calling or swearing allowed. And another rule forbidding kids to hit their siblings, even when they are mad.

What happens when your little darling breaks the rules? That's when you've got to be the family cop and dole out consequences that seem fair and appropriate. If your child was told not to wear ripped jeans to school and he wore them anyway, you could say: "You don't get to wear the jeans for a week."

Avoid making all-or-nothing statements like:

➤ "You can never wear jeans again."

➤ "I'll never buy you ice cream again."

➤ "You can't watch television until you get married!"

Dr. Ellen Says

When you are disciplining your child, strive to be fair. If she is really mad and acts rebellious when you lay down the law of the land, maybe she doesn't understand why you set those limits. Also, cut your kid some slack by not punishing her for EVERY rule that gets broken. Let the small stuff slide so you can focus on the bigger issues.

You probably won't follow through on these threats and your kid will know you're bluffing. And even though you may be mad at your kid for dressing like a slob, don't attack him personally or say: "What's wrong with you? Why are you such a slob?" Attacking him rather than the action can be damaging to your child's self-esteem. You want your child to learn from the consequences, but you still want him to know you love him and care about him.

Keep Your Cool in the Heat of the Moment

Keeping calm is one of the hardest things for parents to do. Don't get discouraged if you fall into your old hysterical self every time your child pushes your buttons. Unlearning old habits takes time and doesn't happen overnight!

But when your child breaks the rule, don't lose your cool! Avoid going on a rampage about how he "never" does this or personalize his action ("How could you do this to me!"). Most kids will tune you out if you deluge them with words. Simply tell your child the consequences of his behavior in a straightforward fashion using a neutral tone of voice.

Some Positive Reinforcement Goes a Long Way

If your kid is being a thorn on your side, try giving him a pat on the back! Positive reinforcement can prevent a lot of misbehavior. I'm not talking about bribery here, where you tell your child: "If you shut up I'll buy you something." The kind of reward I'm talking about is more systematic.

Say, for instance, you want your child to stop fighting with his brother so you target that behavior and tell him: "You've been picking on your brother and that is wrong. If you don't pick on him for seven days, you'll get a present." You can then discuss what that present will be—and negotiate within limits you set for price and appropriateness.

Be very clear about what talking back means. Is talking with a mean tone considered talking back? Remember: Kids don't know what you mean unless you are explicit.

Other types of positive reinforcement include:

➤ Comment on specific great things your child is doing, like being nice to his neighbor or doing his homework without complaining.

➤ Reward your child for following a routine, like getting ready by himself to go to camp in the morning or preparing for bed.

What's Wrong with My Kid?

Many of us feel like we're rotten parents when our kids do rotten things to other kids or treat us badly. But we can also work ourselves into a funk when they refuse to eat healthy foods, reject the new clothes we bought them, or sulk alone in the corner of the room. We see other parents in the park frolicking around with their seemingly happy-go-lucky kids and then look at our own and say: "Why can't you be like that?"

We all know that this isn't the right thing to say. Yet, we can't always help it!

The reality is that some kids are harder to deal with than others. Some children are restless and easily distracted, others react badly to loud noises, and many can't cope with transitions. Each child is born with a different temperament—tendencies to act and react to incidents and people in specific ways. The more you understand your child's quirks, the less frustrated you'll be in dealing with him.

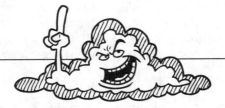

Funk-y Facts

If you think your child is tough to raise, then you'll be happy to know that about 10 percent of normal children studied in a major research project were dubbed "difficult." According to Stanley Turecki, author of *The Difficult Child* (Bantam, 1985), difficult children are normal, but they are hard to raise because of their temperaments. Difficult kids can cause a lot of marital strain and family upset—but if dealt with properly they can also become enthusiastic, optimistic, and very creative people.

Nobody knows for sure what causes a difficult temperament. But research shows that many personality traits are biologically based. We are born with it—and these genes are as important in determining character as the way we are raised. These inborn temperaments make each child unique—but they also present a unique challenge to parents.

All kids break down into nine temperamental traits, first defined by Drs. Alexander Thomas, Stella Chess, and Herbert Birch of New York University in the ground-breaking New York Longitudinal Study, a project that began in 1956 and still continues today. Here are each of the nine traits, along with some questions to help you think about where your child fits in.

➤ *Activity level*. How active is your child? Is he always fidgeting or does he sit quietly?

➤ *Regularity*. Does your child have regular or irregular sleeping patterns or appetite?

➤ *Adaptability*. How does your child deal with change? Is she upset by surprises?

➤ *First reaction*. When presented with a new situation, does your child jump in and participate or wait on the sidelines until he cases out the joint?

➤ *Mood*. Is she generally cranky or happy-go-lucky?

➤ *Intensity*. Are your child's emotional reactions strong? Is he very emotional or distant?

➤ *Persistence*. Does your child have a tough time switching activities? Does she stick to something when the going gets tough?

➤ *Perceptiveness*. How aware is your child to the environment—how does he react to colors, noises, people?

➤ *Sensitivity.* How sensitive is your child to physical things? Is she very aware of noises, scratchy clothing, smells, tastes?

Many of us label our kids "rebellious" when they don't do what we want them to when, in reality, they just simply may not be capable of fulfilling our expectations. Trying to discipline your child without knowing his temperament is like taking shots in the dark—and it's bad for everyone. Your child feels lousy for disappointing you, and you feel like a creep for being so mean.

You'll feel more compassionate—and less angry—at your child if you know that some of her behavior is a function of her temperament. In other words, IT'S NOT YOUR FAULT that your kid won't eat her mashed potatoes if they touched the peas or that she melts down every time you go to a school function with her. And knowing that will make it easier for you to help her.

One of my clients who had constant battles with her son over clothing gave her kid an ultimatum: Either wear the new turtlenecks she bought him or have no dessert for a week. She knew she was being harsh and unreasonable (not wearing a turtleneck is, after all, not a BAD behavior). Her kid cried, stomped, and growled. He just could not wear the turtlenecks, they felt "funny around his neck."

Then she realized that he had a sensitivity to clothing. So instead of insisting that he wear his new turtlenecks (which she got at a great sale!), she started buying him more V-necked shirts. And guess what, no more clothing battles!

Another client used to constantly hound her son for not being polite and for refusing to look people in the face when they talked to him. But after thinking about his temperament, she wondered whether he was rude or just shy. It turned out he *was* shy and felt too embarrassed to make eye-to-eye contact. She now helps him feel more comfortable when he is with people he doesn't know well by trying to engage him in conversation. She may, for instance, ask him a question so he can have a reason to speak, or turn the conversation to a topic that interests him so he can more naturally chime in.

When both of these clients stopped blaming themselves for their kid's temperament, they were better able to think more clearly and cope with discipline more effectively.

What a Temper! Chart Your Child's Moods

You can beat the parent blues by figuring out ways to help your child through his or her difficult moods. Keep a daily mood chart on your child for two weeks, writing down the time of day that your child is upset, cranky, or unhappy and what he is doing when he is feeling that way.

Recording this information will give you a better idea about whether the bad moods are happening at the same time each day and over similar circumstances. Is she grumpy mostly when she wakes up and that's when you get into fights with her about

Dr. Ellen Says

I see a lot of frustrated parents in my practice who complain that "my kid doesn't listen to anybody" and who are convinced that their child is ignoring them just to get them mad. But many times kids don't "listen" because they are, by nature, easily distracted and can't pay attention unless they are really interested. To get their attention, parents should make eye contact with their child when they ask them to do something and speak in a calm but firm voice.

what to wear or what to eat? Does he seem particularly anxious or angry around dinner time? Are there lots of fights about going to bed at night?

Once you isolate the bad moods, you can try to manage your child's behavior. Remember you can only temper his temperament—not change it.

Consider the following suggestions in accommodating your child's temperament:

➤ *"Stop acting so wild and sit still!"* If your child gets revved up before dinner each night and can't sit still at the table after a long day of activities, for instance, try to help him calm down by giving him a bath, reading him a story, or letting him watch his favorite TV program *before* dinner.

➤ *"You've got to get up now or else!"* If morning times are the worst because your child doesn't want to get up, then make sure she goes to bed earlier, and lure her out of bed with a special, favorite breakfast or another nice surprise, such as reading a story or playing a game.

➤ *"Why can't you be like other children?"* If your child tugs at your skirt every time you leave him in a new surrounding, he may have a hard time making transitions. Instead of yelling at him for clinging to you, which will only make him cling more and make you feel worse, try to prepare him so he has time to get used to the new situation. You might say: "This morning you are going to a birthday party, and I know it's hard for you to get used to a new situation, so I'll stay with you for a little while but then I'll have to leave."

➤ *"If you don't eat dinner you don't get dessert!"* You just can't force a kid who isn't hungry to eat when the rest of the family is having dinner if the child is by nature an irregular eater. Like the saying goes, you can lead a horse to water but you can't make him drink. So just save her dinner for when she is hungry and suggest she sit with the family at dinner and participate in conversation.

When All Else Fails

You've tried it all—the rules, consistency, consequences, attention, love. The charts. And still, you and your child are locked in battle. He is disruptive, destructive, and explosive; you are hysterical, desperate, and depleted! The question then becomes: Could his problems be biological?

Could your child have *Attention Deficit Disorder* (ADD) or *Attention Deficit Hyperactive Disorder* (ADHD)? These are the most commonly diagnosed psychiatric illnesses among children, and about 10 percent of all school-age kids are now taking medication for these disorders.

A child with ADD is likely to be impulsive, easily distracted, and have difficulty paying attention. When children are diagnosed with ADHD, they tend to have the same conditions as those with ADD, but they are also hyperactive—easily stimulated and have a hard time sitting still. ADHD can be more problematic and typically requires professional help to treat because it tends to be more disruptive.

For discipline to be effective kids have to pay attention, which is why some kids with ADD/ADHD have so much trouble—and are at high risk for developing learning disorders and behavioral difficulties.

You know your child may have a learning difference if teachers start telling you that he can't pay attention in class, is impulsive, hyperactive, unable to prioritize, and seems preoccupied during class. Kids with these disabilities are easily overwhelmed by stimuli and need careful direction and strong limits.

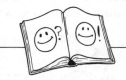

Terms of Encheerment

Attention Deficit Disorder (ADD) is the most common behavior disorder in children, characterized by a short attention span, impulsive behavior, poor concentration, and excessive motor behavior. This condition occurs about 10 times more often in boys than in girls. Children with *Attention Deficit Hyperactive Disorder (ADHD)* display the same symptons, but are also hyperactive.

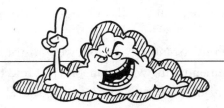

Funk-y Facts

Doctors prescribe three classes of drugs to children with ADD or ADHD: stimulants, tranquilizers, and antidepressants. The most commonly prescribed drug for ADD/ADHD is Ritalin, followed by Dexedrine and Cylert. Studies show that stimulants affect symptoms in up to 80 percent of hyperactive children, making them less aggressive and impulsive and helping them focus their attention. But medication is not a cure and should not be used as the only treatment strategy for ADD. If you suspect your child may have ADD or ADHD, I urge you to see a specialist. Pediatricians are not that familiar with those conditions. An expert is in better position to determine *if* medication is necessary and, if so, what the right dosage would be. For the names of specialists or additional information, contact CHADD (see the last page in this chapter).

Parents are often disappointed when they find out their kids have learning differences. I know I was. When our son was diagnosed with a learning difference, I felt over-whelmed and became depressed. It's very distressing to deal with the fact that your child is not perfect, especially for someone like me whose top priority is learning and education. My son is really bright so this was even more frustrating for him.

After getting the proper diagnosis, which, believe me, wasn't easy, we found out that he was way ahead of his class in reading but he couldn't spell. We transferred him from a public to a private school, where he received special help. He and I also worked together for two or three hours a night making index cards to practice his spelling.

He is now doing really well in school and is a well-adjusted kid.

Learning differences are treatable, but if they are not detected and treated early, they can have a tragic, snowball effect. A child who doesn't learn to multiply in elementary school can't understand algebra in high school and will have trouble with simple math as an adult. A child trying hard to learn becomes more and more frustrated and develops low self-esteem after repeated failures. Some learning-differenced kids misbehave in school because they'd rather be seen as bad than stupid.

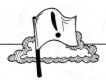

Blues Flag

If your child seems sad all the time, complains of a lot of physical problems, can't enjoy his favorite activities, seems irritated, and acts lethargic and bored all the time, he or she may be experiencing depression. Significant depression exists in about 5 percent of children and adolescents—and kids with learning differences are at higher risk for depression.

Be aware of the most frequent signals of learning differences. Your child might have a learning difference if he or she:

➤ Has difficulty understanding and following instructions

➤ Has trouble remembering what someone just told him

➤ Can't master reading, writing, and/or math skills

➤ Has a tough time distinguishing right from left

➤ Lacks coordination in walking, sports, or small activities like holding a pencil or tying a shoelace

➤ Easily loses homework, school books

➤ Can't understand the concept of time

If you suspect your child is depressed, I urge you to get a proper diagnosis. Go to a physician or other health-care provider as well as a psychologist or psychiatrist to get an evaluation. Many children don't have severe symptoms of learning disabilities until they enter middle school.

Some other suggestions:

➤ Read about ADD and ADHD and talk to other parents.

➤ Contact CHADD (Children and Adults with Attention Deficit Disorder) at 499 N.W. 70th Avenue, Suite 101, Plantation, FL 33317; (800) 233-4050.

Raising children in today's hectic, crazy world is indeed the toughest job in the universe. But for me, this job has also been the most exciting, fulfilling, and creative endeavor I've ever undertaken, and my kids will always come first. I still get slapped with the Pooped-Parent Blues sometimes, but when I do I can beat these bad feelings by applying the action strategies I've described in this chapter. I hope they work for you too. Try them—your relationship with your kids are worth the effort!

The Least You Need to Know

➤ Raising kids today is more complicated than ever because parents often work long hours, reliable child care can be hard to find, and many companies give only lip service to family-friendly policies.

➤ To practice good discipline, parents need to set rules, be consistent in carrying them out, and follow through with consequences.

➤ Positive reinforcement and setting up reward systems can prevent a lot of misbehavior.

➤ Difficult children make the parents' job harder because they need more attention to thrive.

➤ All children are born with temperamental traits that can be managed but not significantly altered.

➤ Parents who try everything and are still constantly fighting with their kids should see a professional to determine whether their child is depressed or has a learning difference.

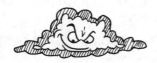

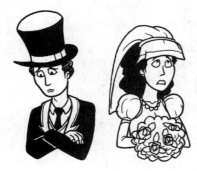

Chapter 17

Battling the Home-Alone Blues

In This Chapter

➤ Is one really a lonely number?

➤ Singles get no respect, but lots of doubts

➤ Let your PC do the walking

➤ Debates over dates

➤ Let's talk, but about what?

➤ The five-date, one-year rule

➤ Success secrets of the happily partnered

If you want to find people to date today, opportunities abound. You can write personal ads, send out e-mail messages, go to singles socials, and hang out in chat rooms giving someone the electronic eye! You can even sit back with popcorn and a beer to review video clippings of eligible candidates and throw the unpopped kernels at the screen if you don't like who you see. With all these opportunities you'd think single people today would be thrilled, inundated with so many choices that they'd have to resort to "eeny, meeny, miny, mo" to choose a Saturday-night date! But that's not what's happening.

Singles today may have more outlets for meeting people than ever before, but they are also having a tougher time developing relationships and maintaining them. The reason: We live in a society that perpetuates the myth that relationships are easy. They should just happen magically and that, once we meet somebody, we no longer have to do anything because that person will take care of all our needs.

Get a grip! Just who is going to fit in that category? Peter Pan and Tinkerbell? No wonder so many singles are joining the chorus to sing, "Another Saturday Night and I Ain't Got Nobody." They feel lonely and bad about themselves or about the world and no matter what they do, they can't seem to avoid another case of the Home-Alone Blues.

To have a healthy, happy, and thriving relationship we must be able to take care of ourselves first, and take responsibility for our own happiness. We need to accept that those who look to others to make them happy end up in unhealthy relationships that often result in abuse or divorce. We must acknowledge that finding and maintaining relationships takes work and often requires learning skills most of us don't naturally have.

All too often, many people marry out of desperation, for fear of being alone in a society that makes singles feel they've veered off course because they haven't walked down the aisle. In this chapter, we'll explore why singles have a hard time finding appropriate companions and how they can go about strengthening themselves, enhancing their self-esteem, and thus increasing the likelihood of finding and keeping that significant other.

Who Is Single?

Well, try about half the population! And that number is growing. Statistics show that people who are single now make up nearly half the U.S. population. In fact, 43 percent of American men and 47.5 percent of American women are single, according to the 1990 U.S. Census. Single-person households grew 35 percent between 1980 and 1992, and will grow another 28 percent between 1990 and 2010, *American Demographics* magazine reports.

Single and married people have more in common with each other now than ever before. Both groups are struggling to keep up with the cost of living, trying to squeeze in workouts, chores, and hobbies along with heavy workloads and so many other responsibilities. We all often feel burned out, complain about having no time to ourselves, and sense that our lives are spinning out of control.

Yet, many singles think married folks have got it made and fantasize that having a mate will solve all their problems. And many marrieds envy the freedom of singles to do what they want when they want to. So what's the answer to the Home-Alone Blues?

When you think of marriage, if the image in your mind is mom staying home making dinner, the family sharing meals and then snuggling up in the den to watch the 1970 version of *Father Knows Best*, then you need to start looking for dates in *Jurassic Park*. And if you buy that fairy tale, you probably also consumed the myth that was spoon-fed to you along with mashed potatoes and pot roast: that there is only one person out there for you, you'll be swept off your feet, and he or she will fulfill your every wish and make you whole. All you have to do is just wait until the relationship presents itself.

These out-of-date fantasies and images spell disaster for modern relationships. As long as we think that someone else is responsible for our happiness, that a relationship will appear magically "when it's time," and that once we find it we don't have to work to maintain it (or even say anything interesting to our partner for the rest of our lives), we'll be susceptible to getting the *Home-Alone Blues*.

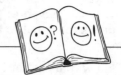

Terms of Encheerment

The *Home-Alone Blues* are the sad, frustrated, desperate feelings we get when we want to find somebody to share our lives but we either don't have the skills to develop and maintain a relationship, or the pickings are slim so we can't find anyone we like. We end up home alone too often with these blues as our only companion.

It makes sense that we'd often get the Home-Alone Blues since society tells us that we are worthless unless we are part of a couple. When you are alone, everything seems made for two—like those two-for-one dinner deals. And just about everywhere you turn advertisements show couples having fun, talking, eating, and laughing together. Yet our social institutions don't teach us skills that allow us to be intimate with people and form healthy relationships.

But don't despair. There's plenty of relationship hope to go around if you learn how to deal with your feelings. Feeling bad about being single can be good if it helps us acknowledge that we need to take charge of our own happiness, be more realistic about what we expect from our partners, and learn the communication skills necessary to make relationships work. Feeling blue is also good if the emotion acts as a motivator for us to develop interpersonal relationship skills so we can find somebody—and keep that person.

Singles Get No Respect

It's hard to be a single in a society geared toward couples (have you ever seen a love seat for one?). If you haven't found somebody by the time you're 32, people wonder what's wrong with you. When your parents call and say: "So, what's new?" you want to hang up because you know what they're really saying is: "Have you finally found somebody?" You avoid going to high-school reunions because the first question from the senior-year prom queen—who has been divorced twice—will be: "Oh, honey. Are you married yet? To whom?" And you definitely want to hide under the blankets during Valentine's Day, the first day of spring—any holiday that entails buying flowers for a sweetheart.

Let's face it, singles get no respect.

When you go to dinner solo, for instance, the waiter shows you to your table—right by the kitchen or near the bathroom. If you are a man vacationing alone and you aren't carrying a cell phone—which signals you're on a business trip—people are leery of you: Are you a pervert or just a giant loser? If you are a woman vacationing alone, people don't know what to think of you: Are you a high-powered career type or a prissy old maid?

I know that it's hard for many singles to meet people because finding someone can feel like a full-time job. So many of my clients are businesspeople who barely have time to change their clothes between business trips, never mind schmooze with people at an ice-cream social. But even those who manage to squeeze in social events have a hard time finding someone they like, and if they are lucky enough to find someone, they have a hard time keeping the person because it's so hard to find the time necessary to invest in growing a relationship.

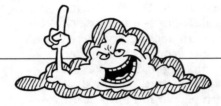

Funk-y Facts

If you think you're pitiful because you have to pop frozen dinners in the microwave for dinner while other families are feasting on home-cooked stews, freshly steamed broccoli, and Key-lime pie, then check out this little fact: The National Restaurant Association says that almost no one makes big, elaborate meals anymore, according to *American Demographics*. American households are increasingly planning their evening meals no more than a half an hour ahead of time, and they often depend on carry-out, home delivery, pizza, and fast-food restaurants for their family meals. And if you think it stinks to watch TV alone night after night, then you'll be happy to hear that so does everybody else. A recent survey of 1,600 households reported in *Metrolina Singles Magazine* said that half of its respondents usually watch TV alone—as a result, some rating services are now reporting TV viewing as per person rather than per household.

Many singles are increasingly disheartened and feel their prospects are grim.

But I have good news that should make you feel hopeful: Throughout my 25 years of clinical practice, I've never had a client who hasn't found somebody appropriate and available after committing himself to changing his attitude and learning interpersonal skills. And when he did find that person, it was someone he freely chose to be with, not someone he settled for out of desperation of being alone. But his secret to success was always the same: He was willing to do the hard work of relationships!

Get Off the Couch and Get on the Wire

Finding a relationship requires a significant commitment of time and effort. The first step is to acknowledge how much you want to meet somebody. I know that this sounds really simplistic, but let me tell you why I'm mentioning it. Many singles are embarrassed to be single. They may feel that their marital status brands them as a failure, a defective product, and they don't want to talk about it, much less advertise it by going to any social event that, well, singles them out.

But to meet somebody worth having, you've got to challenge society's notion of what being single is all about. This means that you may need to figure out what makes you tick, to find out what you like about yourself and what you want to change, and to raise your self-esteem. To attract people you also need to do the following:

➤ Network, network, network!

➤ Present a positive attitude.

➤ Be interesting (though not brilliant) and interested in the other person.

➤ Look good (beautiful or handsome is not necessary) and feel good.

Well, you aren't likely to get a date sitting around your apartment waiting for someone to knock on the door—unless you want to go out with the FedEx delivery guy or gal! So splash some cold water on your face, put on some favorite clothes, make sure to brush your teeth, comb your hair, do all those things your mother used to tell you to do before leaving the house, and start having some real fun!

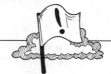

Blues Flag

In your search, beware of settling for addictive relationships! Someone who is addicted to people doesn't *choose* to stay with the partner—she just simply *can't leave* because she's addicted and the partner is her current drug of choice. Genuine love is based on an ability to love freely, *by choice*. According to Dr. Howard M. Halpern, author of the classic *How To Break Your Addiction To A Person* (MJFBooks, 1982), you are in an addictive relationship if you have a compulsive drive to be with your partner, and if you feel withdrawal symptoms when trying to break up (including physical pain, sleep disturbances, weeping, and depression).

You Had to Be There

There are a thousand different ways to network, so pick the way that makes you feel most comfortable and that seems the most fun. The traditional, tried-and-true way is to actually make first contact with people not through e-mail, voice-mail, or any other electronic fashion, but in person.

This wireless, non-technological "I'd like you to meet so-and-so" approach still works. Tell everyone you know that you'd like to meet more people and ask if they know of any good parties, events, or possible blind dates. Almost every organization now offers singles activities as part of its community services. Check out your local club, church, synagogue, or recreation center. Many of these groups offer activities for singles other than parties where everyone stands around contemplating their navels. But most of my clients have not found these single groups useful in meeting people with long-term potential because events designed specifically for singles tend to attract the "broken wings," as one astute client put it. Still, these events are a place to start, build up your confidence, and practice communication skills.

Then when you want to branch out beyond the Planet of the Singles, try the following:

➤ Join a club where people share an activity they love (hiking, biking, running, swimming).

➤ Participate in an organized sport whether or not you're any good at it (softball, volleyball, skiing, golf).

➤ Share the finer things in life (wine-tasting groups, gourmet-food groups, contemporary art, learning Chinese or French).

The best places to meet potential dates are places that you're interested in going to anyhow, because chance are you'll have more in common with the people there. So my advice to you is this: To assure a good time, go to places you'll be happy in even if you don't meet anybody. You'll seem less desperate, which automatically makes you more attractive and more available for a good time.

Many of my single clients love to apply one of my favorite action strategies: The quickest way to help yourself is to help someone else. They've had their best successes meeting quality people by volunteering for their favorite charities, such as the American Cancer Society, church or synagogue groups helping the homeless or other projects, and groups involving the literacy movement and breast cancer research. When people enjoy themselves and are having a good time doing something good for others, they're open to meeting other people and getting to know them and not as desperate to snatch a mate from the madding crowd.

Singles Go Electronic: Let Your PC Do the Walking

If you can't handle going to a singles mingle event to hear a speaker talk about fear of rejection, for instance, you may consider other out-of-sight methods. The Internet, dating services, matchmakers, and personal ads (they are much more creative these days than: "Single white male seeks…") put a layer between you and the person you may meet—so you can think about the candidates, talk to others about them, and decide whether you want to go through with a date. Most of my single clients have had more success with ads and the Internet than any of the dating services because the ads and the Net give you more control to pick and choose from a wider pool of people. They report that working with dating services often feels like a bait-and-switch experience, where what is promised is far different from what the service delivers.

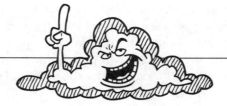

Funk-y Facts

For all those women out there who think that marriage means waiting on your man, doing laundry, washing dishes, cooking dinner, and working full-time while your husband slouches around on the couch after work belching and bellyaching, I've got good news to share with you! A University of Chicago researcher says that marriage brings good tidings and considerable benefits to both women and men, according to *New York Times* reports. In fact, tying the knot may make your life longer, improve your physical and mental state, and give you more dispensable income than you'd have if you were divorced, single, or just lived with a guy. The researcher, Dr. Linda J. Waite, a professor of sociology who presented her findings recently at the second annual Smart Marriages Conferences in Washington, called marriages "a public health issue." She was quoted by the *New York Times* reporter as saying that "people need to know the facts so they can make good decisions. Marriage is good for everyone." The notion that marriage is bad for women stems from a 1972 publication of *The Future of Marriage* (Yale University Press), which reported that married men were better off than single men on four measures of psychological distress: depression, neurotic symptoms, phobic tendency, and passivity. But the study showed women who were married scored higher on the negative traits than single women. So hang in there! Marriage can be great, and once you find the right person you'll feel it was worth all the trouble!

If you're going to go electronic or answer an ad, you should take some safety precautions. I know I sound like a schoolmarm, but I've seen too many clients get into trouble—sometimes serious—by ignoring these warnings, so at least consider the following strategies:

➤ When you finally feel comfortable that the person you are exchanging messages with is trustworthy, arrange to meet him for the first time in a public place with lots of people around, rather than at your home or his. If you feel uncomfortable during the first conversation, you can gracefully exit without having to worry that he knows how to track you down.

➤ I strongly encourage you to meet for coffee before or after work, so if you don't like the person you aren't stuck with her for an entire dinner—which can be especially long if your date is the coffee-drinking, "Sure, I'll have some more" type, dragging out the agony further.

➤ *Never* give out your personal phone number, e-mail address, or actual street address until you feel safe and secure with the person you're considering dating. This means at least several meetings in public places before you give out any personal identifying data. By then you should know who you're making yourself vulnerable to and can't be stalked by the potential serial killer in disguise sitting across from you slowly sipping his wine.

➤ Use the buddy system. Tell a friend or roommate where you're going and when you plan to be home. Leave a number where you'll be, if at all possible. Always carry ID, a credit card, and enough money for cab fare to get home.

➤ Don't let anyone pick you up or bring you home until you know he's earned your "*Good Housekeeping* Stamp of Approval." This means spend time away from home with him in public places until he's shown he's safe enough that you could even bring him home to meet your mother. Then he can be trusted to see where and how you live.

Does "How Are You?" Go Before or After "Hello"?

You finally landed a datewith someone special. You are so nervous that you can't remember your name. Now comes the part that most of us REALLY dread. Having to talk to your date. You need to make a good impression within the first 10 seconds—and you can either use up that precious time babbling incoherently (if this happens, try to smile your way through it), or saying something meaningful—although a "Hello" would do just fine. But what do you say when your heart is pounding so loud you can't hear your thoughts?

First, realize that all of us fear saying something that will sound stupid. We're afraid people will laugh at us if we say: "How are you?" as if nobody in the history of Western civilization has ever said that to another person on the first meeting. The best way to overcome shyness is to fight it with self-confidence, even if it's pretend. You'll realize that all you need to break out of the shell is an attitude adjustment, not a lobotomy or a new personality. And remember: The other person is probably feeling shy too and unsure of what to say.

Before you meet your date, take stock of your personal strengths. Make a list of personal accomplishments on a piece of paper and carry it around with you so you can glance over your attributes to bolster your spirit. You can also do the following:

➤ *Act as if you feel confident until you do.* Put on an act, if you need to, by walking into the room with your shoulders back, chin up. Nobody knows you've been engaged four times and left at the alter once—and they don't have to. Not yet and not ever.

➤ *During the date rely on your good points, find out about your date's, and don't bring up too much of the past.* You aren't filming *True Confessions.* In fact, as a general rule,

220

I don't think it's very helpful to talk about past dates because someone always seems to end up feeling bad.

➤ *Think about the worst-case scenario.* You walk up to a woman to ask her to dance, she catches your glance, makes a horrible face, and runs in the opposite direction. Okay, it's a blow. But it isn't going to make the headline in tomorrow's paper and humiliate you at work and with your family. You were rejected. It's an old story we all know well so try to take it in stride and whatever you do, don't let it stop you from continuing to get back out there and connect to others.

Everybody gets nervous when they first meet, so most dates cut you some slack. The most important quality about yourself that you want to get across is integrity and honesty—don't brag, give pickup lines, or show off and, if you find yourself talking too much, ask the other person questions to engage him in conversation. Keep the discussion light and positive, steer away from heavy topics (like your relationship with your mother)—at least at first. And if you really like the person, show your excitement, but don't lose your cool. You want things to move slowly but steadily.

And if someone makes you nervous and you feel funny but don't know why, always trust your instinct and end the date. Tell her it's better not to see each other again. You don't have to explain why but your request does have to be respected. If someone continues to try to contact you even when you clearly requested no more contact, leave a message on her answering machine or via e-mail or letter that you are serious and please do not contact you anymore. Do not talk to the person directly because it will make you unnecessarily vulnerable and expose you to an unpleasant confrontation. Then ignore any more contacts and if they continue, let the person know you consider her behavior harassing and if she doesn't stop, you'll call the police or you'll tell her mother. That usually does the trick and the contact stops.

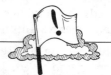

Blues Flag

If you find that you can't overcome your shyness even though you've tried, the shyness could be a form of depression. A sense that constant doom is right around the corner and a feeling that nobody will ever love you could be a sign that shyness is not really the problem—so self-help isn't the answer. See a mental health professional to figure out if what you are experiencing is depression and what you can do to lift it.

The Five-Date, One-Year Rule

Many of my clients are single and, after talking to hundreds of them about sex and commitment, we've come up with a rule of thumb about what works and doesn't work in today's single world: I call it the *five-date, one-year rule.* This means you should go on at least five dates before you have sex; if you don't wait, you increase your emotional vulnerability too much. Sex is one of the most intimate exchanges two people can have and nothing reveals more about who you really are. You don't want some virtual stranger to have that kind of knowledge about you and that power over your essence. You must know who the person really is and if he or she can be trusted before you increase your emotional vulnerability so significantly through sex. There is only one way to really know who someone is: time. You need to see someone over time and in many different situations to see who that someone really is, not who the person wants you to believe he or she is. With this caution in mind, it makes sense to wait about a year before you make a long-term commitment with your partner, so again you won't make a mistake by going too fast too soon and end up a divorce statistic.

Getting Beyond the First Date: Now What?

When you first meet that special someone, you are so in love, you overlook whatever differences you have. In fact, the differences are virtually invisible. There are flowers, poems, cute messages on voice mails. And if you call your friend to share with her the details of the date and she gently asks you how you felt about him being a meat and potato guy while you are a vegetarian…well, then, you just hang up quickly! "Who needs someone like her for a friend?" you mumble to yourself, as you quickly dial your new lover for another fix.

But after the dust settles, a clearer picture emerges and you begin to remember what your friend asked. The guy is not only a carnivore, but he is also fatter than you thought, not to mention rude. You get into fights that don't ever get resolved, and you disagree on everything. One night, you are eating at a restaurant and as his fork sinks into the steak, blood dripping out of the side, your stomach churns. You excuse yourself, escape out of the back door, and hope you have better luck next time around.

Many people can get their foot in the door, but more than a few get their feet stomped on or stuck there. It's one thing to find a relationship, but another thing entirely to maintain it because different sets of skills are involved. When you try to attract somebody, you use your charm, personality, looks, and humor—whatever it takes. But these qualities aren't much help in a long-term relationship when a problem comes up that has to be resolved.

When the going gets tough and the tough stop talking you need to bring other skills to bear. You need the ability to:

➤ Negotiate, compromise, and resolve conflict
➤ Communicate the "tough stuff"
➤ Tolerate ambiguity and ambivalence
➤ Give people space to be who they are
➤ Practice the art of time-outs
➤ Resolve intimacy terrors, yours and theirs

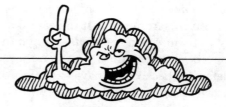

Funk-y Facts

It's not what you say, but how you say it! An article in *Bottom Line* newsletter notes that when it comes to dating, American men are likely to fib about their occupations and incomes, while women tell white lies about their ages and personal histories. So when you go on a date, put on your Sherlock Holmes hat: Keep track of what the person says; then come back later and tactfully ask questions to check out inconsistencies. If your date avoids eye contact, seems stiff and tense, or leans away rather than toward you when talking, he may be telling a fib. If while talking over the phone, she rattles off huge amounts of irrelevant information, she may be trying to distract you. Get the person to slow down by saying: "Would you repeat that?" If the person is lying, he may respond by speaking more slowly, using fewer words, making grammatical mistakes, and speaking at a higher pitch. If you feel the person is not aboveboard, dump him overboard and set sail for healthier seas!

These relationship skills don't come naturally or easily. It takes time and energy to create and built relationships worth having because good partnerships involve shared goals, patience, empathy, compromise, and a commitment to long-range goals. We also need to be able to deal with anger, competition, and conflict. For specific effective communication strategies, look at some of the suggestions in Chapter 14, "The Bedroom Blues: What Happened to Marital Bliss?"

But the first step in maintaining relationships is to acknowledge the fact that it will take time to learn to talk to your partner. You also need to accept each other's differences and give your partner room to be who he or she is. And remember that men and women *are* different and have different ways of communicating. If we understood each other's style, we'd save ourselves a lot of fighting and reach WIN/WIN more quickly.

Here are a few more communication tips:

➤ *Don't hide what you think to please your partner.* Let your partner know how you feel about many issues through casual conversation right from the beginning so that he won't make assumptions about your beliefs—which almost always leads to big misunderstandings further into the relationship.

➤ *When you are arguing and not listening to each other, take a time-out.* Each one of you needs to go to your corner or room or outside and take a deep breath—then decide whether you've cooled off enough to continue the conversation or whether it's time to throw in the towel and try again later.

➤ *When you are arguing, accept that your partner is not trying to hurt you.* Many of us bring all our problems from the past to bear on our new partners and we heap all our anxieties on them. We don't see *them* anymore. Suddenly they've become our critical mothers or abusive fathers. So when they say things that upset us, we get even more defensive because we have to protect ourselves from past and present enemies. We can't communicate effectively when we feel like we have to protect ourselves. When this happens to you, use a time-out to give yourself time to throw out your mother or father from the situation and return to the present to work things out with just your partner.

Rate Your Interpersonal Skills

Now that you know what it takes to develop and maintain a relationship, do an inventory of your interpersonal communication skills. Divide a piece of paper into two columns, labeling one column "Relationship Establishment Skills" and the other "Relationship Maintenance Skills." Then list which skills you think are required for each task. Under "Relationship Establishment Skills" for instance, you might list: learning to go up to strangers and strike up a conversation, or figuring out where to go to meet people. Under the "Relationship Maintenance Skills" you might include: learning to deal with conflict or trying to be more tolerant.

Go over the list carefully and check off the skills you feel you already have—the ones without checkmarks next to them are the skills you need to develop. Ask a trusted friend or relative to rate you too so you get a more accurate picture of where you stand and what you need to do. To build your interpersonal skills, try these suggestions:

➤ Model yourself after people who you think are good at meeting others and maintaining long-term relationships.

➤ Read books on how to communicate effectively in a relationship. There are many excellent relationship books out there that teach you how to build skills. Two good ones are *The Complete Idiot's Guide to a Healthy Relationship* (Alpha Books, 1998) and *The Complete Idiot's Guide to Dating* (Alpha Books, 1996).

➤ Analyze and discuss with your friends the relationships of characters in your favorite movies and TV shows to see how their relationships do or don't work for them.

➤ Ask friends to help you out by letting you know when you're being too negative, or by role-playing a date so you can practice how you'll react to various scenarios.

➤ Ask a friend who you think is a good communicator if you can hang out with her at a party just to see how she handles introductions and small talk.

➤ Find a smart friend who will coach you on building relationship skills. Go to parties with your coach or double date, so later your coach can give you feedback on what you're doing that works and doesn't work. Then do the same for your friend. You can learn together how to win at the dating and relationship game, until each of you scores a winning goal.

Finding and maintaining a healthy relationship is one of the biggest challenges we all face—but once we meet someone who shares our goals, commitment, and passion, it's also one of the greatest rewards. To find that special someone, we must first learn to feel good about ourselves and then be open to meeting other people so that when love appears we'll recognize it and be ready to grow it. And what a smart thing to do, because love is one of the surest strategies to beat the blues!

The Least You Need to Know

➤ Statistics show that people who are single make up nearly half of the U.S. population. Single-person households also grew 35 percent between 1980 and 1992, and will grow another 28 percent between 1990 and 2010.

➤ Many people believe there is one person out there for them, and once they find them, they don't have to do anything to maintain the relationship.

➤ You get the Home-Alone Blues when you want to meet someone but don't have the skills to develop and maintain a relationship.

➤ Finding a relationship requires a big commitment of time, effort, and skills. Maintaining a relationship requires a different set of skills but is just as much work.

➤ Singles can meet people in traditional ways such as parties, singles socials, and joining clubs; but increasingly, they are turning to shared activity groups or electronic media to make a match.

➤ Before you meet a date, take stock of your personal strengths so you will be more confident. During the date, be honest, straightforward, polite, and genuinely interested in the other person.

➤ Acceptance, tolerance, time-outs, and conflict resolution skills are key to making a relationship last.

Part 5
The Worker Blues: Monday-Morning Doldrums

You hate getting out of bed on Monday morning because you know what's ahead—a horrible Tuesday, Wednesday, Thursday, and Friday. Plus, who wants to go to work when your boss is breathing down your neck or when you'll have to face your supervisor to announce you have to leave early—again—to take your child to the doctor?

There are plenty of good reasons today to feel blue about your work life, but you don't have to live with it. This section will give you some tips on finding the job that's right for you so you aren't so stressed out and suggest better ways to communicate with your boss so you aren't at each other's throats. Life is no picnic for today's working parents, so a chapter is devoted solely to the challenges parents face and how they can beat the blues by beating the odds.

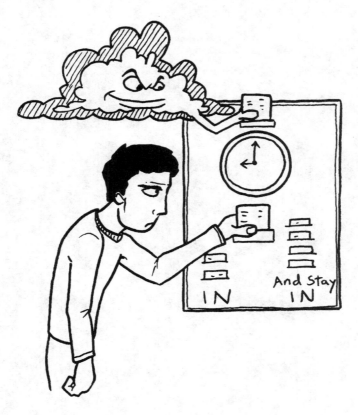

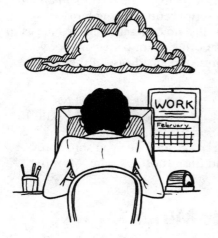

Chapter 18

Licking the Monday-Morning Blues

> ### In This Chapter
>
> ➤ Why you're no longer in charge
>
> ➤ Flexibility is in, stability is out
>
> ➤ Quiz: What job suits you best?
>
> ➤ Change gears: switch careers
>
> ➤ Doing the work you love will bust the blues

The alarm goes off at 6 a.m. and you drag yourself out of bed. It's Monday morning, the beginning of another dreadful week, and the start of five days of full-time worrying. How will you ever get everything done that's waiting on your desk, when you didn't get enough rest on the weekend and you feel like the star of *Night of the Living Dead*? Is this the week you'll get a pink slip after the company announces its plans on "restructuring," "downsizing," or "rightsizing"? Whatever other euphemism is in mode, it essentially means one thing: "You're out of luck, Buck."

Your friends who lost their jobs tell you that you should be happy to have "survived" two other downsizing cycles. But sitting there, sipping coffee from your "I'm the Boss" mug (a mean-spirited present from a manager who has accused you of insubordination), you have mixed feelings: On one hand, losing your job would be terrifying; on the other, nothing could be more liberating.

It sure would be nice to skip analyzing another statistical table. You daydream about working for a publishing company, reviewing manuscripts and meeting famous authors. Only one problem: You've got no writing skills, no contacts, and no clue as to how you'd go about switching careers. So you take another sip of coffee, reboot your computer, and drown yourself in a sea of facts, figures, and a bad case of the Monday-Morning Blues.

If this is your life, then it's a depressingly common one! But work doesn't have to be such a drag if you're willing to learn what you really want to do, develop the skills to do it, and figure out a way to sell your abilities to a company or organization. In this chapter, we'll look at the uncertainty in today's workplace and give you some proven action strategies for how you can smash, thrash, and trash those Monday-Morning Blues, once and for all.

When You Work in the Blue Salt Mines

Millions of Americans roll their eyes and let out a big sigh when they talk about their jobs. If you dread getting up on Monday mornings and life doesn't seem to get much better on Tuesday, Wednesday, Thursday, or Friday, chances are you've got the *Monday-Morning Blues*—those feelings of anger, frustration, or disappointment we get when we hate our jobs but feel stuck in them because we don't have the skills to move up or there is no place in the company to move. Maybe we don't like our profession or the people we work with, or we live in constant fear that we'll see a pink slip on our desks when we come back from lunch. We may be chronically burned out because it takes everything we have to survive this crummy job or the only reason we go down to the blue salt mines every day is to come up with a paycheck every other week.

If you don't have some form of the Monday-Morning Blues, then you probably don't have a job! Who doesn't feel confused, overwhelmed, or even at times incapacitated by the changes in today's workplace? Our expectations are all wrong. We are raised to think that once we find the job we love we'll stay there forever, like many of our parents did. And if we work hard and remain loyal employees, if we follow our job description and do what the boss tells us, the company will take care of us.

But that's not how the world works anymore. Now, we are told *not* to rely on anybody but ourselves, *not* to expect to have a job there the next day, and to be prepared to switch careers at any given point. Instead of climbing the ladder and calling the shots, we are told to sit around the table with a bunch of 23-year-olds and "work as a team" to develop policies. And you're

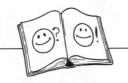

Terms of Encheerment

Monday-Morning Blues are the angry and frustrated feelings we experience when our working arrangement is unhappy or unhealthy. We don't like our jobs, we don't get along with our work mates, we don't feel valued by our bosses, or we fear we'll lose our jobs. Given the unstable nature of today's workplace, almost everyone experiences the Monday-Morning Blues at some point.

thinking: "What do these young kids know about policies? They are so new to the company that they still have to ask for directions to the bathroom!"

So instead of punching the clock, we feel punched in the gut! Is it any wonder we're so stressed out over work and reminded of it every Monday morning?

But feeling bad about hating our job is a sign that something is wrong with the way we think about and do our work and that we need to reevaluate our professional goals. You can beat the Monday-Morning Blues by figuring out what kind of work and work environment is best suited to you and by taking the steps necessary to get a job in that field.

It may take time to figure out what you want to do, and the exercises in this chapter should help you along. But figure it this way: We spend almost 95,000 hours of our lives working, so what's a couple of extra hours doing some soul-searching? If you do it right, you could save yourself thousands of hours of really boring, droning work! If you really do it right, you'll be doing work so passionate and fulfilling that it won't feel like work at all!

Do You Whistle While You Work?

When you are passed over for a promotion or when a coworker you think is a friend goes to lunch with the manager who is trying to sabotage your project, you probably fantasize about how great life would be if you didn't have to make money for a living. But many people choose to work even when their incomes are not essential because work satisfies many of their psychological needs. Meaningful work is one of the best ways to beat the blues.

When we work, we feel good about our abilities, and proud of our accomplishments, and that increases our self-esteem. We also feel more connected to people and make friends so we don't feel as alone and isolated—a major cause of depression. Research has shown that career and work satisfaction are the strongest contributors to mental health. So if you like working, you're way ahead of the game!

But many people find their jobs to be a total bore. They yawn when they answer the phone and are constantly checking the clock to see when it's time to go home. The cause of their dissatisfaction: They don't feel challenged enough at work or they don't feel up to the challenge. They may find the issues they deal with are unimportant, or they may not feel inspired or motivated by the people around them.

Dr. Ellen Says

Employers can enhance the self-esteem of their workers and make them feel more in control by instituting family-friendly policies, including flexible work hours, paternity leave, and other perks. Other ways employers can help employees beat the Monday-Morning Blues is by making them part of the decision-making process so they don't feel controlled by a system that gives orders from the top down.

In my coaching practice called "Bridge Ventures: Executive Coaching Systems," I see many clients who have the Monday-Morning Blues all week long, and believe me, this misery spills into the weekend as well. They've talked themselves out of finding the work they love because they are afraid to take the risk, afraid that they won't get what they want, and feel more disappointed as a result of it. Many of them think it's idealistic to work at a job they love and find that it's perfectly acceptable to complain about their work without intending to make any changes.

My coaching practice emphasizes four steps for helping clients beat the Monday-Morning Blues:

1. Get in touch with your real passions and begin owning and developing those passions as a critical survival strategy for your work and life.

2. Learn to set better boundaries at work for what you can and can't do.

3. Develop and practice a range of communication skills to better express your needs and hear the needs of others.

4. Learn how to connect better with others so you can be part of a productive, strong work team that functions like a healthy family.

The more we build these skills, the more likely we can find a job that's up our alley!

The Retirement Party Has Retired

If you find yourself switching jobs more than you expected, wearing many hats, and constantly on a learning curve, you may feel like you are unstable and unable to hold a down a job. That's probably how your parents view you if they were raised with the company-man mentality. But, actually, you're really on the ball! The days of working for one company for 30 years are over.

In fact, you'll probably change professions at least three times and jobs as often as 10 times, according to the U.S. Bureau of Labor Statistics. Why can't we stay in one place forever? Companies don't have that type of life span anymore. Many are here today and gone tomorrow. The increasing competition among businesses is constantly forcing companies to change the way they operate, and that's why they look for employees who are flexible and able to update their skills.

Instead of hiring 30 full-time employees, for instance, a company may hire a skeleton crew of eight and rely on temporary employees (hired for a short time to do administrative tasks) and independent contractors to provide services such as printing, public relations, payroll, human resources, legal work, and word processing.

The bottom line is that you can't expect to slide by just because you are Mr. or Ms. Nice Guy or Gal. You have to show your company that you can do a lot of things quickly and well, that you can learn to do new things, and switch back and forth between the old and the new. You also have to show your company that you are motivated to learn, eager to take on projects, and willing to be a problem solver. And, of course, you have to do it all with a smile.

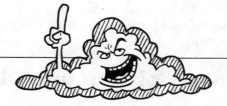

Funk-y Facts

If you want to get in where the job action will be in the future, go into a health-care profession. By the year 2000, one in three people will be 50 or over and health care will become a crucial industry. Other industries projected to boom include computer programming (good computer programmers can write their own ticket); engineering (engineers and technicians will be needed to create the robots now used for Artificial Intelligence); telecommunications; genetic engineering; medical research; and laser technology.

Develop as many skills as possible so that you can market yourself, and be prepared to work full time, part time, or as an independent contractor. Hone your skills and learn new ones so you can offer your services whenever and wherever they are needed. If you're an in-house researcher and you see that your organization is moving toward farming out this function to an outside consultant, develop your writing skills so you can offer your services on publications instead.

Got a Minute? Get a Skill!

Here is a list of the hottest skills employers want today. You'll notice that these skills are the same, whether you are a manager of a Dairy Queen or an accountant for a CPA firm.

➤ Budget management skills

➤ Meeting deadlines

➤ Supervisory skills

➤ Writing skills

➤ Speaking skills

➤ Dependability

➤ Interviewing skills

➤ Communication/public relations skills

➤ Organizing and coordinating skills

➤ Teaching skills

Again, these are basic skills that can be used in any job, so if you don't have them, consider developing some of the skills by taking classes, attending workshops, or reading self-help books.

Take an Inventory of Your Job Skills

Remember that a wide range of skills can be developed. Nobody is born with the innate ability to prepare a budget (although sometimes it seems like some of us were born to spend!). People who work for larger organizations are usually offered the opportunity to take training courses on leadership development, public speaking, and other topics. If it's offered, take the course. Education and relevant skills provide enormous power in today's work world.

But most organizations just leave self-enrichment up to you.

If you want to prepare yourself so the ax doesn't fall on your neck, *read the need!* Anticipate your company's and your profession's changing needs. Look behind the scenes, translate what's beneath the spoken words, keep a lookout for the winds of change. Be proactive about getting training. Network at least once a week for breakfast, lunch, or coffee with those in other departments or companies, so you can scout ahead and figure out where the trail is leading in your area of work before too many others do.

One client who was an administrative assistant, for instance, asked to be trained on the new desktop publishing system so she could help prepare in-house publications. Her manager was thrilled that she took such initiative, and when it came time for layoffs, she was spared because she was the only one who knew how to put out the company newsletter.

To keep current, ask yourself the following questions:

➤ What marketable skills or abilities do I already have?

➤ What skills do I need to develop?

➤ Where can I go or who can I talk with to learn or practice these skills?

➤ Where can I find out what skills employers value?

Developing new skills and honing current ones will help you feel more confident and less vulnerable to getting the blues. But what if you've taken a proposal-writing course, a public-speaking seminar, and a newsletter workshop but still haven't been promoted—or even given a fancier title without a wage increase—because no one is going anywhere in the company?

If You Can't Move Up, Move Over

Many people get the blues because they don't feel challenged by their work and there is no opportunity for them to move up. If you are in this position, it may make you feel better to know that promotions just aren't automatic anymore. The job ladder has collapsed and flattened because of technology and less room at the top. An entire generation of lower- to middle-managers who expected to move up have nowhere to go.

But you don't have to resign yourself to having a dull, unchallenging job. If you can't move up, then move over! Consider a lateral move—that is, move to another position within your department at the same level, transfer to another department, or do the same job at another company. Even if you don't make any more money, you will be helping yourself move toward future promotions because you will gain more skills, contacts, and networking outlets—and you will renew your energy and self-esteem.

If you can't move over, then move out, which has been the most rewarding choice for many of my corporate burned-out clients.

Get Me Outta Here!

I can't tell you how many people come to my practice feeling disappointed with the careers they've chosen. Lawyers tell me how they started out with dreams of making this world more equitable, but all they are doing is making more paperwork. Creative people who've chosen "practical" careers feel they don't fit in with their more conservative coworkers. And many, many clients feel stuck in careers they never actually chose, but rather fell into because that's what their parents expected of them.

But what's wonderful about today's workplace is that you don't have to stick to one job or one profession—nothing is set in stone. Many people switch careers midstream when they realize that they are in the wrong profession, surrounded by people they don't like or can't relate to. It's like being miscast for a slow Victorian romantic movie when you see yourself as the next *Terminator III* hero in a blow-em-up action movie. If you're in this spot, no matter what you do, your job won't fit, and you need to leave.

Many people find that it's far more rewarding to leave corporate America and strike out on their own. They don't strike it rich, but the increased control they feel over their time and work more than compensates for a bigger paycheck. This has been particularly true for women-owned businesses, which compose one of the fastest growing segments of the U.S. economy. In fact, women-owned businesses have recently surpassed the Fortune 500 in how many workers they employ. If we measured their degree of job satisfaction in these businesses, my clients report it's far higher than in the traditional work settings.

What Do You Want to Do?

If that question stumped you, don't worry. Many people—young, middle-aged, and older—don't have a clue about what kind of work they'd enjoy doing, because none of us have been trained to think in that way. Psychologist and researcher, Dr. John Holland, who spends his life helping millions of people choose careers, came up with a map that shows there are six basic personality types in the world of work and six basic work environments.

Dr. Holland found that people are happiest when they work in a setting that most closely fits their personality, with people like themselves who share their interests, values, and abilities.

The following exercise will help you figure out what kind of work you'd like to do. Place an X beside the occupations that best suit your personality; then add up the total at the end. Afterward, read the descriptions of the personality types, focusing on the ones that you had the most checkmarks under in the occupational exercise. This chart appeared in *The Career Guide for Creative and Unconventional People* (by Carol Eikleberry).

What Job Suits You Best?

Artistic

____ Actor

____ Architect

____ Author

____ Dancer

____ Editor

____ Graphic designer

____ Interior designer

____ Photographer

____ Singer

____ Sculptor

____ *Total for Artistic*

Social

____ Clergy member

____ Companion

____ Counselor

____ Nurse

____ Occupational therapist

____ Playground director

____ School principal

____ Social worker

____ Teacher

____ YWCA/YMCA director

____ *Total for Social*

Enterprising

____ Executive

____ Funeral director

____ Lawyer

____ Manager

____ Politician

____ Realtor

____ Retailer

____ Salesperson

____ Stockbroker

____ TV producer

____ *Total for Enterprising*

Investigative

____ Actuary

____ Computer programmer

____ Dentist

____ Mathematician

____ Optometrist

____ Pharmacist

____ Physician

____ Research scientist

____ Surveyor

____ Veterinarian

____ *Total for Investigative*

Realistic

____ Farmer

____ Forester

____ Machinist

____ Mechanic

____ Pilot

____ Plumber

____ Police officer

____ Rancher

____ Repairperson

____ Soldier

____ *Total for Realistic*

Conventional

____ Accountant

____ Banker

____ Cashier

____ Clerk

____ Computer operator

____ Medical records technician

____ Receptionist

____ Secretary

____ Tax preparer

____ Telephone operator

____ *Total for Conventional*

The six personality types are:

➤ *Artistic.* Artistic types like to work in unstructured environments, using their imaginations and creativity. They look for work in libraries, theaters, and museums and want to work with art, drama, painting, or writing.

➤ *Social.* These are the "people who need people." Social types enjoy informing, helping, training, and doing anything that involves working in groups and sharing responsibilities. They like to talk about their feelings and solve problems through interactions with others. You find them in teaching, counseling, or recreation.

➤ *Enterprising.* People who like to be leaders and manage groups of people to reach organizational or economic goals fall in this category. They like convincing others that they're right and like to do social tasks so long as they are the leaders. You find them in business management, sales, or politics.

➤ *Investigative.* If you enjoy scientific and intellectual pursuits, you may fall in this category. Investigative types like gathering information, uncovering new theories, and analyzing data. They often look for work in academia, biology, medicine, or computer-related industries.

➤ *Realistic.* People who fall under this category like to do things that are practical—working outdoors, mastering tools and machines, and using their physical abilities. They tend to venture into the construction industry, the military, or to work outdoors in nature.

➤ *Conventional.* If you like activities that demand attention to accuracy and involve working in an office with an established chain of command, you are probably a conventional type. If so, you'd be better off looking for work in financial institutions, accounting firms, or other large businesses.

Are You in the Right Job?

You may, for instance, fall under artistic and social, and be suited to work as a graphic artist for an advocacy organization. That would be an outlet to be creative and work closely with people.

But are you in the job that fits your type? Where do you fit in? Did you have the most checks under "artistic" even though you drill teeth for a living? Are you stuck selling houses in a "conventional" setting when you'd rather be dissecting worms in a lab—an "investigative" occupation?

If so, guess what, you're in the wrong place at the wrong time, and this situation is a breeding ground for the Monday-Morning Blues!

Looking for That Hand-in-Glove Fit

Choosing work that fits your personality is crucial to your mental health. When you choose to do work that is meaningful to you and with people who have similar interests, you are more likely to feel happy and successful at your job and less likely to hop around from one career to another. But you also need to develop skills that make you more desirable to an employer in the area compatible with your work personality.

Do you know what are the top 10 skills valued for CEOs and potential leaders in their companies? In the book *How To Think Like A CEO* by D. A. Benton (Warner, 1996), the top 10 skills in order of importance are:

1. Secure in self
2. In control of attitude
3. Tenacious
4. Continuously improving
5. Honest and ethical
6. Thinking before talking
7. Original
8. Publicly modest
9. Aware of style
10. Gutsy/a little wild

How many of these qualities do you have? Make a list of the top 10 skills and rate yourself on a 1 to 10 scale to see how strong that skill is in you (with "1" representing "very weak" and "10" representing "very strong"). Have a coworker you can trust also rate you on these qualities. This feedback will help guide you on which areas you need to learn and practice and which are the strengths you can emphasize and use more at work.

Doing What You Want Even When Money Doesn't Follow

Taking a job doing the work you like at the organization of your choice is the preferable first option for most everyone. But if that's not possible, consider the following alternatives:

➤ Take a job you aren't crazy about so you can pay the bills, while doing what you love as a hobby. A writer, for instance, may be an editor at a microbiology association by day and write fiction by night. Sometimes hobbies metamorphose into careers. The key is to do something you love, regardless of whether a paycheck is attached—the money may come later when you least expect it.

➤ Take a temporary job to support yourself while you establish the business you've always dreamed of owning. Temporary

Blues Flag

We may choose to take jobs that we are overqualified for just because we like the people who work there and the politics of the organization. But *beware*: While you may enjoy palling around with your colleagues, you'll probably be down in the dumps over not feeling challenged. When you don't use your skills, you don't enjoy your job as much, so your self-esteem drops and you are more vulnerable to getting the Monday-Morning Blues. To find a job you love, follow your passion—then you'll always beat the blues because you'll feel challenged and fully alive!

Dr. Ellen Says

If you still can't figure out what profession would make you happy, try hiring a professional coach or career counselor. Just like a physical trainer helps you train your body, a coach can help you train your mind for success, guiding you toward possibilities that are right for you based on your skills, talents, preferences, and potential. These experienced career trainers can suggest ways to improve your personal style and help you identify and remove your obstacles to success. Give it a try!

agencies can give you daily assignments so you don't have to dig up customers yourself, or you could work as a part-time clerk, waitress, bartender, telephone operator, or in the fast food industry. One of my cousins, Kathy, has the talent and drive to be an opera singer. To support herself while she is in training, she is a bartender at a hot downtown restaurant. Madame Butterfly by day; martinis by night.

➤ Do freelance work in your field. Be prepared for a less stable income and more working hours, but what you get in exchange is more freedom and the ability to set your own schedule and choose your own projects.

Wouldn't it be wonderful to be in a good mood on Sunday night, knowing that the next day you're going to be doing something you love? But if you're the type who dreads going into the office and drags yourself out of bed on Monday morning, recognize that your bad job is bad for your health and believe you can and will change it. Start with trashing those Monday-Morning Blues by committing to one action strategy a week until you find the work you love!

The Least You Need to Know

➤ Many of us feel confused, overwhelmed, and frightened by the changes in today's workplace, and that's why we get the Monday-Morning Blues.

➤ Work is important because it increases our self-esteem and makes us feel connected to others. Research shows that career and work satisfaction are the strongest contributors to mental health.

➤ Flexibility, not stability, is the name of the game in today's corporate world.

➤ Statistics show that you'll probably change professions at least three times and jobs as often as 10 times.

➤ The best way to stay afloat in the workplace is to hone your skills and constantly develop new ones so you can be viewed as a resource to your company in many areas.

➤ Before you switch jobs, find out which type of work your personality is best suited for.

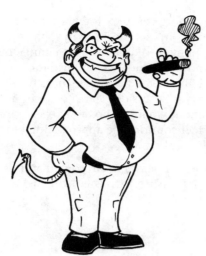

Chapter 19

The Bad-Boss Blues

In This Chapter

➤ Bad bosses can really make you sick

➤ Quiz: Do you have the Bad–Boss Blues?

➤ "Boss" is out, "facilitator" is in

➤ Bad bosses are not born, they're made

➤ Take your share of the blame: the 50-50 deal on responsibility

➤ Recording your bad-boss problems in a journal can help you solve them

➤ Got a problem? Get a coach!

Can you guess the number one problem presented to business coaches these days? It's no longer how to break through the glass ceiling or generate more money to better support a family. The number one work problem we now see concerns bad bosses and unsatisfying jobs. We discussed how to cope with the Monday-Morning Blues in the previous chapter. But is it possible to fix a bad-boss situation?

The chances have never been better! At every level, people are worried about their jobs because jobs are more uncertain now than at any time in history. And for the first time bosses are as worried as the workers. They're also coming in for coaching on how to become better bosses because they know that a bad boss is bad business, and these days neither the boss nor the business will survive the crushing competition of today's workplace. This kind of anxiety has produced an unprecedented window of opportunity for growth, learning, and improvement for both bosses and employees.

The relationship between employer and employee is more complex today than ever before because the roles aren't cast in stone any longer. In fact, nothing in today's business world is cast in stone because everything changes so quickly. This change in the workplace gives subordinates more flexibility and independence but also more responsibility to take care of themselves because Big Brother is no longer there to protect them. But this partnership can work well only if both sides learn to communicate effectively. As employees, we need to be clear about what our bosses expect from us and what we can give to them. We also need to feel comfortable approaching our bosses as problems arise and be proactive about solving them.

In this chapter, we'll examine what the changing roles of bosses mean to you and explore tips on what you can do to improve your relationship with the people who can make or break your job!

Coping with a Bad Boss

We hear about bad bosses all the time. Friends and family members who can't believe their supervisors are so nasty, self-righteous, controlling, or just jerks. The bosses who pound their fists on their subordinates' desks demanding that a proposal be done NOW, the ones who call attention to your inadequacies in public, or those who call you names or make sexist jokes. Then there's the *Jurassic Park* micromanagers who can't get into the swing of team leadership spirit, and the young Gen-Xers who think you're an old fart because you aren't eager to learn PageMaker. There's the slave driver who expects you to work until midnight and won't even pay for the Chinese takeout, and the bosses who scare you half to death with their glare and icy hearts.

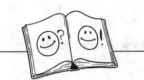

Terms of Encheerment

The *Bad-Boss Blues* are the frustrating, disturbing, and vulnerable feelings we get when our bosses treat us badly and disrespectfully and we feel too powerless to do anything about it. Supervisors from the old school of management may use a command and control style of leadership, which results in their employees feeling unimportant, depressed, and therefore less productive.

Most people have horror stories to share about their bosses and most of us have fantasized (at least once) about ways we could inflict excruciating pain on them, or at the very least, just tell them off. Why do we have such strong feelings about our bosses? Because we often confuse them with our parents and see our controlling mom or withholding dad when we look at them, and because they have so much control over our jobs, our livelihoods, and often our emotions. We often give them more power than they really have, but they certainly have the power to decide one critical issue that determines the direction of our future: whether we'll be axed or spared!

Many of these horror stories involve bosses who wield power the old-fashioned way, by telling their workers what to do, how to do it, and when to do it. Some of our bosses may be inconsiderate, aloof, careless, or even incompetent, but few are downright abusive. Still, dealing with difficult bosses can make your life pure hell and give you a case of the *Bad-Boss Blues*.

The best way to beat these blues is to become an empowered employee—find and follow your own passions during or after work, develop and stay up to date with marketable skills, volunteer for an indispensable job at work, or become an active part of the management teams that make policy decisions and solve the organization's problems. If the Bad-Boss Blues cannot be resolved, the key is to always be able to walk away because you maintained the emotional independence and the skill base to move onto another job.

Your Boss Can Make You Sick

When you say "My boss makes me sick," you probably don't realize just how right you are! Studies show that having a bad relationship with your boss is detrimental to your health. When we feel used or abused by our supervisors, our self-esteem drops, we get depressed and anxious, and often convert our distress into physical symptoms such as stomachaches, headaches, and sexual dysfunction.

If your stomach gets tied up in knots when you think about your boss, and you dread going into work because your boss makes you feel like scum, you've probably got the Bad-Boss Blues. But don't feel bad—almost everybody who drags themselves out of bed in the morning and schleps their briefcases or backpacks to work can relate to you. In fact, a survey conducted by *American Demographics Magazine* showed that having bad bosses is the second most common complaint in the workplace. The first complaint is being stuck at a boring job.

But you and your boss can get along much better. Recognizing your bad feelings can be empowering because it gives you a chance to examine the dynamics of your relationship with your boss and find ways to improve it. Most times you'll see that just making time to talk to your boss at crucial junctures of a project's development will improve your relationship. Or asking the boss right away to clarify what she meant by something she said may avoid a misunderstanding that can unnecessarily grow into a big deal and waste everyone's energy.

The important thing, though, is to be proactive and not let your anger build up. If you're mad at your supervisor because he is breathing down your neck as you try to crank out letters at the computer, don't just sit there and sigh, hoping he'll get the message. Tell him, diplomatically, that you'll bring the letters to him when you're finished: "I appreciate your making yourself accessible in case I need you. But to be productive right now I need to have a little space to concentrate."

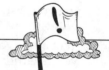

Blues Flag

If you've got the kind of boss who treats you disrespectfully, who never asks for your opinion, or who humiliates you in front of your coworkers—and you've tried to tell him that this behavior is upsetting, but to no avail—it may be time to either report the supervisor to a higher-up or look for a new job. Remember, working with an abusive boss is bad for your health and may make you sick. There are plenty of better bosses out there!

Most bosses are reasonable—they'll realize that you want them out of sight, apologize, and walk away. With this example, you can learn a very important lesson about the Bad-Boss Blues. It's usually not the boss who's the biggest problem. The problem is more often in ourselves: our fear of authority, our lack of communication skills, our discomfort with conflict, our need to please, our taking everything personally, our immaturity, our disorganization. The bad news is that these problems fuel the Bad-Boss Blues because they cause so much frustration and disappointment; but the good news is that they can be more easily changed because they reside in you and you can control them.

Is Your Boss That Bad?

We all complain about our bosses to some degree—it's the social thing to do, like rolling your eyes when you're talking about your in-laws. But just how bad is your boss? Take the following test and see for yourself.

Do You Have the Bad-Boss Blues?

Answer the following questions (T) for true and (F) for false.

1. Most of the time you go into work feeling like your head is going to explode or feeling anxious and uneasy. ___

2. When you talk about your boss at home, you sometimes find yourself clenching your fist, your stomach tightens up, and you fantasize about how you're going to "really give it to him" next time he yells at you. ___

3. Whenever you make a work-related suggestion, your boss looks at you like you're either speaking in tongues or like you're an idiot. ___

4. When a coworker asks what you would like for Christmas, you tell him a dartboard with a picture of your boss's face on it that you can use for target practice. ___

5. Your favorite activity at work is getting away from your supervisor or surfing the Internet to plan your next vacation. ___

6. You think your boss is monitoring your calls and e-mail but you can't prove it. ___

7. You become a clock watcher and can't wait to get out of the office. ___

8. You snap at your spouse, your kid, and your cat on Sunday night because you are bummed about going to work the next day. ___

9. Your boss acts in public like team management is the greatest thing next to sliced bread, but in private she still expects you to say, "Yes ma'am" and shut up. ___

10. You feel helpless about making any real changes in your boss or the organization. ___

If you marked five or more of these questions "True," you've probably got a case of the Bad-Boss Blues. You need to either improve your relationship with your boss by communicating your needs and expectations, or set a time line to get out before your motivation is squelched and your self-esteem is squashed.

This is a good time to use the Blues Scale we showed you in Chapter 1. Every day before and after work, monitor your progress or lack of progress by finding your rating on that 1 to 10 scale. If your self-esteem and identity are on the line and they are being damaged by a bad boss who can't or won't change, then you have no choice but to move on and leave the abuser. Your self-worth is more important than any particular job. Sometimes the best action strategy is just to leave, but only after you've exhausted every other alternative to make it work. If you just quit because it's unpleasant, your self-esteem will be damaged because you'll see yourself as a quitter and you'll miss the opportunity to learn precious skills about coping and conflict resolution that will help you secure a better job next time around.

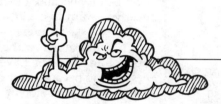

Funk-y Facts

How mean can your bosses get? Pretty mean, according to the authors of *Driving Fear Out Of The Workplace* (Jossey-Bass Publishers, 1991). This book lists the many ways in which bosses can threaten you—ranging from the more subtle forms of control to physical abuse. *Silence*, for instance, is one weapon. If you've ever found yourself fumbling for something to say while your boss sits quietly, staring at you with cool eyes, the boss is probably trying to intimidate you and make you feel like your judgment and worth is in question. When your boss uses *brevity*, short sharp answers to your questions, he is cutting you off. Other forms of abuse include ignoring employees, putting them down, blaming them for things going wrong, discrediting them, yelling and shouting, and finally, physical threats. You don't have to put up with this kind of abuse from anyone. The first step in stopping it is to identify what's going on. Then make a commitment that you're no longer willing to be a battered employee and try the action strategies in this chapter for coping with the Bad-Boss Blues.

Nobody Knows the Trouble They've Seen

Nobody is born being a bad boss, although it does seem like some come by it more naturally than others. And when you think about it, supervisors aren't really "bad," they may just be ineffective because they don't know how to motivate people to work, how to reach out to others when they need help, or how to talk to their subordinates.

245

Many of today's managers were raised in the old corporate model of top-down management, where they bark orders at their underlings and their underlings go fetch. They just don't know how to do it any other way. And it's in your best interest to understand this and stop judging them. Instead, empathize and put yourself in their place. You don't have to agree for one second with what they do, but it gives you power to know *why* they do it. This knowledge helps you understand how to better speak their language, know when and how to approach them with issues, and how much potential they have to change or whether it's hopeless and you're the one who needs to do the changing by leaving.

First of all, understand that your boss faces more daily pressure than anything in the history of modern business. Bosses are under the gun to produce more than ever before, because downsizing, rightsizing, or whatever you want to call it has left many companies with virtually a skeleton crew—and the same amount of work, if not more. At the same time, supervisors are being told that they have to stop bossing their employees around because that doesn't motivate them, and must, instead, sit side by side with them as equal partners in the decision-making process.

To help you understand the difference between the old guard and the new guard, take a look at the following distinctions. You'll notice that titles such as "boss," "supervisor," "manager," and the like are out of fashion, and "facilitator," "coordinator," and "sponsor" are now the "in" terms. These different titles reflect different attitudes in management—from command management to team management.

Dr. Ellen Says

If you're the boss and want to begin building more positive relationships with your subordinates, ask them how supervisors should act to get their employee's cooperation, interest, and enthusiasm. Your job: Listen to employees and let go of preconceived notions of how to do things; share the power to make things happen and everyone wins; give them the benefit of the doubt, pat them on the back for small accomplishments; and coach people to success by helping them remove the obstacles to their best performance.

Bosses issue commands and expect obedience. They view themselves as decision-makers in an organizational structure that is run by the chain of command with little, if any, flexibility. Their management style: Subordinates must follow the rules. Bosses are often leftovers from World War II, the Korean War, or the Vietnam War, where military orders were their only alternative to survive.

Facilitators help self-managed teams make decisions, expecting that subordinates who participate in this process will feel more motivated, empowered, and committed to the organization. They see organizational structure as flexible so that it can address the changing needs of their workers. The problem here is that facilitators often don't provide enough structure and direction, and everyone feels they're floating in a sea of stress without a compass or map.

Bosses ensure that their employees will meet their performance standards by telling them what to do, how to do it, and when it needs to be done. They also prefer payment to be based on seniority and rank. This style can lead to promoting incompetence and overlooking talent that doesn't conform to the party line.

Facilitators create an environment for quality performance by working with subordinates to clarify job expectations, build a cooperative team, solicit input on ways to improve quality, give feedback, and establish work standards. Facilitators would rather have a flattened hierarchy, in which people are paid and acknowledged for their skills. The problem here can be that there are too many frustrated, underachieving people in the middle and nowhere to go since up is no longer an option.

Bosses tend to micromanage, control, and tell subordinates what to do, with little or no regard for how they sound or the effect they're having on others.

Facilitators are expected to be visionaries, able to articulate goals that the organization should move toward and guide subordinates in that direction by supporting, teaching, coaching, and developing teamwork. They are often expected to communicate at a higher level but not trained as to how to do it, so there's often a significant gap between what's expected and needed and what actually happens.

Negotiate a 50–50 Power Deal

So how do we improve our relationships with our bosses?

For starters, we can stop blaming our bosses for everything that goes wrong and admit when we're wrong. It's the first step toward regaining our power. When we stick to our guns and feel convinced that we are right and our bosses are wrong, we never actually hear what our supervisors have to say—and we miss the opportunity to learn and to solve the problem. These are critical skills and if you don't learn them at your present job, you'll just repeat the problems at the next job where even more will be expected of you because you're more experienced.

Yet employers and employees are locked in fruitless power struggles all the time. Why don't we just accept that half of what happens in an argument is our responsibility? For one thing, it's embarrassing to admit that we're wrong. Also, acknowledging that we're wrong may mean we need to learn new skills so we can do a better job, and there are a hundred reasons we don't like that solution. Our favorite solution to the Bad-Boss Blues is to get the boss to change, much like a marriage where we expect our spouses to change and forget that the best way to make that happen is to change ourselves first.

Once you own up to your 50 percent of the problem, however, you can do something about it and you'll ultimately feel more empowered. Try this action strategy: Whenever you find yourself locked in battle with your boss, stop and think: "What have I done to contribute to this?" "What am I getting out of continuing this?" Answer the questions as fairly and completely as you can without judging yourself or being negative to yourself. Judgments get in the way of solving problems, so check them at the office door when you arrive at work each day and work on being a problem solver, not a victim.

Keep a Journal

If you don't get along with your boss but you aren't sure why, keep a week-long journal and note all the negative incidents that take place between you and your boss. In your journal entry, be sure to include what lead to the incident or misunderstanding and what happened right afterward.

Over the weekend, go over your journal and figure out what types of arguments you and your boss had: Are there any particular issues that triggered the arguments? Do they happen at the same time during the week? Then talk to coworkers about these incidents and get their take on it—how did they think you reacted?

After getting their feedback, ask them what they would have done if they were in your shoes to get a sense for different ways of handling similar incidents in the future. One client, for instance, did this exercise and found that she often got mad at her boss when he asked her to take over the telephone switchboard at the front desk while the secretary went to lunch.

Instead of making a snide remark about the situation by saying to him: "You didn't need to hire someone with a master's degree in media relations to answer phones!" she said in a calm tone of voice, "I don't mind answering phones once in a while, but I can contribute more to the firm by assessing our communication needs and working out a new communication plan. Maybe we could get an intern to come in and answer the phones at noon. Would you like me to look into it?"

Three rules of thumb:

➤ Try to frame your comments in terms of what would work best for the firm, not what works best for you. This is not the time to say "I need…" but instead phrase it "The company needs…" or "This position would work better if…"

➤ Don't complain about something to your boss until you can suggest a reasonable solution.

➤ Never whine or act like a victim. Even if you're right, your style is so wrong that you'll lose power no matter what you try to do.

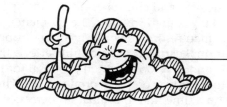

Funk-y Facts

How do you talk to your boss so he hears you? According to Roger Fisher and William Ury, authors of *Getting to YES* (Penguin Books, 1991), "Without communication there is no negotiation." The three big problems with communications, the authors say, is that negotiators may not be talking to each other clearly, may not be hearing each other, or may be misinterpreting what the other says. The solution: Listen actively and acknowledge what is being said, speak to be understood, speak about your own motivations and intentions and not theirs (for example, say "I feel let down, instead of "You broke your word"), and speak specifically about the problem and suggest how to solve it, while being open to hearing and entertaining the differences in your proposed solutions.

Coaching Away the Bad-Boss Blues

One of the most exciting new trends in today's workplace is the growth in coaching services for employees. Businesses and employees increasingly turn to coaching as a way to help employees remove their obstacles to success.

According to one of the most respected senior coaches in the field, Robert Hargrove, author of *Masterful Coaching* (Jossey-Bass, 1995), the coach is a "vision builder and value shaper"—that is, someone who helps you clarify your vision and sort out your values so you are more likely to achieve your goals. The coach then guides you through what Hargrove calls "personal transformation and reinvention," helping you get to the next level of your career. To take this step, you may have to go back to school to develop skills in certain areas or learn certain new skills on the job, such as becoming a more effective team player.

Example: A bright, energetic college graduate who is an Internet lover starts to work in his uncle's company, an old-fashioned manufacturing business. He has all kinds of ideas about how to improve the plant, boost workers' morale, and enhance productivity to bring the company into the 21st century—but nobody wants to listen to him. They hate computers, and they see him as a punk with a stupid earring in his ear. He goes to a coach to figure out what he should do, and together they go over the options: He could try to look for a new job, talk to his uncle about changing his position within the company, or put out a proposal to his uncle detailing how the changes he suggests will affect the company's bottom line.

After talking over the pros and cons of each option, he may decide he wants to talk to his uncle about working something out. The problem is, every time he is alone with his uncle the young man resorts to whining and pouting, and his uncle doesn't take him seriously. Solution: Learn better communications skills so he can initiate discussions with his uncle and develop a written proposal for his uncle with five bullet points about how to improve company productivity. The young manager and the coach then decide on a time line to evaluate progress. They meet again at a later date to determine the next steps necessary toward achieving success.

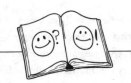

Terms of Encheerment

Executive coaching is a professional service offered to women and men in business who need to overcome personal and professional obstacles in order to reach their career goals. In sessions with the coach, the businessperson's goals are mutually established and converted into a detailed action plan. Follow-up and further skill training occurs subsequently to ensure success. Coaching is a newly emerging profession which blends psychology and business consultation by helping individuals learn to balance both work and personal needs in order to make their lives more productive and profitable.

The need has grown so much that recently I developed a new business to organize an employee and *executive coaching* service from the growing number of requests I've been receiving. The new coaching firm is called "Bridge Ventures: Executive Coaching Systems," and the logo is a graphic of the Brooklyn Bridge. The Brooklyn Bridge is a powerful symbol to me of the link between my home in Brooklyn Heights and my work in Manhattan and the constant need for me and my clients to keep the two, work and home, in balance. The Bridge also symbolizes integrating beauty and power in our work lives, and since I often run or walk across the Bridge for exercise, it has also come to mean a bridge to both inner and outer strength.

A bridge has become a helpful way to think about the purpose of coaching and what we need to do to succeed in today's workplace. In our coaching program, we have developed systems to do three things: evaluation, feedback, and coaching skills. Sometimes we go on site and work with businesses to evaluate the executives and employees on their job performances and obstacles to success. Then we help the business develop a coaching plan by building whatever skills they need. Mostly, we work with individuals who typically come for two to six coaching sessions. Sometimes the sessions are held over the phone or through video conferencing if the person lives far away or in another country.

After years of trial and error, here are the coaching steps that my company takes to help executives define their goals and work toward reaching them.

1. *Identify the problem* the client is having at work and look at the obstacles to his or her success.

2. *Briefly evaluate* the emotional impact of these problems and offer a lot of support and reassurance.

3. *Move into action.* Agree upon two action strategies to deal with solving the problem. Make a commitment as to when these strategies will be accomplished and do coaching to build skills to accomplish the action strategies. Write out the strategies and the time line for accomplishment and have a copy available for the client and the coach.

4. *Follow up.* Talk again at the designated time to evaluate how it's going and fix what's not working. Build more skills to get to the next level of goals.

These steps have been particularly helpful to encourage bad bosses to learn new communication skills. We teach them very specific skills to respond to the poor feedback they received from employees. To gather this kind of feedback, we use a tool called "360-degree Feedback," an evaluation method that allows employees to be critiqued by various people who work with them at their level, above them, and below them. As a subordinate, you can rate your boss through this form anonymously. The great thing about a 360 is that the boss finally gets feedback, too—he is not immune, not anymore—and the playing field between boss and employee is suddenly more level. For more information about Bridge Ventures: Executive Coaching Systems, see the end of the book.

Co-Coaching

If you can't find or afford a professional coach to deal with the Bad-Boss Blues or how to change a boring job, you can follow the *co-coaching* model, which is really a more formal structure for friends or acquaintances helping each other out by trading knowledge in their areas of expertise. Find people who have good relationships with their bosses and ask them how they developed them—what worked and what didn't. Then ask them to be your coach as you try different communication approaches with your boss. In return, figure out what topic would be of value for the other person to receive coaching and take turns coaching each other using essentially the same steps. Remember, this is coaching, not therapy, so the emphasis is on changing behavior, not on process and history.

Terms of Encheerment

Co-coaching is an informal bartering of information among two people who each have expertise in different areas and can exchange knowledge to further each person's goals. You can form a co-coaching partnership with a friend, acquaintance, or relative—the only criteria is that the other person have expertise in an area that you need help with in order to get ahead.

Co-coaching can be done over the phone, and the partners can set up any type of arrangement that best suits them, such as setting aside an hour a week during which each partner gets to talk for 30 minutes or taking turns each week. Make sure you schedule the appointments in the way you would any other appointment, and don't change it unless you absolutely have to.

My co-coach is a partner in a financial consulting firm who is helping me organize and grow my finances. She is the only woman partner in a male firm so I help her find ways to be more effective in that setting. She doesn't want to be a bad boss or work for one. So we talk every Tuesday morning at the same time. We've been doing this for over a year now and it's worked far better than either of us had expected. Plus it has really been fun to have the built-in time each week to have coaching on whatever is bothering me about work or finances.

There will always be some glitches in the dynamics between supervisor and subordinate—that's just the nature of power relationships with anyone. But employees have more power today than ever before to choose what they want to do professionally and how they want to do it. To benefit from this freedom, employees need to form partnerships with their bosses and communicate openly, honestly, and frequently. Both boss and employee need to learn new communication skills to meet the challenges of work today; but there's never been a better time to learn them because the rewards are tremendous when you do.

The Least You Need to Know

➤ Studies show that having a bad relationship with your boss can make you physically sick.

➤ The Bad-Boss Blues are the frustrating, disturbing, and vulnerable feelings we get when our bosses treat us badly and/or disrespectfully and we feel powerless to do anything about it.

➤ Most supervisors aren't really "bad." They are not effective simply because they don't know how to motivate people to work or how to talk to their subordinates.

➤ To improve our relationships with our supervisors, we need to accept 50 percent of the responsibility for the existing problem.

➤ Keep a journal to record when you have the most problems with your boss and over what issues—then talk to friends or a coach about better ways of handling the situation.

➤ Get a professional coach to teach you how to communicate better with your boss, or develop a co-coaching arrangement with a friend or coworker.

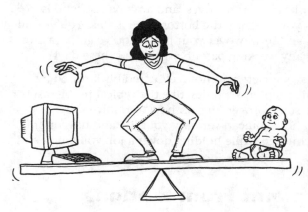

Chapter 20

The Working-Parents Blues: Life on the Balance Beam

In This Chapter

➤ Working parents: the gymnasts of the new culture

➤ Is your company family-friendly?

➤ Give me flexibility or give me death

➤ Getting your house in order

➤ Delegate: the Exchange/Loss/Gain formula

➤ Do you know how your kid is doing?

Your boss yelled at you because the proposal is full of typos, your child is mad at you for missing the "make your own taco" party after the game, your spouse wants to know if you ever plan to have sex with him again, you can't remember where you put this month's bills, and your babysitter is shaking her head as you boil water to make macaroni and cheese for the third time this week!

There's so much to do at work, you're coming home later and later at night, your wife seems to be doing better at her career than you are, you're worried about your son and his "F" in math, your teenage daughter now thinks it's cool to smoke so she can stay thin, college bills loom as your bank account shrinks, and lately you've noticed that your pot belly has expanded so much that you can't touch (or even see) your toes anymore.

You feel like a terrible mother or father, a careless professional, an irresponsible spouse—and all you want is literally a room of your own, preferably with a large-screen

TV and a fridge full of beer or chocolate ice cream. The further away, the better, from your husband or wife, your kids, your boss, your relatives, and anyone else who is going to place any more demands on you. Because the bottom line is this: You've had it! You're overworked, overwhelmed, and in way over your head. You've got a case of the Working-Parents Blues. Are there any working parents who don't these days?

You can't be a working parent in today's society and not feel incredibly stressed by all the demands placed on you. In this chapter, we'll describe the typical problems working parents face today and share some proven tips on how to resolve the Working-Parents Blues. We'll tell you how you can simplify your life and have more meaningful relationships with your children while holding down a job you enjoy and *not go bonkers*.

The Number-One Complaint From Working Parents

As working parents, many of us feel out of control and out of balance. We are swamped with work but afraid to cut back or complain for fear of losing our jobs. We don't have much time to spend with our children and when we do, we're often so grouchy, grumpy, and tired that we can't give them the support, love, or patience they need to grow into happy, healthy adults.

Our houses are a health hazard because we don't have time to really clean them, our hair is a disgrace because we can't get to the beauty parlor or barber, and our spouses are in distress because they feel neglected by us and overwhelmed by their own work demands. Let's face it, folks: As working parents, we've fallen off the balance beam so many times that we've become the laughing stock at the gym of life. But just because we often fall, that's no reason to stop trying!

With the *Working-Parents Blues*, we often feel that shaky, precarious feeling that we've got too many balls up in the air and they're all about to crash down over our heads! It makes sense these blues would be among the most common, since we live in a society that expects us to be ambitious, successful professionals and dedicated, hands-on parents, yet provides little support to meet any of these expectations.

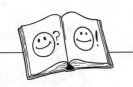

Terms of Encheerment

Working-Parents Blues are the frustrated, angry, guilty, upset feelings we get when we try to do what's best for our children and our jobs. But long hours at work, chores, and responsibilities get in the way of our spending quality time with the kids. These days men get Working-Parent Blues about as often as women because more and more men deeply yearn for the opportunity to really be there for their children.

Family-Friendly Workplaces: Sing It Again, Sam

Despite all the companiessinging the tune of family-friendly workplaces, many companies still look down on employees who actually try the policy and have the nerve to take time off to be with their kids. Although moms who leave work early to do car pool may get dirty looks from their supervisors and childless coworkers, they're getting off easy compared to dads who get labeled slackers if they are the ones who take the kids to the doctor or who stay home to do the nursing when their kids get sick.

The workplace just hasn't caught up with the reality of working parents. A recent survey conducted by the Center for Work and Family, published in *Business Week*, showed that many corporate work-and-family programs are only half-heartedly applied, serving more as window dressing than offering employees relief from real work-family conflicts.

Yet, the reality is that moms and dads are on the job for the long haul. While some women work because they enjoy the intellectual challenge, most women log in the hours just to get a paycheck for the family. It's nearly impossible these days to get by on one salary. With millions of people laid off from work due to corporate downsizing —and the increasing uncertainty of the job market—it often makes sense for all members of the family to be able to earn an income and contribute what they can.

But you don't have to get stuck working for an inflexible, rigid, 9-to-5 kind of boss who sees your little darlings as interlopers ruining your work and undermining the company's profits. Increasingly, working parents are seeking employment in more flexible work environments where they can create their own schedules, work from home, or make other arrangements to accommodate their children's or aging parents' needs.

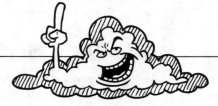

Funk-y Facts

Working parents are slowly changing the workplace by demanding that they have time to meet their family needs. It's not just the women who are forcing companies to rethink their family and work policies. The men are becoming just as vocal. According to Dr. James A. Levine, author of *Working Fathers* (Addison Wesley, 1997), fathers increasingly want the ability to both provide for and spend time with their children. Although work is definitely a powerful source of male identity, family is equally as strong. Dr. Levine quotes a 1991 Gallup poll which found that 59 percent of American men get more satisfaction from taking care of their families than from doing a good job at work. He also quotes a 1996 Consumer Survey Center poll of men in their 30s and 40s that shows that 84 percent of baby-boomer men say that "success" means being a good father.

Recognizing that working parents are here to stay and companies need them to compete effectively in a tight job market, many companies are giving employees more leeway in where and how they want to work. It makes better business sense to make workers happy because happy employees mean more productive employees. Consider the following statistics:

➤ At Bell Atlantic, productivity among telecommuters (employees who work at home or at satellite sites closer to home) rose to 27 percent.

➤ Happier employees are also more likely to show up at work. According to the American Management Association, companies with flexible scheduling options report absenteeism is cut by as much as 50 percent.

There is nothing more depressing than sitting at a meeting listening to a bunch of colleagues drone on about some boring project when you know your kid is up at bat and you're not there to cheer her on. Most of us are trained to just dismiss these gut-wrenching feelings and accept guilt as part of what we all must pay to be a professional in today's world; but it doesn't have to be that way.

You can beat the Working-Parents Blues by taking more control of your working environment and choosing a job that will give you the freedom to fulfill your professional duties and your parental responsibilities. In your personal life, you can learn to hire or trade for household help, delegate more effectively, prioritize what really needs to get done, and learn how to say "NO"—all skills that help beat the Working-Parents Blues.

Dr. Ellen Says

A dear friend of mine who was a very successful, but very tired, advertising executive wanted to spend more time with his newborn, a beautiful baby girl named Eve. So he quit advertising and started a new service business that gives him more flexibility with his time and the opportunity to apply all the advertising and marketing ideas he's learned but used to give away to others. He still wakes up early but instead of rushing into the morning commuter traffic, he turns on the computer and reads his e-mail to his baby while holding her in his lap.

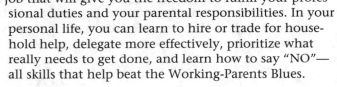

We Work Hard for Our Money

Back in the olden days, yougot dressed up to go to work and punched in from 9 to 5. Today, many employees can make up their own schedule and work at dawn, dusk, or the dark of night, whenever they want—so long as they get the work done on time and do it well.

This more relaxed management approach works well for working parents, who are better able to juggle their schedules so they can spend more time with their kids and get more done around the house. One client, for instance, convinced her boss to let her work from 7 a.m. to 3 p.m. So now, instead of racing out of work at 5 p.m. so she can get to aftercare by 5:30, then rushing home to whip up dinner in 15 minutes so the whole family can eat together, she can pick up the kids earlier and spend more time with them before making a healthy dinner together.

Flex time is one of many different job options employees can take advantage of or request. A few other common arrangements include:

➤ *Part time/job sharing.* Many people are working just three or four days a week or shorter days throughout the week. Others have found another working parent who wishes to job share, and they split a full time job in half so each person has half the responsibility but many of the same interesting challenges. These working parents may not be making as much money, but they are realizing savings by not sending the kids to an after-school program—and by preserving their sanity.

➤ *Compressed work weeks.* Another option is working 10 hours a day, Monday through Thursday, and getting Fridays off. Many people, working moms especially, use Fridays to go grocery shopping and do the laundry or other chores so the weekend is free for family time and fun.

➤ *Flex time.* Coming in earlier and leaving earlier is one of the most popular forms of alternative scheduling.

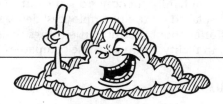

Funk-y Facts

Increasingly, couples are working at home together as home-based work becomes more popular. Susan Crites Price and Tom Price, authors of *The Working Parents Help Book* (Peterson's, 1996), offer the following pros and cons of working at home:

➤ **Pros:** You are there when your kids come home from school; you're there for homework questions; you don't have to commute or get dressed up; you can be more productive because there are fewer distractions; your kids can learn more about work by seeing you do it and older ones can get work experience by helping you out with stuffing envelopes and other gopher work.

➤ **Cons:** Kids can be a distraction, even when you have a babysitter; they may be upset by seeing you but not being able to be with you; you may miss the social interaction of an office; you may let some work slip by doing household chores instead; you have no support staff; you can end up working more than full time if you let projects flow into nights and weekends. "If you don't find it easier to spend time with your family," the authors say, "you've defeated the purpose of working at home."

➤ *Telecommuting or working from home or a remote site.* Many companies and government agencies now have satellite offices that their employees, who work from home, can use for meetings or computer equipment. In some cases, agencies set up telecommuting sites where employees can work every day and save themselves long, increasingly stressful commutes. This allows parents to get home in time to have dinner with their kids and return to the office after dinner, if necessary.

➤ *Virtual office.* This option occurs when an entire group of employees can work from remote sites. These offices are becoming more popular as technology allows people to do virtually everything from home that they would normally do from the office.

What's in a Company?

Many companies seem family-friendly from the outside. Pictures of family members are prominently displayed on top of employees' desks and people gather by the water cooler swapping stories about the cute little things their children or grandchildren did last weekend. But, in reality, many of these companies have lousy family and work policies.

So how do you tell?

Look at the following factors:

➤ See if the company recognizes that different employees have different needs and find out whether it offers a range of programs and resources to serve family and home life situations.

➤ Ask whether managers consider arrangements other than the normal 9 to 5, Monday through Friday work schedule.

➤ Ask whether the company measures performance by outcome rather than number of hours you clocked, and how and when performance is measured.

➤ Make sure that the company supports employees' efforts to remain involved in their children's education without penalizing employees for being absent.

Get Your House in Order for Order in Your Life

If you're like me, you're always searching through piles of stuff around the house to find the shirt you want to wear, a letter you have to answer, or your kid's lunch box. But you know things have gotten REALLY bad when you take your son to a birthday party on the wrong day because you couldn't find the invitation, or you drop off your daughter at ballet class (dressed in her tutu)—a week after the last session.

It's not that we are intentionally careless...we're just busy. And distracted. It's hard to keep track of the details of your kid's life when you're plotting your next move at work, angling to be promoted over your colleague. But you can reduce your stress significantly—and avoid other embarrassing mistakes—by just getting better organized and planning ahead. The following are some tips that have helped my clients, friends, and me get our acts together when our brains are on intermission:

➤ *Keep kids' papers together.* Ever find yourself shuffling through shoe boxes, piles of mail, and stashes of newspapers to find the notice for your son's Boy Scout meetings or your daughter's school supply lists? Have a folder with each child's name on it where you can throw in school calendars, camp notices, and whatever else comes in the mail for your child. Have your child go through this folder once every two weeks to update it.

➤ *Avoid morning madness.* Mornings are the worst time for parents because, in addition to getting themselves together, they've got to hustle their kids out of bed, rush them through breakfast, and get them out the door—all on time! Do everything you can the night before, including setting the breakfast table, making the lunches, and laying out your child's clothes for tomorrow.

➤ *Designate some area on your stair landing or by the front door as the Family Launch Pad.* All backpacks, musical instruments, sports equipment, school projects, and the like are to be placed on the Launch Pad *before* the child goes to bed at night, so in the morning he can find everything he needs and be launched with minimal stress.

➤ *Encourage your children to do more for themselves in the morning.* For instance, use an alarm clock for children over eight years old so they get up by themselves. If someone gets up before you, have them fix their own breakfast (cereal with milk) and then clear the breakfast table and put the dishes in the dishwasher so you can attend to last-minute details.

➤ *Keep everyone's schedule on a calendar.* On Sunday night, get everyone in the family together to set the schedule for the week. Use a different color pen for each child and write in the week's activities, including any birthday parties, gymnastics lessons, music classes, and play dates. Make copies on Monday at the office for both parents and any childcare help; then keep the calendar by the phone so you can glance at it while talking on the phone to make arrangements.

➤ *Reject the culture's yearly calendar and do your own.* Our culture has established a holiday and commercial calendar which is deadly for working parents. We are supposed to do all our holiday shopping in the three weeks between Thanksgiving and Christmas, even though it's one of the most exhausting times of the year with kids and relatives. In the summer, as we rush home from vacation in August, we are expected to do all the back-to-school shopping in one weekend.

Since there are three particularly high stress times for working parents each year—when school begins, when school ends, and the Thanksgiving and Christmas/Hanukkah holidays—lower your stress by changing the calendar. Do your holiday shopping in October and be done by mid November when everyone else is just starting. All year long when you see something a child or relative would like, buy it and put it away until the holiday. Buy school supplies and clothes in July when there are sales and more time. Organize camp supplies and schedule camp physicals for April or early May, not early June just before school is out when you're so busy with end of the school year activities. Think through one year at a time and make up a calendar for annual chores that works best for you, not for the stores at your local mall.

➤ *Do all your food shopping at once.* Take one night to look in your cabinets and see what you've got; then plan the week's meals and jot down what you need at the supermarket. Keep lots of frozen vegetables and easy-to-prepare foods on hand for those times when you can't spend much time in your kitchen.

➤ *Combine chores.* Be strategic and plan your chore day like a military maneuver for maximum efficiency and effectiveness. Plan to drop off your books at the library, on the way to the dry cleaners, after stopping at the bakery to pick up the birthday cake. Make haircut appointments for your kids at the mall and use that opportunity to go shopping for clothes and buy those birthday presents. If the kids get grumpy from being dragged around too much, buy off their patience by offering to take everyone for pizza afterwards—a win/win for all since you don't have to cook!

Delegate Chores or Get the To-Do Blues

It's bad enough that there's so much for working parents to do and so few hours in the day to do it—but it's REALLY bad if you're stuck doing the cooking, cleaning, shopping, and other chores yourself! Working moms especially tend to take on too many responsibilities because they feel it's their responsibility to meet their family's emotional and physical needs. The end result: Burnout Blues + Working-Parents Blues = the To-Do Blues.

The answer to keeping yourself sane is: DELEGATE! And avoid those To-Do Blues altogether.

Make a list of all the tasks that need to be done around the house (making dinner, washing dishes, doing laundry, vacuuming, mowing the lawn, and so on) and then divide them up among the family. Everybody should do something to contribute to the family. Even the little kids! In many households, working parents feel guilty for spending so little time with their kids that they overindulge them by not giving them any responsibilities. I'm guilty of that too! But I think it's important for kids to feel like they are part of a family team. Doing chores teaches them responsibility and makes them feel like they're truly contributing to the family. And delegating tasks to them (as long as they are age-appropriate tasks) will free up some of your time and take a load off your shoulders so you really can spend some quality time with them because you're not half dead with exhaustion!

So delegate and direct *all* the helping hands at home to whip through that to-do list together.

Besides delegating to the family, consider delegating to hired help to do the basics for you. Women especially may feel guilty hiring a cleaning service, for instance, because they feel it's their duty to clean the house even after putting in an eight-hour shift at the office. Somehow they still equate cleaning and doing laundry with feeling adequate as a woman. But wouldn't it be nice to have someone else clean your house so you could have extra time to spend with your son at the park or your daughter while she's playing dress up? You might feel even better about yourself as a woman and a mom.

But how does a working parent make the decisions about the best way to spend limited resources of time and money? A technique that has worked well for many of my clients is applying the Exchange/Loss/Gain formula. The strategy is to write down what's really important to us, what we're willing to exchange to get it, and the losses and gains we're likely to experience as a result of the exchange. Here are some examples of exchanges from clients who have used this solution successfully:

Exchange: Hire a weekly or monthly cleaning service.

Loss: Money. I may not be able to afford my Starbucks cup of coffee each morning.

Gain: Time, energy, peace of mind. I'll no longer have to do Saturday cleaning, and won't worry about a dirty home for the rest of the day.

Exchange: Limit the kids' after-school activities and have them help with the household grunt work.

Loss: Feel guilty about not doing it all myself and dragging them into this mess. They'll be mad at me in the short run, and it will take more of my time to train them how to do the chores.

Gain: More time and energy available for me in the long run. I'll be less exhausted, available for more talks and to help with homework. Kids will learn more about home responsibilities. Might even stop one of them from entering the Prince- or Princess-in-Training Syndrome and becoming a spoiled brat adult.

Making the cost and benefit clear helps working parents make far wiser decisions about how to balance everyone's needs. If you don't write them down, you'll probably see just the loss but not the gain—and that will make you feel blue and even more out of control. Use this formula whenever you need to make a big decision or know something has to give but are too overwhelmed to decide what it is.

Keep Your Hand on Your Kid's Pulse

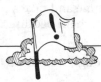

Blues Flag

To cope with the blues—and stop them from turning into black moods—I urge you to join a parent's support group. To find a support group, call your child's school, PTA committee, local YMCA, or your community center. You need someone to share war stories with, get advice and support. I remember when each of my boys was born I went to a "Mommy and Me" class. I still have close friends from those classes. And if you can't leave the house, join a group on the Internet: 24-hour support and company with other working parents. One especially helpful site for women is http://www.iVillage.com. Women are now about half of the new Internet users; they were only a third of new Net users just two years ago.

You may be bummed out because you were passed over for a promotion, but nothing feels worse than learning something is wrong for your child. Nobody likes to admit their child needs help—much less working parents, who are likely to minimize or deny any problems because it's upsetting, it takes time to resolve, and it just seems like one more thing.

But I urge parents to go after their kids' problems, to catch them early on and nip them in the bud—if parents ignore their children's cries for help the consequences become much more serious and time consuming later. Believe me, I know how hard it is to face up to the fact that something is a real problem for your child. One of my children has a learning disability, and, as soon as he was diagnosed, we felt terrible but launched into action to give him a school and training that respected his different style of learning and also appreciated his brightness and creativity.

It was the greatest educational investment we made because our son's self-esteem has improved dramatically and the tutoring empowered him with new skills. If we hadn't gotten him help, all of us would have felt genuinely handicapped by something that didn't have to be a handicap. So don't wait for the school to pick up on a problem because often they miss it or there are too many kids to offer the kind of help your child needs. If you think something is wrong with your child, follow your gut, find out, and get professional help to fix or lessen the problem.

Staying Connected with Your Kids

As working parents, few of us have extra time to volunteer. Most of us dread that call from the home-room mother (undoubtedly a stay-at-home mom) asking if we can come in and help make costumes for the play, bake brownies, or serve lunch. But it's a good thing they call because most of us feel too guilty saying no so we shuffle our work schedule around to make time to go, and then we're so glad we went!

Volunteering at school is the best way to find out what is really going on with your child. You're also much more likely to feel connected if you meet the teachers, the principals, and your child's classmates, and more able to spot problems your child may be having. So don't wait for the guilt-inducing call from the room mother, volunteer to go into the class and read stories once a month (if the kids are young) or to teach the kids a skill (if the children are older). Your child will feel really special having you there (at least until they become teenagers, in which case they'll pretend they have no idea who you are and then you'll really know they're doing just fine).

These days, the Working-Parents Blues are unavoidable. But if you believe you can beat these blues, you can. You must be willing to learn new delegation skills, take risks at work by asking for what you need, and understand that no matter what you do or how well you do it, you'll fall off the balance beam more often than not. But when you try these strategies, you earn the best of both worlds: satisfying parenting and the opportunity to do meaningful work. Even your mental health will improve. Although working parents, especially single parents, are the most stressed, they're typically the least depressed because they have so much joy and so many alternatives in a very full life.

Dr. Ellen Says

When we come home from work sometimes, all we want to do is collapse on the couch. Why not let some of your kids collapse with you? To feel connected to your children you don't have to always talk to them. Just sitting side by side watching TV after dinner or reading the paper while they do a puzzle will make your children feel physically close to you—and safe. It's the simple joys in life that will help lift the Working-Parents Blues!

The Least You Need to Know

➤ The number one complaint from working parents today is that their life is out of balance.

➤ Despite all the hype about family-friendly workplaces, many companies are still operating on a 9-to-5 schedule. However, more and more companies are offering arrangements like flexible hours, compressed work weeks, and telecommuting to help working parents.

➤ To get better organized, avoid morning hassles by getting everything ready the night before, designate a Family Launch Pad, do your weekly grocery shopping in one trip, join a support group, and combine chores.

➤ Delegate household chores to your kids, and, if necessary, hire a cleaning staff to keep your house neat and organized.

➤ No matter how busy you are, take time to volunteer at your child's school because it is a good way to stay connected with your child.

Part 6
Mind Your Body to Mend Your Mind

The blues don't just make you feel bad, sad, or mad. If they go unchecked for too long, they could turn into a depression and make you feel sick as well.

The blues, for instance, help create heart disease and slow down recovery after heart surgery. The blues are also connected to cancer. The chapters in this section describe the different stages of recovery that people with heart disease and cancer go through and what the family can do to cope with the blues during tough times. This section also covers the range of antidepressant medication on the market and highlights natural therapies such as St. John's Wort that many people are using to overcome mild to moderate depression. Finally, you'll learn the long-term strategies you can take to protect yourself against getting the blues.

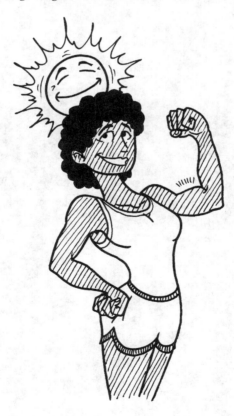

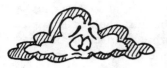

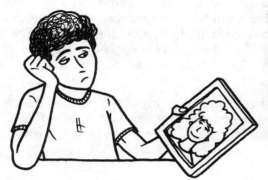

Chapter 21

Good Morning Heartache: The Cardiovascular Blues

In This Chapter

➤ It's all in your mind—and goes to your heart

➤ Hostility humbles your heart

➤ To heal your heart, banish loneliness and stress

➤ Coping with homecoming blues after heart surgery

➤ Caregivers get sick hearts too

Heart disease is a subject that literally pains my heart. Too many of us have sad stories to tell about someone we love suffering a heart attack. My father, a charming, sweet Irishman who loved to smoke, drink, and carry on, suffered two heart attacks before the age of 50. At the time, his heart attacks were a gut-wrenching surprise. Had I known more about depression then, I wouldn't have been shocked, because anyone with genetic vulnerability and as much unresolved depression as he had would probably have a heart attack.

Men typically hide their depression with the kinds of things my Dad did: deny there's any problem; smoke, drink, and work too much; and not talk about their feelings. Even though he hid it well, I now realize my Dad was depressed most of his adult life. He was divorced unwillingly, worked for the IRS (now there's an occupation where the blues can flourish), and was separated for weeks at a time from the children and relatives he loved. Stress, isolation, and loneliness played a major role in weakening his heart. His unnamed and unrecognized bad feelings grew into the Cardiovascular Blues and later into a clinical depression.

Research confirms that stress, hostility, and lack of meaningful social contact cause a heart attack or make a heart condition worse. And beware, because the Cardiovascular Blues tend to run in families. Sure enough, many years later my younger brother had a severe heart attack at the age of 43. Luckily, he survived, and he learned from my father's mistakes: The first heart attack is a warning to shape up and if you don't listen, the second one usually kills you. My brother heard his calling the first time and with a will and lucidity that my dad never had, he turned his life around. It was amazing to watch his transformation from being a machinist who dreaded punching in the clock every day to a public school tutor who freely gave whatever heart he had left to emotionally troubled kids.

In this chapter, we'll explore information I've learned from my family history and from my clients about how your mind deeply affects your body and vice versa. I'm now more convinced than ever that the blues fuel heart disease—but I also feel encouraged knowing that there is a lot we can do to combat the Cardiovascular Blues and strengthen our hearts with love and health.

"Say It Ain't So" to America's #1 Killer

Heart disease loves to make its grand entrance with a dramatic heart attack, and this accounts for nearly half of all deaths in the U.S.—twice as many as are caused by all forms of cancer. Heart disease seems to be everywhere and the high risk factors are by now well known: high blood pressure, high cholesterol, obesity, smoking, and other self-destructive behaviors. But did you know that many of us are in complete denial about these risk factors?

"Say it ain't so" is our favorite motto, as we continue to gobble Big Macs with fries and pretend everything's fine. Why? Because acknowledging our risk means making big changes in our lifestyles and that's one of the hardest things any of us can do.

If you've been living high on the hog, hearing that you have to switch to alfalfa sprouts and 1 percent cottage cheese and then run three miles a day to boot, you're not going to be delighted with the news.

It's easy to say "cut back on stressful activities," but who can get out of the rat race when you've been locked up in that maze for so long? The fact is that most of us don't even know where to start taking care of ourselves when our doctor tells us we have to change our attitudes about health and fitness and our philosophies about life. And when we realize that our old lives have come to an end and new ones must begin, we get the *Cardiovascular Blues*—but we also get the opportunity to change our lives in ways that are far more satisfying.

Terms of Encheerment

Cardiovascular Blues are the anxious, fearful, helpless, and frustrated feelings we get when we are told we have heart disease and must fundamentally change our lives in order to continue living. Cardiovascular Blues also include the heart disease caused by unresolved stress and depression.

Getting to the Heart of Heart Disease

If you've been following health reports over the years, the physical factors leading to heart disease have probably been pounded into your head. For years, people ridiculed suggestions by alternative medicine types (those "out there" guys who are into crystals and Kitaro) that the mind played a role in making your heart sick.

But recent research shows that feeling hostile, having no social support, and being stressed out all the time can also set the stage for developing heart disease or making it worse if you've already been diagnosed with a problem. In other words, your mind can make your body sick!

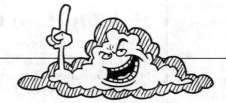

Funk-y Facts

FOR WOMEN ONLY! The notion that cardiovascular disease is a man's disease is a destructive myth for women. Men suffer heart attacks about 10 years before women, so they are at higher risk when they are younger. But as women approach menopause, the risk of heart disease begins to rise. Surveys show that most women are more afraid of breast cancer than cardiovascular disease, even though 1 in 26 women will die of breast cancer while almost 1 in 2 will die of heart disease. The first sign of a heart attack for women is usually chest pain when resting. Other common symptoms include pain or pressure from the jaw to the diaphragm, breathlessness, heartburn, nausea, and intense fatigue—symptoms that become much worse when there's also a depression.

How Hostility, Loneliness, and Stress Hurt Your Heart

The mind/body connection in heart disease received much attention in the 1960s when San Francisco cardiologists Meyer Friedman and Ray Rosenman set out to show that Type A behavior—people who are constantly rushed, have a lot of hostility, and are intensely competitive—was present in most of their patients with heart disease.

Over a period of eight years, the men who scored as Type A developed heart disease twice as often as those who were labeled Type B—calm, cool, collected types. What's interesting is that those with Type A behavior were at high risk of getting heart disease even if they didn't have the physical symptoms that make people susceptible to cardiovascular problems.

269

In the 1980s, Dr. Redford Williams, author of *The Trusting Heart: Great News About Type A Behavior* (NY Times Books, 1989) and director of the Behavioral Medicine Research Center at Duke University Medical Center, further developed this theory and discovered that not all Type A behavior can result in heart disease. Being competitive and getting things done quickly, he found, could be good because these qualities can help you accomplish goals. But hostility and anger, he found, had little redeeming value. Dr. Williams developed a hostility test that men can take to gauge where you stand.

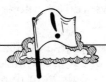

Blues Flag

Symptoms of heart disease often mimic the symptoms of depression, and doctors diagnosing your condition may overlook the depression altogether! Studies show that as many as 32 percent of all medical patients also suffer from serious depression that goes unidentified in up to half the cases. If you are diagnosed with heart disease, visit a mental health professional in addition to your cardiologist to determine if you are also depressed and, if you are, the nature and extent of your depression.

Hostility Hurts Healthy Hearts

The fact that hostility is bad for your heart isn't totally shocking. Researchers have suspected for some time that bottling up anger contributes to heart disease because the level of stress hormones circulating in your blood goes way up and stays elevated when you're really angry.

But it's worse than anyone guessed. In another long-term, well-designed study, it was found that those hotheads who scored in the top 20 percent of the hostility scale were 42 percent more likely to be dead 20 years later than those calm souls who scored in the lower 20 percent of the hostility scale. So your heart's health depends on your hostility, and the less hostility you carry, the better your heart.

How Hostile Are You?

I know I can get hostile sometimes, especially when I've had a bad day and I'm under a lot of stress. And that may be why I love to box, because I can release so much hostility. But sometimes there is so much going on in our lives that it's hard to tell what we are feeling, except irritation and a short fuse. When I find myself scowling or being irritable with others, I take the hostility test that Dr. Williams developed to see where I stand.

This way I can determine whether I'm just having a bad hair day or whether my heart is hostile enough (and therefore too vulnerable) to warrant a change of behavior. I encourage you to take the following quiz, which is excerpted from his book, to see where you stand.

How Hostile Are You? (from *The Trusting Heart: Great News About Type A Behavior*)

Circle the answer that best describes you.

1. When family members or even persons I don't know do things (or fail to do things) that hold me up or prevent me from doing something I wish to do, I begin to think that they are selfish, mean, inconsiderate, and the like.

   NEVER   SOMETIMES   OFTEN   ALWAYS

2. When strangers, friends, or members of my family do things that seem incompetent, messy, selfish, or inconsiderate, I quickly experience feelings of frustration, anger, irritation, and even rage; at the same time I become aware of these feelings, I notice unpleasant bodily sensations, like trouble getting enough breath, my heart pounding rapidly in my chest, my palms sweating, and the like.

   NEVER   SOMETIMES   OFTEN   ALWAYS

3. When I have the thoughts, feelings, and bodily sensations just described, I am very likely to express my feelings in some way—whether by words, gestures, tone of voice, or facial expressions—to the other person or persons who I see as responsible for my unpleasant thoughts and feelings.

   NEVER   SOMETIMES   OFTEN   ALWAYS

According to Dr. Williams, if you answer "OFTEN" or "ALWAYS" to at least two of these questions, your hostility level is elevated enough to cause some worry. This means that your hostile feelings are placing your mind and your heart at risk.

Ways and Means to Ward Off Hostility

Scoring in the "hostile" category can make you feel more hostility! But don't beat up on yourself (or someone else). Take heart from these words: Most of us act mean to others sometimes and then feel terrible about it. But the good news is that once you know you're being hostile, you can change your thoughts and behaviors by taking small steps.

A few suggestions to become Mr. Nice Guy or Ms. Nice Gal:

➤ Get yourself a pet. Recent studies found that people with pets have lower "cardiovascular reactivity," says Dr. Dean Ornish, in his ground-breaking book *Love and Survival: The Scientific Basis For The Healing Power of Intimacy* (HarperCollins, 1998). Only 6 percent of pet owners died more than a year after being hospitalized with a heart attack, as compared to the 28 percent without pets who died at around the same time. One study showed that a dog had a much better effect on lowering blood pressure on its owner than a friend who was considered judgmental. It's generally hard to stay hostile when you're petting a cuddly animal.

➤ Tell your friends that you know you are acting hostile and you are trying to change that. Ask them for feedback and suggestions about what you can do to stop the behavior.

➤ When you get angry and snap at people, stop reacting with your gut and give yourself a break from the intense feelings. Take time out to get control of yourself and try to talk yourself through the cause of your hostility. Develop an action plan for dealing with it. Just keep reminding yourself: You may be right, but is it practical to hold onto being right? Usually the answer is NO because the anger, no matter how justified, will serve as a major obstacle to your success and relationships.

➤ When hostility hits, take a deep breath through your nose and slowly count to 10, then forcefully exhale through your mouth. This provides your brain with more oxygen so it will think better and triggers a greater relaxation response throughout your body. When you feel more in control you can decide whether or not to nail the other guy (with words of course).

➤ Helping others also reduces your hostility because volunteer work or lending a helping hand dissipates anger and gets your focus on someone else instead of your miseries and rages. In his book, Dr. Dean Ornish quotes a study revealing that people who volunteer at least once a week are two and a half times less likely to die during the nine- to 12-year study as those who never volunteered. Another study found that women who were members of volunteer organizations lived longer than those who were unaffiliated.

➤ You'd be amazed at how hostility melts away when you forgive somebody who has hurt you. Try not to hold a grudge against people by realizing that everyone is human and makes mistakes and it's in the interest of better health for you that you let go of the anger.

➤ Instead of isolating yourself from people when you're feeling angry, try to connect with friends and share the burden.

➤ Remember that hostility is often a cover for loneliness and/or depression, especially for men. If you're living with Attila the Hun, in pint size or giant size, check under the hostility hood to see if the blues are lurking in there. If you find them, reread Chapter 4, "Decoronation Blues: Even Kings, Jocks, and Cowboys Get the Blues," to remind yourself about effective action strategies that help men beat their blues.

When the Heart Is a Lonely Hunter

You simply can't afford to have a lonely heart. Consider the following, reported in Dr. Ornish's book:

➤ Want to die prematurely? Then damage, destroy, or fail to develop your social system. One study conducted by Dr. D. G. Blazer of 331 men and women over 65 found that those who did not have good social systems were *386 percent* more likely to die early.

➤ At Duke University, Dr. Redford Williams studied 1,400 men and women who had coronary angiography for a blocked artery. Five years later, the unmarried, lonely ones were *three times* more likely to be dead than the married patients who had a confidant to talk to.

➤ Dr. Thomas Oxman of University of Texas Medical School found that among men and women who had open heart surgery, the patients who were not part of an organized social group were *four times* more likely to die within six months after surgery.

➤ At Case Western Reserve University, 10,000 men were studied for risk factors for developing chest pain (angina). The men who reported that their wives "did not show their love" were nearly *twice* as likely to get angina in the next five years as those men who felt their wives showed their love.

All of the studies suggest that loneliness is just as harmful as an illness. So to keep your heart healthy, connect, connect, connect. Give to others, be useful, love well, and you'll protect yourself much better from the Cardiovascular Blues.

Managing the Stress Mess

In addition to loneliness, the other major enemy to your healthy heart is prolonged stress. Having too much stress will substantially raise your risk of cardiovascular disease because you're bathing your cardiovascular system too often in the toxic chemicals generated by stress. Producing these chemicals is like pouring Drano through your veins, arteries, and heart every day. Not exactly a good thing. In fact it's just a matter of time before it's a disaster to your heart.

So for the health of your heart, it's non-negotiable that you identify and reduce your level of stress. If relationships stress you, then do a relationship inventory and assess the quality and quantity of your relationships. Accept that something's wrong and it's up to you to find out what it is and take the steps necessary to correct the problem. Either change your expectations, learn new communication skills, or ditch the relationship that's causing you stress and build new, more satisfying ones.

If your career is the source of your stress and you just hate the daily grind, consider changing careers (see Chapter 18, "Licking the Monday-Morning Blues." People, usually men, who've been diagnosed with heart disease are often forced to change professions to slow down and reduce the stress. For many people, this is a blessing in disguise. The reason my brother started tutoring after his heart attack was that he couldn't physically handle the work he was doing before. He is the happiest and calmest he has ever been!

What do you know, second chances can give you the best choices of your lifetime!

Homecoming Blues—Back From the Hospital

Depression is so commonafter you come home from heart surgery that doctors traditionally expected it and did very little about it. No antidepressants, no counseling, no comfort. More of an impatient attitude like "What do you expect?" Of course, that attitude just made the homecoming blues even worse. Now doctors understand that depression following surgery isn't inevitable and if the depression is treated, the patient recovers more quickly, both mentally and physically.

During the first week in the hospital, most heart attack survivors go through a wide range of emotions:

➤ Some can't believe they've had such serious, life-threatening surgery, and they feel angry, asking themselves: "Why me?"

➤ Others deny that anything is wrong with them and pretend that undergoing bypass surgery was no different than getting your tonsils out.

➤ Many feel anxious about what this operation means for their future. Will they be all right? Will they ever be themselves again?

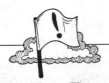

Blues Flag

If your doctor makes you feel uncomfortable or unimportant, I urge you to find a different physician. You need to be able to talk to your doctor safely and freely. Many people have a hard time beating the Cardiovascular Blues because they don't trust their medical care, and this distrust feeds their feelings of helplessness. So if your doctor gets you down, find a more understanding and respectful physician partner.

And everyone gets the Cardiovascular Blues for a number of reasons: They've been through significant trauma; they now face a painful, slow recovery period; they stared death in the face; and even worse, they have to CHANGE to stay alive. Not just a little change, but a lifestyle change. That makes many people feel quite blue. There were many reasons they didn't make the changes before and now they don't have any choice but to make the changes now, so it feels even worse.

For about half of all people who survive a heart attack the condition is more serious and they go through a period of clinical depression afterward. This is definitely a time for "better living through chemistry" when antidepressants can substantially speed up recovery (see Chapter 23, "Better Living Through Chemistry"). In most cases, the depression should resolve itself within four months. If it lingers longer, they need to get professional help and counseling. Chronic depression takes a huge toll on the heart, and people who remain depressed after a heart attack are more likely to suffer another one which is usually worse.

Plus, people who pretend that the first heart attack was no big deal are not likely to take their medication, modify their lifestyle, or pay attention to any symptoms of heart problems—placing them at higher risk for another heart attack.

Coping with Your Own Recovery

If you are ill or recovering from an operation, it's natural to feel helpless, dependent, and out of control. But even if you're physically limited in what you can do, you can regain a sense of control and beat the Cardiovascular Blues by following these suggestions:

➤ *Readjust your expectations.* Accept the reality that you're in recovery and you just suffered a major physical disruption. It's going to take your body some time to heal. Try to focus on your gains rather than losses. Your pain depletes the chemicals in the brain that help us feel good, so pain control and positive thinking is crucial for keeping a balance in our biochemistry and psychology that helps us in recovery.

➤ *Remind yourself that every step counts.* Even the smallest step is a move toward recovery. Progress may be something as simple as sitting up in bed, or reaching out to touch a visitor, or taking a first step. Steps grow bigger, but recovery has its own speed. You can't hurry your recovery, but you can continue to believe in it and it will happen if you let it.

➤ *Stay in touch with other people.* We've discussed how destructive a lonely heart can be, but it bears repeating because it's so crucial to your recovery. Stay connected to other people! A study of heart patients showed that those who received the amount of attention they wanted got better in one month—as opposed to four months—and showed higher self-esteem and less anxiety than people who didn't get attention.

➤ *Learn to communicate with people who care about you.* You'll have a lot more influence and control over your environment if you learn to ask the people you love for what you need. Be very specific and don't apologize for having needs. But don't present your needs as a demand or command or you'll burn out the people who would like to meet your needs and you'll end up with little need satisfaction.

➤ *Use positive visualization techniques.* Using positive visualization techniques helps reduce depression (see Chapter 6, "Quick Strategies for You to Beat the Blues"). In one study, men and women volunteers were told to visualize their white blood cells as strong, powerful sharks swimming through the bloodstream, attacking the germs that caused colds—and there was, in fact, an increase in the effectiveness of the white blood cells! So think long, hard, and good about clean arteries and a strong heart!

Caregiver Blues

If your loved onehad the heart attack, you can expect to be blue too. It's natural for you to have concerns and fears and you should talk about your feelings to others and gather as much information as you can. Here are a few of the feelings you may be experiencing:

➤ You may feel guilty, as if you caused the heart attack, even though it's not true.

➤ You may be afraid that your loved one will die and feel overwhelmed by that thought.

If you are feeling this way, I strongly urge you to join your local Mended Hearts or other support groups for heart and stroke patients and their families so you don't feel so isolated. When someone in the family gets sick, it affects everybody and changes the dynamics of the household. This is especially true when the person develops heart disease because a change of lifestyle is in order.

Guiltless Pleasures

If you are holding down the fort while your spouse is recovering from heart surgery, you need to take care of yourself too. Take time every day to do things you enjoy—and don't let guilt interfere. Remember, you've got to be in good spirits to help your spouse. So go out and buy yourself some flowers, sit at an outdoor cafe and watch the people walk by, or take a walk in a beautiful park.

Heart disease is a fact of life and death. But knowing that feeling angry, stressed out, and isolated makes us more vulnerable to developing heart disease gives us a heads-up about what we can do to protect ourselves. My father lost his heart because he got stuck in a depression and didn't know how to take care of himself. After his first heart attack, he stayed depressed and refused to take his medication and continued to smoke and drink to lessen his bad feelings. That behavior nearly guaranteed he'd have a second, far more serious heart attack, and he did.

I remember how worried I was about him, scouring hospitals nearby looking for him when he didn't show up for the weekend visits after my parents divorced. I wish I could go back in time and help him resolve his depression. But I can't, so the best I can do is apply in my life the lessons he taught me and share them with you. *Realize that the quality of your social relationships and whatever is on your mind will significantly affect the health of your heart.* The heart is too precious to waste, so listen to it and when things get too rough, take action and beat those Cardiovascular Blues before they beat you.

The Least You Need to Know

➤ Unresolved depression significantly contributes to heart disease and slower recovery time, and can even lead to death.

➤ When we are diagnosed with heart disease, a complete change in lifestyle is necessary: Slow down, increase the quality of our relationships, do meaningful work, exercise, and eat right.

➤ It's normal to get the Cardiovascular Blues when we have heart disease or to feel helpless watching a loved one get sick, but these blues can be resolved.

➤ Recent research shows that feelings of hostility, loneliness, and prolonged stress can set the stage for developing heart disease or worsening an existing heart problem.

➤ To deal with the homecoming blues, accept that your recovery will take time, tell yourself that every little improvement counts, stay in touch with people, and use positive visualization techniques.

➤ Caregivers may feel guilty for their loved one being sick and be afraid of losing that person; joining a support group can help.

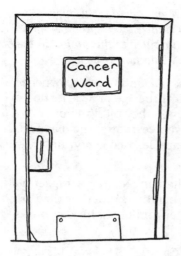

Chapter 22

Conquering the Cancer Blues

In This Chapter

➤ Meet a cancer hero and his family

➤ Positive attitudes = positive results

➤ "Your days are numbered"—NOT!

➤ Let laughter lift your spirits

➤ Take control of your condition to beat the hospital blues

➤ Coping with breast cancer and prostate cancer

➤ Relaxation, visualization/imagery, biofeedback, and other techniques

➤ Survival tips for cancer caregivers

How people face their deaths tells you volumes about how they lived their lives and a great deal about how to live ours. Death teaches us more about life than any other experience; so to hide from death and avoid it means you'll lose some of life's best lessons and moments. Don't believe me? Meet the Silverstein family from New Haven, Connecticut, and listen to their story of how they beat the Cancer Blues. The family has generously allowed me to share their experience to give comfort and hope to other families facing the Cancer Blues.

The family and their experience are real. They contributed and approved every word of the following story. Only their names and identity have been changed to respect their privacy. I am deeply grateful for the enormous time and energy they contributed to this project in the hope of helping others face a cancer crisis with more information about how to cope.

The father of the clan, Sam Silverstein—an upbeat, social, and friendly owner of a retail store—was first diagnosed with colon cancer in 1988 at the age of 58. The doctors didn't give him a time line for how long he had to live—they didn't know... *What they did know is that it didn't look good.* But he lived for seven years after the diagnosis. He staked a claim over his life, took control of his care, and learned everything possible about beating the Cancer Blues.

His healing journey was the most enlightening, challenging, empowering, and affirming experience in his life and the lives of his family members. When he died at home the day after Thanksgiving in 1995, his adult daughter Annie said his death was "...one of the most honorable things I've seen in my life."

What kept Sam alive—and helped him conquer the Cancer Blues—was his consistent positive attitude; his eagerness to stay connected to people and to resolve any conflicts between him and others; his involvement in making decisions regarding his care; his superb sense of humor; his willingness to try new therapies, both traditional and alternative; and his ability to share his feelings, from the lightest to the darkest, with other people, especially his family.

Sam and his family are what cancer specialist and author Dr. Bernie Siegel calls "ECaPs"—Exceptional Cancer Patients who fight with everything they have against their illness. Unfortunately, only 15 to 20 percent of cancer patients are ECaPs. The rest tend to be passive, pleasing to their doctor, and resigned to their fate, so their life expectancy is often shorter than the ECaPs'. The bottom 15 to 20 percent of cancer patients seem to give up when they hear their diagnosis and use the cancer as a good excuse to check out early because life had been too much anyway.

The Silverstein family and I also hope that by sharing Sam's story, we can encourage more cancer patients and their families to move out of the middle group of pleasing, passive patients into the dynamic, powerful ECaP group. As you read Sam's story, you'll see why being a ECaP can be so rewarding for the cancer patient and the family, and why the ECaP strategies are the best available for beating the Cancer Blues.

Sam and his family's coping strategies apply to all the cancers, but since there are issues specific to other cancers, such as breast cancer and prostate cancer, these issues will be addressed at the end of this chapter.

The Start of a Remarkable Journey

Sam Silverstein came into my life through his daughter Annie, a sweet, creative, wonderfully spirited coaching client of mine. Annie is a gifted artist whose passion is painting and the creative arts. She was young and very talented but very depressed that she couldn't make a living at what she loved to do, so she initially came to me for help in developing new career strategies. Annie always got along well with her dad, but after he was diagnosed with cancer in 1988, they both wanted to resolve several issues in their relationship before he was no longer able. So Annie asked her dad and mom if they would like to see me so everyone could better communicate the issues.

There was only one problem: Seeing a therapist was a very big deal for Sam. He was a traditional guy who didn't want to have to deal with therapy. Coming to see Dr. Ellen was strong psychological chemo for him. But Sam loved his children so deeply that he was even willing to see a "witch doctor" for them to try to resolve whatever they could so they could feel as strong and loved as possible. Only later did he concede that part of him had also come for himself, because, as he said, "Every little bit helps."

Seeing Sam and his wife Sarah was the beginning of a remarkable journey for me too. Hearing about the Silverstein's experience dissolved the deep fear that I had when I thought of someone I love or myself getting cancer. I eventually lost my fear of death and began to see it as the most natural process in the world, full of joy and sadness and wonderment.

Seven More Years

"When we got Dad's cancer diagnosis," says his daughter Annie, "they didn't tell us how long he had to live. They said they didn't know. That was actually good, I think, because we didn't have that time reference hanging over us. However, we were operating with a lot of unknowns. That was hard. We didn't know what to expect. But we had a choice then about how to deal with it."

Sam chose not to give in. He chose to survive—and survive he did, for seven more years. All but the last six months were really great years.

His daughter Annie remembers the day Sam received the call from the doctor with the cancer diagnosis. Her younger brother had just been married the day before, and the family and a few close friends were enjoying the afterglow of a terrific wedding. After Sam hung up the phone he told everyone. Annie says, "We were stunned and scared. Dad was shaking. It sunk in very slowly. And after a while, Dad looked around and said: 'I'm going to beat this sucker.'"

"When he said that, the tone was set," adds Annie, who just a week before had seen her dad looking gray and shaky one morning, and later that day

Blues Flag

After a scary diagnosis or medical procedure, if your mental pain is so intense that you want to die and the feeling lasts for two or more weeks, it is very likely you're clinically depressed. IT'S NOT NORMAL TO FEEL THIS BAD, even when the disease is at an advanced stage. You can be successfully treated for this kind of depression with medication and counseling. As the depression lifts, you'll be better able to cope with the pain, resume control over your care at every stage of the illness, and feel more able to give and receive love when you need it most.

learned from her mom that he had bled into the toilet. "We had an attitude. If he could be that way, then I could too. Part of the tension was not knowing how he was going to react. I heard him decide to fight. It would have been very different if he had surrendered to the disease at that point. If he gave up, I might have too."

The Art of the Positive

The word "surrender" was not in Sam's lexicon—although he had his share of depressing moments. He didn't buckle under when he first suspected he had cancer, nor when he learned he needed to have a colostomy. He refused to give up when the doctor told him he'd probably be impotent or while undergoing chemotherapy, when everyone told him his chances of long-term survival were slim.

Annie remembers Sam's reaction when Sarah told him that 90 percent of the people didn't make it beyond the point he was at. "Dad said, 'Isn't that *neat*, I'm going to be in that 10 percent!' That was amazing. I don't know that I believed him, but I wasn't going to discourage him. I didn't want to get my hopes up too high, either. But that's what kept him going. That's why he survived longer than most people."

Many people who get cancer start digging their graves soon after they are diagnosed—some actually welcome the diagnosis as a way to end their problems. They assume that the rest of their lives will be full of despair, loneliness, and pain, and the thought of knowing their death date may be prematurely set in stone is just too much to bear.

Research shows again and again that having a positive outlook slows down the progression of the disease and makes a difference in the quality of the person's life. The patients who survive stronger and longer are the ones who fight for the right to live, who look cancer right in the face, and who leave no stone unturned in trying to find cures. They argue with doctors, fight insurance companies, try out new alternative therapies, share their feelings with others, and stay connected.

A social man who was very active in a wine-tasting society, Sam loved people. So he refused to feel alone and keep cancer as his dirty little secret. He talked at length to friends and family about it, keeping it quiet only in business circles where knowledge of his cancer would have influenced business deals.

Cancer, Annie said, deeply touched the whole family. "We talked about it a lot," she says. "I learned from my dad that you've got to make it real, grab it by the lapels and say, 'You are cancer, I'm me, and we have a relationship now.' As soon as it's real it can be dealt with. It's hard because it throws mortality right in your face...and in the face of others who would love to run as quickly as possible in the opposite direction."

You bet we want to run away from cancer as fast as possible! We're no fools. The bottom line is that cancer is a mean, nasty enemy. Sometimes, *no matter what you do*, cancer will not negotiate any compromise or take any hostages. In addition to taking your life, cancer first robs you of your sexual desire. Then it snuffs you out, often with a Clint Eastwood kind of snarl: "Make my day!"

For this reason, people who get cancer often feel their bodies and their God have betrayed them. They feel so deeply alone and forsaken because they have been banned from the village of the well and exiled to the village of the sick, where people constantly live under a cloud of immense fear and potential darkness. Communication is the only bridge between the land of the well and the land of the sick. And most of us don't have a clue how to communicate about something as dreadful as having cancer, so we usually don't say anything at all.

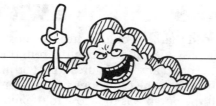

Funk-y Facts

In *Love, Medicine and Miracles* (Harper Perennial, 1990), Dr. Bernie Siegel talks about the nature of exceptional patients—the ones who take control of their care and need to know everything about their X-ray reports, entries in their charts, and courses of treatment. Physicians, he says, don't realize that the patients they consider "difficult" or "uncooperative" are the ones most likely to get well because they're the best fighters. He quotes a study by psychologist Dr. Leonard Derogatis, revealing that women with metastatic breast cancer who lived the longest had lousy relationships with their doctors, *as reported by the doctors.* These feisty patients asked a lot of questions and expressed their emotions freely. Many of their doctors were not pleased. NCI psychologist Dr. Sandra Levy also showed that seriously ill breast-cancer patients who talked about how depressed and anxious they were lived longer than those who showed little distress. She found that feisty "bad" patients tend to have more killer T cells, cells that seek and destroy cancer cells, than the more mellow "good" patients." So, to beat the Cancer Blues, be "bad," bold, and brave; bond and barter but never, ever bow.

Sam was a great communicator when it came to business matters. But he didn't share his personal feelings with many people. After the surgery, however, he felt a need to talk about cancer and the colostomy. Although at first many of his discussions were focused on the disease itself, treatment, and other related topics, he gradually opened up to share his personal feelings as well.

But it was over the last six months to a year of his life that Sam took a huge communications leap. "Sam had already taken care of the will and many of the business matters," said Sarah. "But there were a lot of personal family issues that were still unresolved. So Sam, Annie, and I went to see Ellen to figure out how to go about communicating at that level. She suggested that he make an appointment with every one of his kids to talk about his relationship with them."

When I met Sam in the later stages of his illness, he was astonishingly clear and inspirational in expressing his feelings and needs and made me feel very connected and caring toward him. But I could tell he had developed this communication skill gradually over the years as his disease progressed.

The major blow to Sam's self-esteem, though, and his biggest coping challenge was having to get a permanent colostomy.

Life Down Under: This Time Without My Tube

Sam desperately hoped that he wouldn't need a colostomy (defined by *Webster's* as the "surgical construction of an artificial opening from the colon to the outside of the body"). Doesn't that sound absolutely dreadful? Fortunately, the doctors told him that they may be able to remove the cancerous polyp from his colon without interrupting his functions. But if the polyp was too close to the muscle, they'd have to remove the muscle, the sphincter muscle, which would require a colostomy—an operation that entailed, as Annie explains in more understandable terms, "opening you up from front to back and rerouting your colon so you wear a bag on your lower belly, where you poop."

Everything happened so quickly that the family barely had time to think about the consequences of surgery. On Monday, Sam got the cancer report. On Tuesday, he talked to a surgeon who put him in the hospital right away and scheduled the operation for the next day. The family was told that if the operation was short it meant the doctors were able to just remove the polyp. But if surgery went on for longer that meant they'd have to do a colostomy. So when a nurse came out into the waiting area while Sam was in surgery, the family knew what was in store. "If that's what they had to do to keep my father alive," Annie says, "then do it. That's how the family felt. Dad felt the same way. Everyone understood and accepted the facts and we knew life would be different. But we'd deal with it."

The specter of dealing with cancer is one thing. But dealing with the colostomy was the immediate hurdle. Sam was a private, very neat man. Losing a major body function was difficult. "The thought of a leak or a smell or having gas embarrassed him," Annie explained. "It took him a while to learn to live with it. A terrific colostomy nurse came to help him and educate both Dad and Mom on to handle the colostomy. Mom said three things happened to my dad all at once," Annie continues. "He had a colostomy, he became impotent, and he got cancer."

Dr. Ellen Says

Your state of mind can influence the course of cancer. To beat the Cancer Blues, you need to be able to accept your new body. Denying that your body has changed can have serious repercussions. People who withdraw and become depressed about losing a breast or penis function can lead a terrible life—not because their looks have changed, but because they don't have any more intimacy. Learning how to take care of yourself, doing relaxation exercises, and joining a support group will make you feel less scared and more in control.

That's a lot to handle, even for someone as optimistic as Sam.

Sometimes there are physical reasons for becoming impotent, other times the reasons are psychological, and often it's a combination of the two. What's important is to get the proper diagnosis. But partners have to talk honestly with each other so they can find a way to be close and give each other pleasure—despite the new challenges.

Some people get referrals to a sexual rehabilitation program in a cancer center, sexual dysfunction clinic, urologist, or sex therapist. Sam overcame his aversion to therapists, and he asked the fabulous colostomy nurse to find him a good sex therapist. He decided it was more important to get help than to live with impotency.

Laughter Fuels Health: "Horny Flicks"

Sam went to see a sex therapist and psychiatrist, and Sarah thought it was great. "Our sex life changed after that," Sarah points out. "We had constructive things to work on, instead of frustrations." Annie adds, "My mother said that the sex therapist gave them back a sex life, not the same one that they had before, but at least they had another one."

Part of the treatment, adds Sarah, was that she and Sam had to make a date to allow a certain amount of time for sex. "We had to go to bed at 9 p.m.," Sarah explains. "This gave us permission to go to bed much earlier than we normally did. Usually, we worked until 11 or 12. So, in a sense, going to bed at 9 felt like we were on a vacation."

The key to sexual health, the therapist said, was for Sam to stop thinking about his impotence and to take action. His prescription: **horny flicks**. "Our sex therapist gave us six names of porno flicks that he suggested we get," says Sarah, who went out to buy a video cassette player for their bedroom television. "He explained that the films had to have a plot and a story line. The idea was that Sam should concentrate on the movie and not worry about whether he could get an erection. When I went to get them at the video store, I couldn't find them. I think they were too old and didn't exist anymore."

Sarah didn't have time to go to another video store. So Annie's sister Kate headed out to a REAL adult video store downtown—not just a store with a room in the back for porno flicks like the one Sarah went to. Once there, she explained to the employees her father's predicament and asked for their help in finding her videos that had a plot—not just those gratuitous wham-bam-thank-you-ma'am flicks. The guys searched high and low and came up with six videos. She bought five, and they gave her one for free.

"My sister came home with the six videos and we were all giggling," Annie says. "We never talked about sex with my dad, it just wasn't on the menu. My mom wrapped each film in a plain brown paper and put a different bow on each one. Then she hid them all over the place throughout the house: under the pillow, in his sock drawer, on the counter next to the toilet.

"Dad would disappear and we'd hear him laughing because he had found another brown paper package," Annie continues. "It was a scream. That was a great moment. It became okay to know that Dad had a problem and we could all offer him support about it."

In the end, Sam's humor—a crucial coping mechanism when you've got cancer—was his saving grace. Even while in the midst of great pain, he retained his humor. Annie remembers that after the surgery, the colostomy, and everything that came with it, Sam kept the whole situation in perspective. "Well," he said, "No one can call me an asshole anymore!" Annie adds. "We just cracked up. I couldn't believe he said it."

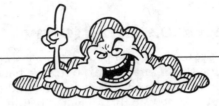

Funk-y Facts

Humor is a crucial coping mechanism when you've got cancer. A hearty laugh relaxes your diaphragm, exercises the lungs, and increases the blood's oxygen level. Studies show that laughter also physiologically reduces pain because of the change it produces in brain chemicals. Humor distracts and helps us reduce pain by redirecting our attention. Norman Cousins found that laughing for 10 minutes while watching *Candid Camera* reruns or *Marx Brothers* movies gave him two hours of pain-free sleep. Laughter is truly one of the best medicines, whether or not you're beating the Cancer Blues, so make sure you have some each day.

In fact the family feels so strongly about the presence of humor that Sarah has decided to fund a humor and educational library at one of the cancer clinics in their area. It will be filled with funny videos, books, and pamphlets, including the Norman Cousins books and the Bernie Siegel tapes in memory of Sam and to combat the memory of the many empty hours their family spent in their waiting room, battling their own version of the hospital blues.

The Hospital Blues: It's Not Just the Bad Food

Dr. Bernie Siegel reminds us that "hospital" evolved from the Latin word for "guest." Can you believe it? Is there a more inhospitable place than a hospital? It's not just the bad food, but often a bad attitude by an overworked staff and a feeling of death, not life. And then there's always that institutional waiting area where there's nothing to do but indulge in unhealthy behavior, like smoke, overeat, watch too much TV, or fight with loved ones to release stress. Just when you need the most support, you get the least. Instead, you're hit with a case of the hospital blues and feel worse and more out of control than when you came into the hospital. But it doesn't have to be that way.

Sam beat the hospital blues by becoming the CEO of his own health-care system. He and Sarah coordinated communication between specialists, learned everything possible at each stage of treatment, and were very proactive in developing partnerships with the various health-care providers. He took control over his treatment and stayed directly involved in the decision-making process.

For example, after Sam got the colostomy, he had to get checkups at the hospital regularly to determine whether there was any rise in cancer activity in his blood—which did rise over the course of the next five years. On the way to the hospital, Sam and Sarah would make notes and talk about what questions to ask the doctors and how to phrase the questions. The doctors, however, were simply not that forthcoming.

"The doctors were the best, but they think that their way is the only way," Sarah says. "Most of our visits to the hospital with the doctors were sparring matches. We wanted information and they didn't want to give it to us. Or maybe they thought we shouldn't know everything and they were just trying to protect us. It was hard to know and figure out."

It didn't take long for Sam and Sarah to figure where the real power was in the cancer unit—the nurse. "Exceptional people will be drawn to each other," Sarah continues. "The head nurse is an exceptional person and the three of us became friends. She could honestly answer questions that were puzzling us. She also helped Sam by telling him how he could take care of his feet, which hurt a lot, and what to do about the sores in his mouth from the chemo."

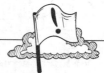

Blues Flag

To avoid the hospital blues, plan your hospital visit in advance and make sure you bring things with you that you enjoy, like a good book or a portable cassette player. Listening to a compelling book on tape can be a great distraction while waiting or during the ride to and from the hospital. Sometimes, Sam and Sarah listened to Hawaiian or country and western music on the way up to the hospital and back, because that kind of music was a "funky" family favorite and made Sam smile. Avoid the waiting area and head to the chapel, the outside grounds, or the cafeteria while waiting for your appointment. Frequent 10-minute walks outside are also mood boosters and stress reducers.

The High Road, the Low Road, or No Road at All

While continuing with the recommended medical treatment, Sam began to search for other roads to wellness. His cancer cells were returning, but the doctors didn't want to treat them aggressively with more chemotherapy for fear of the treatment's toxic effects. A friend of Sam's suggested he try *biofeedback*—a technique that allows a person to regulate his or her body's sensations. It worked for the friend to help him stop smoking.

Sam regained his spirits because he regained his control. "This was an option that was not invasive or chemical and it was another empowering thing he could do," Annie says. "It gave him a sense that he may be able to control what's going on. Doctors don't have all the answers. My dad was willing to beat it, however he could. Watching him was great. You just wanted to say: 'Go for it, it's cool.'"

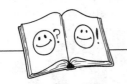

Terms of Encheerment

Biofeedback is a technique of monitoring the physiological system so a person can regulate certain body sensations. Through this technique, people learn, for instance, to tighten the muscles at the neck of their bladder so they can better control impaired bladder function. Biofeedback is often used with visual imagery and has been shown in research to reduce nausea and anxiety before, during, and after chemotherapy because it increases the person's feeling of control over his or her body.

Biofeedback taught Sam to become more aware of his body and to breathe deeply for relaxation. He put stickers all over the house and office that said "BREATHE!" to remind himself to slow down and take control. In a state of deep relaxation, he could visualize little Pac-Men eating up the bad guys (cancer cells). "He even had a dream about that," Sarah says. "I think his CEA went back down for a while."

Sarah says that, in retrospect, she wishes they had tried more alternative therapies—like yoga, acupuncture, massage, nutritional supplements, herbal medicine, tai chi—and working on balancing "chi." He did use some nutritional supplements and Sarah had him on a regimen of vitamins and minerals.

Had they tried more alternative healing roads, her family would be traveling in good company. In 1992, a Harvard Medical School study found that Americans in one year go more often to alternative practitioners than to traditional doctors; in the past year, over a third of the adult population has seen an alternative therapist.

These alternative mind-body therapies fall under two general categories:

➤ *Physical.* The body-centered therapies include deep relaxation, deep breathing, acupuncture, body manipulation, dance therapy, and massage—all of which relieve tension associated with anxiety.

➤ *Mental.* These exercises draw on the link between positive thoughts and healing so that you can change your perception of pain and improve your mood. Techniques like hypnosis, imagery, meditation, distraction, and music therapy all let you mentally rehearse uncomfortable situations until they feel less threatening.

Cancer Creates Closeness, If...

Cancer can break families apart or bring them closer together.

In Sam's family, everyone got closer (and remain closer to this day). Annie started working with her father to give him time off to do other activities and take care of his personal business. "My decision to help my dad was about wanting to get to know him as an adult. I admired him, and at that point I realized this was my opportunity. If you don't have something like this facing you it's easy to say, 'I'll get to him later,' and later never comes.

"Ironically, cancer is the worst and best thing that has ever happened to me," she adds. "A lot of things in my life wouldn't have happened if Dad didn't get cancer. I wouldn't have gotten help for my own depression and career problems." She also wouldn't have had the chance to have the heart-to-heart talks she finally had with her dad to iron out issues from the past that had been bothering her. Sam met with Annie and her sisters separately to talk about and resolve their relationships. "I have the conversation on tape," Annie muses, "I don't think I'll ever let them go. We didn't solve and resolve everything, but we started to, and that was enough for me to continue, even when he couldn't any longer."

Stay Connected: It's Never Too Late for a Party

Many people who get cancer isolate themselves by withdrawing from friends and family. While this is a natural reaction when the illness is first diagnosed, it will make the patient feel worse and may throw him into a major clinical depression later on. Sam rejected the blues; he kept up his social life until the end.

By October 1995, it was clear that Sam wasn't doing well. He was thinner and tired. Everyone knew that the time was near and they threw him a party to "celebrate" him. "He understood what we were doing," Annie says, "and we invited the people he wanted to see. He still rewrote our invitations to get the tone just the way he wanted it! People came down to spend time with him and he accepted them being there. It was just a really great day."

Sam also wanted one more chance to participate in a national meeting of one of his groups, and he managed to lead an all-day group through lunch. But shortly after, he was driven to the hospital, where he stayed for two nights.

Sam's Pilgrimage Ends on Thanksgiving

When it became clear to his family that the end was near, they wanted to take him home—that's where Sam said he wanted to die. Again, the doctors were against this plan, suggesting that he'd be more comfortable staying at the hospital, and that it would be easier on Sarah and their children. The family fought with the doctors and wouldn't take no for an answer. A doctor friend of the family called an ambulance to take Sam home.

People at the hospital said a tearful good-bye, and Sarah rode home with Sam in the ambulance—staying in touch with her children via cell phone. During the ride home, Sarah sang Sam all his favorite songs. Annie says, "I was talking to Mom, suggesting what other songs to sing to Dad. It was spooky how it all came together, how coordinated we all were, how it felt like a 'meant to be.'"

Within a certain window, people seem able to choose when they will die. Sam clearly thought so and he had no intention of ruining Thanksgiving for his family by dying on that day. So on this holiday, all of his relatives who had come to visit—including aunts, sisters, nephews—gathered around Sam, whose bed was placed in the living room in plain view of the Thanksgiving meal.

"We were ready to do whatever we could for him," says Annie, who explained they had hired hospice nurses—who were terrific—to administer pain medication and teach the family how to keep Sam comfortable. "So we had our Thanksgiving dinner with all the relatives, and Mom fed him sips of wine and little tastes of food. At one point my brother helped Dad out of his bed to walk him to the bathroom. When he came back, my brother had his arm under Dad's elbow to steer him back to bed. But Dad bolted across the living room to sit on the couch. I said, 'I guess you didn't want to go to bed Dad, did you?' He weakly and defiantly grinned. It was another little victory. We cried a lot that day, also we also laughed a lot. My younger sister couldn't leave his side. Not easy to watch."

Dr. Ellen Says

Families experiencing cancer often ask me: "How can we possibly manage this?" I tell them: "Fight the cancer *together*, communicate needs without judgment, and help the cancer patient gain and retain as much control and dignity as possible, even if it's over the tiniest details. Also, appreciate that everyone in the family will handle the crisis differently. And each person has something special and unique to contribute. Since nearly 25 percent of cancer patients succumb to clinical depression, so keep an eye out for the signs, and insist that your loved one get professional help if he or she seems depressed.

He spent a restless night with Sarah in the hospital bed with him, to comfort him as much as she could. And when the time came, the children and Sarah gathered next to him to support his letting go. Soon Sarah felt for his heartbeat and his breath faded away.

"We were all crying," Annie remembers. "We kissed him good-bye and kept saying good-bye and how much we loved him and to have a good trip. The hospice people had said we could keep him as long as we wanted (after he died). So we did. We cried and laughed and friends came to visit with us and with him all day and we remembered things and told stories. We all felt incredibly bonded. I'll never forget that feeling of intimacy and closeness and connection in and through Dad."

As sad as it was, the family felt relieved too. Says Annie: "We'd check in with each other and say, 'Do you feel okay?' and the person would say, 'I feel okay.'" It's been over two years now since Sam has died, and Sarah and the family still feel his spirit, as do I. Joining her father during his last moments of life was one of the best experiences Annie ever had. "If you can be there at the death, it's a good thing. It's one of the best things I've ever done. I felt so connected. It was like witnessing a birth, one of the most powerful moments in life."

It's been an honor and a privilege to learn how Sam Silverstein and his family beat the Cancer Blues, and I will always be deeply grateful that they allowed me to share some of their experience. They are one kind of cancer heroes. There are others out there too who we also need to visit because each hero is unique, and each cancer brings its own set of problems and life lessons.

Let's turn our attention now to two of the biggest killers of men and women, respectively: prostate cancer and breast cancer.

Prostate Cancer: A Gigantic Case of Denial

Denial kills.

And nowhere is this statement more true than in the case of men with prostate cancer. According to Dr. Barbara Rubin Wainrib and Dr. Sandra Haber, the authors of *Prostate Cancer: A Guide for Women and the Men They Love* (Dell, 1996), 43 percent of doctors surveyed by the American Medical Association in 1992 claimed that men with prostate cancer go untreated only because they don't want to bring it up with their doctors.

Even more shocking is that 85 percent of doctors surveyed said that even those men who do talk about prostate cancer aren't prepared to cope with it. Yet, this year alone, over 40,000 American men will die of prostate cancer and 175,000 new cases will be diagnosed. Men don't want to talk about prostate cancer because they can't deal with the thought of getting a disease that attacks their sexual capabilities and manhood. And our culture supports their denial because it's seen as so unmanly to have the "family jewels" threatened in such a awful way.

Another cancer hero is former U.S. Senate Majority Leader Bob Dole, who had prostate cancer in 1992. He shared his struggle and triumph with the public and helped bring prostate cancer out of the male closet. Other public figures have also gone all out on awareness campaigns alerting men to the importance of early detection. They have made it clear that the manly thing to do is to face your denial and probe that prostate whenever vulnerability appears.

Editor and writer Michael Korda recently wrote an excellent book on his experience with prostate cancer, called *Man To Man: Surviving Prostate Cancer* (Random House, 1996). In the book, he describes the ultimate macho denier, John Wayne, who bragged that his proudest achievement was that he had "licked the Big C." As Michael Korda explains: "Of course, he hadn't. The Big C came back and licked him, in the end. Nobody is a match for cancer, not even the Duke." But you have a good chance for recovery from prostate cancer if you don't let denial get in your way of detecting and fighting it.

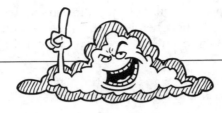

Funk-y Facts

When American writer Cornelius Ryan discovered he had prostate cancer in 1974, he started keeping a journal of his experiences, say Dr. Barbara Rubin Wainrib and Dr. Sandra Haber, authors of a very helpful book for those living with a cancer patient, *Prostate Cancer: A Guide for Women and the Men They Love* (Dell, 1996). "It served a therapeutic use," Ryan said. "To record unsettling thoughts and feelings in the journal, away from the presence of others, eased the awful feeling that I was under a sentence of death." His journal, the author continues, became *A Private Battle*, a best-seller, which was published by his wife after he died. Ryan's experience reminds us that writing out our feelings in a journal is one of the best ways to beat the Cancer Blues—or any kind of blues.

Breast Cancer Blues

Every woman is at risk of getting breast cancer, the leading cause of cancer death for women 15 to 52 years old. More than one in a half million women have been diagnosed with breast cancer, and another million have it but don't know it yet. However, despite the amount of press breast cancer has been getting, it is treated pretty much the same way it was 50 years ago.

Although there is no single cause for breast cancer, certain risk factors include age and family history of breast cancer. One in 200 women inherit the breast cancer gene and face up to an 80- to 90-percent risk of developing the disease. Researchers are getting close to figuring out which gene causes breast cancer, at which point the high-risk population will get genetic counseling.

Every day scientists are also discovering new preventive measures women can take to reduce the risk of getting breast cancer. Last year, a *New England Journal of Medicine* study revealed that women who exercise or have physically demanding jobs are less likely to develop breast cancer. The study was based on over 25,000 women for a period of 14 years. Those who exercised at least four hours a week had 37 percent less chance of getting breast cancer than those who watched TV or read in their spare time. The leanest women cut their risk by 72 percent if they exercised four or more times per week. This was one of the clearest studies showing the link between the increase in breast cancer and the lack of exercise.

The other clear link is between social support and breast cancer. If you've got breast cancer, one good way to beat the Cancer Blues is to join a support group. A landmark study conducted at Stanford University by Dr. David Spiegel showed that women with metastatic breast cancer who were in a support group lived nearly twice as long after the study began, and were much happier than those who did not belong to a support group.

Remember one of the primary action strategies to beat all of the blues: The more connected we are, the healthier we are? Well, it's never been more true than when you're trying to beat the Cancer Blues. Connect, connect, CONNECT! If there's a group, join it no matter how shy or reluctant you feel. Groups almost always help, yet sadly, only 10 percent of cancer patients participate in these support groups. If only they knew, they would consider a support group one of the most important medications they could take for treating their cancer. And support groups are very helpful to family members of cancer patients in beating the Cancer Blues and hospital blues.

Dr. Ellen Says

I urge my clients to get tested for breast and prostate cancer, but I also urge them to talk to their doctors about when to get tested and how often. I suggest you to stay on top of the emerging research on both prostate and breast cancer. Read up on these topics in health journals and magazines, call the American Cancer Society at (800) ACS-2345, or check out the Society's web site at http://www.cancer.org. For more resources, turn to Appendix B.

More Coping Strategies for Beating the Cancer Blues

Here are some additional coping strategies for beating any of the Cancer Blues:

➤ *Relaxation.* Being able to relax your body and mind is one of the most useful skills for dealing with stress and discomfort. Studies show that when you are relaxed you need less pain medication. Meditation, focused breathing, and deep breathing are all relaxation techniques.

➤ *Visualization/Imagery.* A mental process in which patients envision positive situations so they can improve their moods, attitudes, behaviors, and even physiological responses. Since the body doesn't know the difference between a real and an imagined response, positive visualization gives you more control over your mind and body. As one example, Dr. Bernie Siegel, author of *Love, Medicine and Miracles*, recommends that his cancer patients use imagery to "see" their immune systems defeating cancer cells.

➤ *Express your feelings.* Take time each day to explore your feelings and write them down in a journal. In one research study, breast cancer patients who expressed

Dr. Ellen Says

We don't know exactly what causes cancer, but we do know that certain attitudes and behaviors put us more at risk: depression, recent losses, too much change too fast, powerlessness, no emotional outlets, being too nice. The research backs this up. Depressed men in one study were two times more likely to get cancer than non-depressed men. In a study of identical twins, the twin with significant depression was the one likely to get cancer while the other stayed healthy. "Housewives get 54 percent more cancer than the general population and 157 percent more than women who work outside the home," according to Dr. Bernie Siegel, reporting on research from the University of Oregon. In the *Will to Live*, Arnold Hutschnecker summarized it when he wrote: "Depression is a partial surrender to death...cancer is despair experienced at the cellular level."

their fear, anger, depression, and guilt lived far longer than those who refused to feel or to deal with their feelings. Write about feelings in your journal, not just what happened during the day. And move from writing, which is associated with left-brain functioning, to drawing, which is right-brain–based, so you can see and understand your experience from all sides.

By the way, drawing (and it doesn't matter how it looks) is a very powerful way to beat the Cancer Blues. In one study of 200 cancer patients, the researchers could predict with 95 percent accuracy who would be dead in two months and who would experience remission, based on the patient's drawing. So get out those pens and markers, use color when you can, and draw anything you feel or think about your cancer experience. Stick figures and scribbles are fine—just show in pictures how you feel and don't rely solely on words to express yourself.

Caregivers Need Care Too

If you are taking care of someone who has cancer, you are probably tired, stressed out, scared, upset that you never do enough, and angry a lot of the time. You may resent the sick person because you have to take care of everything now, and feel guilt, depression, even physical illness.

It's crucial to recognize the importance of taking a break and resisting guilt for having these normal feelings. Action strategies that other cancer families have tried include delegating responsibilities to others, asking friends for support, and accepting that you can do only so much for your loved one.

Here are some additional tips for coping with cancer patients from two of the most knowledgeable psychologists I know, Dr. Sandra Haber and Dr. Barbara Wainrib, who specialize in working with cancer patients. More tips can be found in their book *Prostate Cancer: A Guide for Women and the Men They Love.*

1. Make a "goody contract" with yourself. Write a list of specific ways that you can treat yourself, and then commit to giving yourself at least one of these goodies a week.

2. Tune into parts of your body that are feeling tense and do something specific to relieve that tension. Ask a friend to give you a rubdown, get a professional massage, take an especially long, hot, luxurious bath or shower.

3. Eat something outrageous! Try an item from the exotic foods aisle of your supermarket or a comfort food from your childhood that you haven't had for years. Set a truly fantastic table or have a freestyle picnic on the floor.

4. If someone volunteers to do something, let that person do it. If a casual acquaintance suggests doing your laundry, say "Yes!"

5. Focus on the positive. Ask yourself, "What was the high point of the past week for me? How or why did I have that experience? Is there anything I can do to have the experience—or a similar one—again?"

When cancer strikes someone in the family, the entire family is stricken with the disease. Cancer changes more than cells—it changes hopes, dreams, relationships, and abilities. But the change does not have to be all bad, as the Silverstein family has shown us. In fact, they, and so many other cancer heroes, have taught us another critical life lesson: *It is possible to beat the Cancer Blues, whether or not you beat the cancer,* and the struggle makes life get richer rather than poorer for everyone involved.

The Least You Need to Know

➤ Research shows that having a positive outlook slows down the progression of cancer and makes a difference in the quality of a person's life.

➤ Patients who are considered difficult or uncooperative are often most likely to do well because they're the best fighters.

➤ Humor is a crucial coping mechanism to beat the Cancer Blues.

➤ Taking control of your medical condition will empower you.

➤ Prostate and breast cancer can be treated if detected early on.

➤ A good way to beat the Cancer Blues is to join a support group and exercise four times a week.

➤ Relaxation, visualization/imagery, biofeedback, and other techniques can help reduce the stress of being ill or caring for someone who is ill and improve your attitude about life.

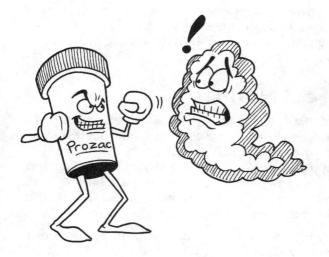

Chapter 23

Better Living Through Chemistry

In This Chapter

➤ Drugs that can actually chase away depression

➤ What are antidepressants, how do they work, and how can they work for you?

➤ The pros and cons of the "wonder drug" Prozac

➤ The terrific trio of neurotransmitters: serotonin, dopamine, and norepinephrine

➤ How tricycles, MAOIs, and SSRIs can keep depression away

Every morning it's the same thing. You drag yourself out of bed and dread everything about your day. You dread having to work, to socialize, to talk to your family. And when this dreadful feeling lasts more than two weeks, your doctor prescribes an antidepressant, but you don't want to take drugs because you're afraid you'll get addicted to them.

But there are drugs that don't make you high or low. They just make you feel normal. These kinds of drugs feed your brain vital chemicals it needs for you to feel good and for your brain to function effectively when stress has worn it out. These drugs are called antidepressants, and they really do produce "better living through chemistry" for those who need them.

In this chapter, we'll talk about some of these drugs and how they work. We'll also describe the different types of medication available today. The good news is this:

If there were ever a "good" time to experience depression—this is it! Scientists are hard at work coming up with better medications all the time so that no matter how depressed you feel, if you keep working at it, you can find the right answers for your mind and body and live better through chemistry!

Drugs That Make You Feel Normal

I would be the last person to suggest that you take drugs—unless you *really* need them. And some people *really* do need antidepressants to get well. Now I know some of you may be saying: "Yeah, yeah, yeah! I won't go near that junk, no matter what that nutsy Dr. Ellen says. You hear about people goin' off the deep end on this stuff all the time." I used to think like that too. I thought I really would be nutsy Dr. Ellen if I encouraged my therapy clients to work with a physician for antidepressants. I thought we could fix whatever was wrong through therapy. I was wrong. Really wrong.

What I didn't know and what is very hard to learn is how deeply the mind and body are connected when you have the blues and depression. When the mind is blue, it makes the brain blue and vice versa. So it makes sense that if the brain is drained of "feel-good" chemicals, there's no way you can feel good with any amount of therapy until the brain is filled up again.

So how do you know if you or someone you love needs these drugs? In Chapter 2, you took a quiz to determine whether the feelings of sadness, anxiety, and frustration you or a loved one are experiencing are the result of everyday blues or depression. If it's just a funk, the self-help exercises in this book will help you or your loved one beat the blues.

But if you're clinically depressed, then it's very important that you get help from a psychologist, social worker, psychiatrist, or other mental health practitioner who specializes in the treatment of depression. (See Chapter 9 for a discussion of therapy options.) The best treatment for depression involves some type of talk therapy, often combined with the use of *antidepressants*: drugs that balance the chemicals in your brain responsible for controlling behavior and mood.

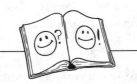

Terms of Encheerment

Antidepressants are prescription medications that help depleted mood chemicals in the brain return to normal, balanced levels.

Most therapists work closely with a psychiatrist or family physician to find the antidepressant that's best for you. The client, therapist, and psychiatrist keep talking with each other and experimenting until they find which medicine works for you.

One antidepressant you've probably heard mentioned is Prozac, because that was one of the first of a new class of antidepressants (called Selective Serotonin Reuptake Inhibitors or SSRIs) that treats depression with the fewest side effects. The bloom is off the rose on Prozac and the other common SSRIs (Paxil and Zoloft), however, because of the sexual dysfunction that some people experience when they are taking these drugs.

These side effects are troublesome, for sure, but when you consider that depression is a life-threatening illness, some side effects may be worth it. The bottom line is these medicines can save your life or the life of someone you love. Learn about antidepressants if you have any vulnerability to depression, because your life may depend on it.

And, don't worry, you're not stuck giving up your sex life, either. There are over 20 medications on the market that help alleviate depression, and various combinations can reduce or eliminate side effects.

Antidepressant News You Can Use

When the chemicals in your brain are in balance, so are you—you feel happy, energized, and hopeful. When these brain chemicals are out of balance, you feel unhappy, tired, and despairing, no matter what you try to do to help yourself feel better.

So if you are depressed, and you have been in therapy for three months or more, then you probably need an antidepressant as well as therapy. If you think or talk about suicide or have wanted to try it, then you need an antidepressant because you have a serious clinical depression. You can feel great relief from taking antidepressants—and today, there are many to choose from. Many of the newer ones (such as Prozac, Zoloft, Paxil, Serzone, and Wellbutrin) have fewer side effects and are easy to take, so you are more likely to stick with them until they effectively treat your condition.

Nearly all antidepressants have about the same cure rate and people usually fall into one of two groups:

➤ *The Buster Category.* Sixty to 70 percent of all patients taking antidepressants report significant improvement in their mood, which, in clinical terms, means that they experience less than half as many symptoms as they did without the drugs. A lucky few bust through their depression in one to two months and lose all their symptoms. For most people in this category the change is more gradual but eventually most or all of the depression symptoms recede, if the person is also in therapy at the same time they are taking medication.

➤ *The Bummer Category.* About a third of the people who try antidepressants find they do not work. Then we move into a complicated phase of trial and error, with various combinations of drugs and talk therapy, until we find something that works. If you hang in there long enough, you and your physician will almost always find a recipe that works.

Most people get prescriptions for antidepressants from their general practitioners, since these are the doctors they go to first when something is wrong and they aren't feeling well. Once your doctor rules out physical problems, she may ask you questions about your mental health and then suggest you take antidepressants. Although your family doctor will likely have some basic knowledge about how antidepressants work, the real experts in the field are psychiatrists or psychopharmacologists—a fancy name for a medical specialist who studies a drug's effect on the brain. Many of these medical specialists study the effects of antidepressants on the behavior of depressed people and examine how the naturally occurring substances within the brain, like serotonin, affect the part of the brain that deals with emotions and regulates our mood. They can help you find what works for your particular chemistry.

These experts—who will work directly with your family doctor or your mental health professional—are particularly helpful if the first antidepressant you took didn't work and you are having trouble finding the right medication. They've successfully treated hundreds of patients with different drug combinations, fine-tuning dosages and tinkering with regimens, until they come up with what works.

Dr. Ellen Says

Be a CEO and take charge of your own health care. If you're not satisfied with your doctor's opinion or if your general practitioner refuses to try a different antidepressant after the first one didn't work well, ask to see a psychiatrist or psychopharma-cologist who specializes in the treatment of depression. Many physicians won't refer out to mental health professionals, so insist on it if you are not happy with the treat-ment you're getting, or turn to other medical practitioners for suggestions on whom they recommend you see. There are drugs that will treat your particular brain chemistry, but you need to work with an expert to find them.

Finding the Right Rx: If at First You Don't Succeed...

A psychiatrist or pharmacologist will be in a better position than a general practitioner to suggest which drug you should try first. But identifying the right antidepressant is an art, not a science. Experts say that up to 40 percent of the people don't respond to the first drug that's prescribed to them.

And please don't despair if the first drug did little for you but give you a headache or nausea! I've seen this happen many times to men and women in my practices in both New York and California. Seeing these effects so often has made me deeply respect how each of us is different in the make-up of our brain chemistry and how these differences must be respected. Depression medication is one place you can bet that one size does *not* fit all. For example, women and certain ethnic groups respond differently from Caucasian males to antidepressants, and they need a different dosage.

The chances that you'll respond to the second antide-pressant prescribed are 50-50. The 20 percent of those who still don't respond after the second attempt can still get a shot at beating depression because a combination of drugs that your doctor prescribes usually does the trick.

Clients who don't respond to the first or second drug often become disillusioned and feel hopeless, which only makes them feel more depressed. But when they come across the right antidepressant, their whole outlook changes. Once they are on the right medication, they can think more clearly, take charge of their lives, and use talk therapy far more effectively.

So hang in there and never stop believing that you can and will feel better!

Prozac Country: Why Doctors Often Start Out with Prozac

Doctors often start by prescribing Prozac—a member of the Selective Serotonin Reuptake Inhibitors (SSRIs) drug group. These drugs are easier to take than the older antidepressants, because the dose regimen is easy to follow, and they have fewer side effects than antidepressants on the market. Many of the older drugs required the patient to take anywhere between one to 12 tablets a day. At least one-half of the new antidepressants require patients to take only one pill a day. Prozac is the best known antidepressant and for most people the one that has the fewest initial side effects.

Antidepressants' Lag Time and Side Effects

Although antidepressants have improved greatly over the past two decades, they are still far from perfect. The major problem is still lag time. It can take these drugs anywhere between three to six weeks to achieve full effect; but I have seen people start to feel better right away. Doctors will encourage you to continue taking the drug during the start-up period to see if the drug works, even if the side effects are bothersome. When you're depressed to begin with, it's no fun walking around feeling nauseous, spaced-out, and lethargic. But the good news is that these side effects usually disappear within a few days to a week, so the wait is easier to tolerate.

Those who are severely depressed and can't function—that is, they can't get out of bed, go to work, or take care of their families—need medication that will take hold right away. So far, no one medication has been proven to act any faster than any other. It just takes the brain some time to adjust to the change and absorb the new chemicals that antidepressants provide. Working with a therapist is especially helpful at this phase of treatment, because the therapist tells you what to expect and offers hope and support.

Even the wonder drug Prozac can't perform miracles—but the help provided by close, supportive relationships can make all the difference.

The other major problem with the antidepressants is side effects. The most common antidepressant side effects I've seen in my clients over 20 years of practice include the following:

➤ *Headaches*. This is the most common symptom I hear about; taking an over-the-counter pain reliever such as aspirin usually brings relief.

➤ *Trouble sleeping or sleeping too much*. This is the second most common symptom. You may have trouble going to sleep or find you have to take a nap in the afternoon—you hit a "wall of tiredness" and can't function until you sleep.

➤ *Feeling restless or antsy.* This is not the energizing kind, but an uncomfortable, hyper feeling.

➤ *Constipation or diarrhea.* A product like Ex-Lax or Pepto-Bismol will bring relief.

➤ *Dry mouth.* Try chewing gum or sucking on hard candy to release more saliva.

➤ *Weight loss/gain.* Some people gain or lose a few pounds (but they don't lose enough for this to be considered a weight loss aid—darn!).

➤ *Skin rashes.* One client had a red rash crawl up her arm and down into places we can't mention. Hydrocortisone may bring some relief.

➤ *Sexual dysfunction.* Some men report having trouble with erections and ejaculations, while some women experience trouble having orgasms and may lose interest in sex.

With this many side effects, it's easy to see that these drugs have not hit the miracle category yet. The side effects also make most of us wonder how these drugs really work and why there are still so many problems with them. But even with these side effects it's worth trying out medications if you need them because they're the best thing we've got to relieve clinical depression.

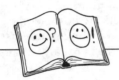

Terms of Encheerment

Neurotransmitters are chemicals in the brain and nervous system that carry messages across the gaps between neurons. The three main neurotransmitters involved in the development of depression are serotonin, dopamine, and norepinephrine. Depressed people have a significant depletion of these chemicals in the brain. The antidepressants restore these neurotransmitters to the level they should be so you can feel good again.

The Three Stooges: When Chemicals in the Brain Go Nuts

Scientists aren't sure how antidepressants work—the more we learn about the brain, the less we know and the more complicated its inner workings seem. We do know that antidepressants correct a chemical imbalance in the brain. The medication elevates the numbers of *neurotransmitters*—chemicals in the nervous system that carry messages throughout the cells—which are responsible for fighting depression and producing a good mood.

There are over 100 different kinds of neurotransmitters in our bodies. Three seem especially crucial to our well-being (aren't you glad you have to learn about only three of them?) These are:

➤ Serotonin

➤ Dopamine

➤ Norepinephrine

When we feel depressed, we don't have enough of these chemicals circulating through our brain and the shortage of this good stuff affects our sleep, appetite, mood, and sexual interest. We become grumpy, worn down, and anxious—and are not happy campers under any circumstances.

More specifically, this is what happens when our brain chemistry is out of whack:

➤ When you have low levels of serotonin, you are likely to experience mild to major depression, aggression, violence, and, in extreme cases, you may even have thoughts of suicide. Several autopsy studies have shown that the levels of serotonin are significantly lower in the brains of people who committed suicide than in normal brains. When your brain's serotonin is replenished, you feel better overall—more confident, focused, and relaxed.

➤ When you're low on dopamine, you're down and out. You feel lethargic, weak, and have trouble paying attention and focusing. Once the levels are back up, you regain a sense of strength, focus, energy, and personal power.

➤ Having too little norepinephrine will make your brain work more slowly, so you won't be able to think quickly on your feet. This chemical is necessary for all muscle activity.

The Booming Market for Depression-Busters

Today, there are three major classes of antidepressants, as well as new individual ones that are in a league of their own. Each type of medication affects the different neurotransmitter systems in different ways. The three classes are:

1. *Tricyclics.* These are the older class of antidepressants that boost our neurotransmitters by blocking their reabsorption. The problem is tricyclics are nonspecific, so they are not generally as effective as antidepressants, such as SSRIs, that target specific neurotransmitters.

2. *Monoamine Oxidase Inhibitors (MAOIs).* These are our heroes, the freedom fighters, that keep up the count of the three neurotransmitters affecting depression by destroying the nasty enzymes that burn up these crucial chemicals.

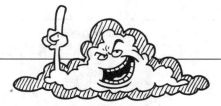

Funk-y Facts

Before researchers developed antidepressants, drugs that improved emotion and behavior came about by sheer chance. The antituberculosis agent Iproniazid, for instance, elevated the moods of people with tuberculosis, so the drug was given to psychiatric patients in 1957. Shortly after, monoamine oxidase inhibitors (MAOIs) were introduced to the public as a treatment for depression, but they carried so many dietary restrictions in their use that they were never that popular.

3. *Selective Serotonin Reuptake Inhibitors (SSRIs).* Prozac, Paxil, and Zoloft are in this class—they work by interfering with the reabsorption of mainly serotonin, ensuring that more of that neurotransmitter remains in the brain.

Tricyclics: Traditional Depression-Busters

Tricyclics are among the oldest antidepressants on the market. Until this class of medications was developed, psychiatrists treating severely depressed patients had three choices: prescribe amphetamines, give electroshock treatment, or admit the patients to psychiatric hospitals or keep them in such places as described in the movie *Snake Pit* or the more recent movie *One Flew Over the Cuckoo's Nest*. The tricyclics offered a far more attractive option than the snake or cuckoo approach to depression treatment.

These drugs beef up the brain's supply of norepinephrine and serotonin and have been used to cure other conditions such as panic attacks, migraine headaches, chronic pain, and bulimia. Although the drugs are still effective, they are not exact in the areas they target, so many physicians and psychiatrists prescribe them only if the newer ones have too many side effects or just don't work.

Tricyclics have the general side effects we have already described and can speed up your heart rate by 20 or more beats for minutes. They can lower your blood pressure and in extreme cases, significantly contribute to suicidal feelings. The following table lists some tricyclics. If your doctor prescribes a drug from this list, make sure you thoroughly discuss the possible side effects with him.

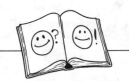

Terms of Encheerment

Tricyclics are a class of traditional drugs that treat depression by blocking the reabsorption of several different neurotransmitters and thereby raising their level so the brain can use them to produce positive moods.

Tricyclics

Generic Name	Brand Name
Imipramine	Tofranil
Amitriptyline	Elavil
Trimipramine	Surmontil
Doxepin	Sinequan
Amoxapine	Asendin
Clomipramine	Anafranil
Desipramine	Norpramin
Nortriptyline	Aventyl, Pamelor
Protriptyline	Vivactil
Maprotiline	Ludiomil

The Makings of MAOIs

Soon after the tricyclics were developed, scientists came up with another class of antidepressant—*Monoamine Oxidase Inhibitors* or MAOIs (try saying that three times really fast, or even just once!). These drugs stop the enzyme monoamine oxidase from breaking down the three neurotransmitters that we need for well-being—serotonin, dopamine, and norepinephrine—so each of them rises and keeps our brain happy.

MAOIs aren't likely to be your doctor's first choice of antidepressants either because of their possible side effects, which include the usual ones previously described and one really juicy one: There are certain foods you can't eat if you're on an MAOI. According to Dr. Ronald Fieve in his book *Prozac* (Avon Books, 1994), these include cheese, Chianti wine (darn), yogurt, lima beans, pickled herring, smoked meats, liver, and large amounts of caffeine or chocolate.

These foods contain a chemical called tyramine, which interacts with the MAOI, that can cause a rapid rise in blood pressure so fast the blood vessels in the brain can burst, causing a stroke or occasionally death. This gruesome process has the weird name of the "cheese effect" and while very rare, it does happen, so watch what you eat if your doctor prescribes one of the following MAOIs for you.

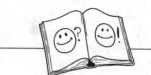

Terms of Encheerment

Monoamine Oxidase Inhibitors (MAOIs) are a class of antidepressants that stop the enzyme monoamine oxidase from breaking down, which boosts the levels of serotonin, dopamine, and norepinephrine in the brain and improves mood.

Monoamine Oxidase Inhibitors

Generic Name	Brand Name
Phenelzine	Nardil
Tranylcypromine	Parnate

SSRIs Win the Gold for Least Side Effects

Scientists hit the jackpot when they developed the *Selective Serotonin Reuptake Inhibitors (SSRIs)*. Prozac and the other drugs in this class (see the following table) are popular because they have fewer side effects than the older antidepressants and you don't have to watch what you eat like you do with the MAOIs.

When developing the drugs, scientists were able to zero in on serotonin alone without affecting any other chemicals in the brain. Older antidepressants, on the other hand, have more side effects because they use a kind of shotgun effect to achieve chemical balance in the brain. At the expense of interfering with neurotransmitters, the older antidepressants hit receptor sites all over the brain, and their impact is less specific.

Selective Serotonin Reuptake Inhibitors

Generic Name	Brand Name
Fluvoxamine Maleate	Luvox
Paroxetine	Paxil
Fluoxetine	Prozac
Sertraline	Zoloft

An SSRI alters serotonin balance, and in so doing is involved in controlling aggression, sexual functioning, and maintenance of mood. About 60 to 70 percent of depressed people who are taking Prozac or another SSRI will experience remission within two to six weeks; the rest either can't deal with the side effects of the first few days or just don't respond to the drug.

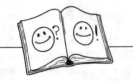

Terms of Encheerment

Selective Serotonin Reuptake Inhibitors (SSRIs) are one of the newest classes of antidepressants—including Prozac, Zoloft, and Paxil—that improve mood by blocking the reabsorption of serotonin in the brain that causes depression. They have fewer side effects, overall, than any of the other existing antidepressants at this time.

This class of drugs has been used to successfully treat depression and a host of other conditions, including:

➤ Panic disorders

➤ Social phobias

➤ Obsessive-compulsive disorder

➤ Bulimia and other eating disorders

➤ Impulsive behavior disorder

Studies show that SSRIs are ideal for people who have a variety of depressive illnesses and are especially helpful in tackling depression in its early stages, before the condition takes root. According to Carol Turkington and Eliot F. Kaplan, authors of *Making the Prozac Decision* (Lowell House, 1995), SSRIs work so well that doctors may someday start recommending early screening for depression, like they do for breast cancer and high blood pressure.

Prozac: First SSRI to Reach Market, Not Necessarily Best

Even though Prozac is only one of the SSRIs, it's the best known antidepressant because it was the first to hit the market and be marketed successfully. Millions of people heard about and marveled at the potential benefits of this wonder drug—so much so that even those who weren't depressed wondered if they should take it, too, so they can become, in the words of Dr. Peter Kramer, author of *Listening to Prozac* (Penguin, 1997) "better than well."

Some people who take Prozac may feel "better than well," especially at first, as the serotonin levels begin to rise. And sometimes people feel like different people when their depression is lifted. But eventually they realize that this positive feeling is simply a natural part of feeling good, not a lobotomy or personality transformation. The medication won't eliminate your problems—you will still be the same you, warts and beauty marks and all—but it will help you better cope with these problems. But although Prozac is among the first antidepressants doctors will write a prescription for, it isn't always the best for everyone. Some people don't respond well to Prozac and need to try other antidepressants.

The Pits About Prozac

Prozac has its drawbacks. Like all antidepressants, it has some side effects, including nausea, insomnia, anxiety, and sexual dysfunction. The latter is the number one reason people stop taking Prozac. It is now estimated that nearly 30 to 50 percent of those who take the drug experience some sexual difficulty, decrease in sexual desire, and absence of orgasms. However, experts say that many of these side effects can disappear after the person gets used to the drug.

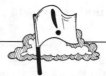

Blues Flag

Experts warn people NOT to take Prozac or other SSRIs with MAOIs (Nardil, Marplan, or Parnate) because this combination could be very dangerous—involving vomiting, high blood pressure, shock, and even death. Follow your doctor's instructions. Wait at least two weeks after taking an MAOI before you start on Prozac, and at least five weeks after taking Prozac before you start on a MAOI.

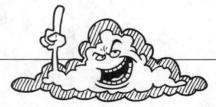

Funk-y Facts

Current research, some of it conducted by drug companies, suggests that people taking Prozac have less suicidal risks than people taking some of the older antidepressants. Reason: People can't commit suicide by overdosing on Prozac as easily as they could by taking an overdose of the older antidepressants.

Another drawback to the drug Prozac is cost, which can average about $1.50 per capsule. All SSRIs are more expensive because their patents are still in force and they have are no generic versions as there are for the old antidepressants, whose patents have expired. Many insurance companies cover all medications except for those affecting mental health, and many others only pay for generic drugs.

Another problem is the length of time the drug stays in the body. It takes Prozac up to six weeks to leave your body after you stop taking it. So if you have an adverse reaction to this medication, you're basically stuck with some lousy feelings for a month or so after your last dose; but usually the symptoms are not serious or that much of a hassle and they fade away.

New Drugs on the Horizon

The future holds bright promise for treatment of depression. Every year, more scientists are hard at work trying to find new drugs that can treat depression. In addition to the tricyclics, MAOIs, and SRRIs, there are four other antidepressants currently available. Each has its benefits and drawbacks—and each will give people who can't tolerate or can't be helped by SSRIs another shot at well-being. These include:

➤ *Wellbutrin.* This drug works really well for some clients and not at all for others.

➤ *Effexor.* This is a very effective drug, but be careful if you have high blood pressure. You'll need to monitor your pressure more than usual.

➤ *Serzone.* This drug is sometimes called son of Deseryl, and like its papa, can make some clients mighty sleepy; other clients couldn't feel better.

➤ *Remerson.* This is another promising drug; it's still too new to evaluate its side effects.

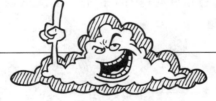

Funk-y Facts

The United States system of drug approvals is among the toughest in the world and companies cough up about $359 million to bring a drug to market, according to authors *of Making the Prozac Decision.* It takes companies about 12 years to get an experimental drug approved by the FDA.

No Shame/No Blame: When to Start and Stop the Meds

Just how long should you be taking any of these drugs? The length of treatment is a controversial subject. Many people are told to take antidepressants for at least six months to a year after the end of a depressive episode, tapering off the dosage over several weeks. But, increasingly, some experts suggest that recurrent depressions are chronic—if you've had more than one episode, chances are you'll have many more—so you're probably better off going on and off antidepressants for the rest of your life, as soon as you start to experience the symptoms of a clinical depression again.

Don't quit too soon. It's important to take the antidepressants for the full course of treatment. And *always* discuss going on or off the medication with your doctor!

Research shows that 70 percent of patients who stop taking their meds too early (five weeks or less after their symptoms stop), become depressed again. The relapse rate drops to 14 percent among people who continue taking them at for at least five months after the signs of depression have abated. And yet other studies find that the longer patients are on antidepressants, the less likely they'll be to get depressed again.

If you do get off the meds and find that you're getting depressed again, don't beat yourself up. Needing medication is not a sign of weakness—it's a sign of strength, courage, and the will to lead a happier, healthier life. And don't make the mistake I did, thinking I or my clients were not "sick" enough to take these medications. It has nothing to do with being sick or weak. It has to do with a chemical imbalance in the brain that isn't your fault. So if you and your doctor agree that's the way to go, reach for the chemical support if you get caught in the grip of a real depression.

The Least You Need to Know

➤ Today, there are about 20 antidepressants on the market; many of the newer ones have few side effects and are easy to take.

➤ While your family doctor has some knowledge of antidepressants and can write the prescription, see a psychiatrist or psychopharmacologist for an expert opinion if you have any questions on dosage or combining medications.

➤ Identifying the right antidepressant is an art, not a science. About 40 percent of the people who take antidepressants don't respond to the first drug, but they have a 50–50 chance of doing well on the second drug.

➤ Tricyclics, MAOIs, and SSRIs are antidepressants that boost the level of one or more of the neurotransmitters (serotonin, dopamine, and norepinephrine) in your brain, fighting off depression.

➤ Prozac gets more attention than the rest of the SSRIs because it was the first drug of its kind to hit the market and be marketed successfully to mainstream America.

➤ Research shows that 70 percent of patients who stop taking their meds too early can have a relapse and become depressed all over again, sometimes more severely.

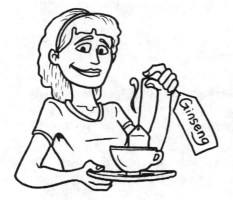

Chapter 24

Let Mother Nature Help: Natural Therapies for the Blues

> **In This Chapter**
>
> ➤ Boomers and seniors bloom on the new kind of weed
>
> ➤ St. John's Wort is "nature's Prozac"
>
> ➤ So few side effects, so many benefits
>
> ➤ How St. John's Wort can take the place of an antidepressant in some cases
>
> ➤ Taking care against drug interactions
>
> ➤ The benefits of ginseng, ginkgo biloba, and other unpronounceable herbs

If you'd have asked me 15 years ago whether I'd ever consider taking a shrubby wild herb to treat my own blues and depression, I would have gulped and said: "Me, do you think I'm *that* crazy?" After all, I was supposed to be a respected, educated psychologist who meticulously footnoted all my journal articles, spoke before hundreds of other colleagues at symposiums, and scoured through publications in hopes of finding new drug treatments for depression signed, sealed, and delivered by the FDA. Herbs were for the birds, as far as I was concerned.

Well, now I have to "eat crow"—I've become one of the growing millions of Americans and Europeans who are joining the Asian cultures to see medicinal herbs in a new light. Believe me, I was *very* skeptical when I first tried St. John's Wort—the herb that has been proven to treat the blues and mild to moderate depression in ways similar to Prozac and other antidepressants. But after six weeks, I was sold on the herb!

The herb took away my lows but not the highs, and it's provided me with a safety net for my moods so I don't crash into the dark pit of depression like I used to. And the best part was that I didn't have the drowsy, doped-up feeling I had when I was taking

Prozac, I could buy it off the shelf at a health food store, and I didn't have to lose my shirt to be able to afford the medicine!

You are probably thinking, "Dr. Ellen really is crazy. She's selling out to a fad!" But herbal medicines are not fads. In fact, they are becoming so mainstream that you can find them in any health food store or supermarket.

In this chapter, I'd like to share with you my experience with St. John's Wort—what is now generally known as "nature's Prozac"—and give you the latest information on the herbs du jour that treat anxiety, enhance memory, boost your immune system, and address other popular concerns.

But before we get started, a couple of caveats: I am not any kind of expert on medicinal herbs and their uses. In terms of my training as a psychologist, herbal remedies are considered outside my area of expertise. My knowledge is based on reports I've read about St. John's Wort and other herbs, the experiences of my clients who take these remedies, and my own mood change since I've been taking these herbs to beat my blues and depression.

Educating yourself regarding alternative medicines can be a very helpful action strategy to beat the blues. But I urge you to consult your doctor before taking any of these remedies and stay connected with her or him throughout the course of your experience. Natural or not, these are mood-altering substances, so you need to be careful using them.

Also, it's very important to remember that although St. John's Wort is often called nature's Prozac, it is recommended only for the blues and mild to moderate depression, *not* significant clinical depressions or if you're feeling suicidal or vegetative (you've become such a big couch potato you can't function in regular life). For severe depression it's recommended that you use a prescription antidepressant until the clinical depression has lifted (as we discuss in the previous chapter). Sadly, Mother Nature doesn't seem quite strong enough to successfully battle the enormous dark force of the clinical depressions.

From Beatlemania to Vitamania: Americans Go Botanical

Walk up and down the aisles of a health food store (don't be turned off by the smell—it's simply Mother Nature's B.O.!) and you'll see rows and rows of minerals, vitamins, and herbal medicines jumping off the shelf. One promises you a stronger heart, another a longer life, the third provides better moods, less stress, enhanced memory, heightened sexual powers—everything but the kitchen sink and someday they might throw in one of those too.

Wake up America, and smell the herbs!

"Vitamania," as some critics call it, is sweeping the country, as everybody and their brother is buying vitamins and minerals. The herbal business is booming. Last year, sales of dietary supplements—including herbal products such as vitamins, minerals, and amino acids—were estimated to be $11.8 billion, and that number is growing at a rate of 8 to 10 percent annually, according to *Nutrition Business Journal*.

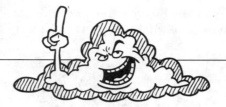

Funk-y Facts

Mother Nature recently gave me a terrible surprise and later came to the rescue. Pushing me into menopause early was her terrible trick. My body began to rock and roll with flashes and memory lapses. A friend, Dr. Robert Portman, had started a natural therapies company called Pacific Health Laboratories. He urged me to try their new product called *ProSol Plus*, a combination of St. John's Wort, gingko biloba, and other vitamins. Because I trust his quality control, I followed his advice, although skeptically. To my amazement, my mood lightened (the St. John's Wort), I could remember things again (the gingko biloba), my energy increased, and I was able to sleep better than I had in months (the way all the herbs interact). If you want more information about ProSol Plus, see their Web site at http://www.prosolplus.com or visit the General Nutrition Center (GNC) in your community.

What's spurring the botanical growth: baby boomers who are seeking to live longer and better. They are enthusiastically embracing alternative medicine to find answers that traditional science has failed to provide. In fact, the *Journal of the American Medical Association* (JAMA) reports that 40 percent of Americans now use alternative medicine to treat a variety of illnesses and to maintain their general health and well-being.

Americans are just now discovering what Europeans have known for centuries. Well, it's about time! We may be the most technologically advanced nation in the world, but we're practically clueless about the medicinal power of plants growing right under our feet! And it's not like we haven't had time to study them—these plants have been around for thousands of years.

The herb that has received the most attention is St. John's Wort (or Hypericum). This herb has provided relief for millions of Americans suffering from mild depression who can't stand the antidepressant drugs they've been taking or who haven't tried anything at all because they're afraid of medication or feel ashamed to be depressed—and they don't want anybody, including their doctors,

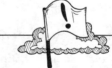

Blues Flag

DO NOT take St. John's Wort if you suffer from severe depression. If you aren't sure whether what you are feeling is a clinical depression or just the blues, take the quiz in Chapter 2 to find out and consult with a psychologist or psychiatrist. Research shows that St. John's Wort works effectively to treat mild to moderate depression—not major depression.

to know. The many folks who have tried the antidepressants and been turned off by all the side effects have been a vital and growing force in the acceptance of these natural therapies.

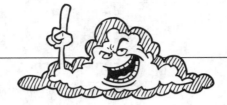

Funk-y Facts

Herbal medicines in Germany are so popular that they now account for 30 percent of all the over-the-counter (OTC) health products purchased there, according to the *Financial Times*. One reason for their popularity: People can buy them off the shelf without a prescription and avoid having to rush to the doctor every time they have a minor ailment. Germany has also taken the lead in researching Hypericum (St. John's Wort)—the herb that has been proven to treat mild to moderate depression. In fact, Hypericum products account for more than 50 percent of the German antidepressant market. It's hard to believe, but "nature's Prozac" beats synthetic Prozac in German sales for those who no longer want to bear the blues.

Terms of Encheerment

St. John's Wort is an herb that has been proven effective in treating mild to moderate depression—as successful as prescription antidepressants in most patients. St. John's Wort is the most extensively researched and used herbal antidepressant known. It has no real reported side effects beyond the potential sun-sensitivity for some people and occasional reports of mild headaches, nausea, or tiredness, which seem to quickly dissipate.

The Wonders of St. John's Wort

Almost everyone has heard of *St. John's Wort*. (For those of you who haven't, I'll give you a hint: It's not a new line of make-up or a drug that gets rid of small rounded protuberances on your face.) This medicinal herb has been written up in hundreds of magazines, discussed on TV shows, and talked about at parties because of its effective treatment of mild depression.

News about this herb's effectiveness doesn't come from just accounts of a bunch of scraggly, laid-back hippies still stuck in the '60s, smoking that other kind of weed. Bona-fide medical studies have shown that people with mild to moderate depression who took St. John's Wort reported fewer symptoms and a feeling of well-being— and had virtually none of the side effects that many patients get when they take chemical antidepressants.

Interestingly, about a hundred years ago, it was reported that sheep and cattle who overdosed on St. John's Wort became photosensitive and died of sunburn. Since no human has yet binged on the herb and had his or her sunblock fail, St. John's Wort seems to be a safe alternative for beating the blues.

In 1996, the *British Medical Journal* summarized the findings of 23 well-designed studies regarding St. John's Wort. There were over 1,700 people in these studies, which is 1,500 to 1,600 more subjects than are typically used in drug studies in the U.S. What did all the studies show? St. John's Wort works just as well as antidepressants—that is, 50 to 80 percent of mildly depressed people who take it feel better. And it affects the brain in much the same way antidepressants do, by blocking the breakdown of key neurotransmitters like serotonin, but it seems to do it in a gentler, more natural manner.

It's hard to believe: Scientists have labored in their labs for decades to find medication that treats depression, companies have spent millions of dollars doing research and testing the drugs so they can safely be brought to market—and here is this wild weed that ranchers in the Northwest tried to kill because they considered it a pest. And that pesky weed can do the job just as well if not better than the products of all those laboratories.

And you don't even have to go to your doc to get it! You have a different ally this time around: Mother Nature and her power to beat the blues.

It's easy to see why the news of St. John's Wort spread like wildfire. In 1997, in fact, St. John's Wort got such good press for treating mild to moderate depression that it moved from the 100th to the fifth best-selling herb in the nation in only a few years. No wonder so many are courting the wort!

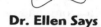

Dr. Ellen Says

St. John's Wort is the most extensively researched and used herbal antidepressant—and it looks like it may become a major option for treating mild to moderate depression, which can feel like long-term, low-grade blues. This herbal medicine is already benefiting many of the 18 million Americans who are depressed—12 million of whom had not been getting any treatment of any kind.

The Wort's Humble Beginnings

But where does this beautiful herb with such an ugly name come from? ("Wort," by the way, is an archaic word for "plant.")

St. John's Wort comes from a weed with bright yellow flowers that grows wild in the northwestern United States and much of Europe. When the black dots from the flower petals are squeezed, a red liquid is released, which represents the blood of St. John, according to the ancient stories. It typically starts blooming around June 25, during the traditional celebration of St. John's Day, hence its name. But its use dates back to ancient Greece (doesn't everything?) when Hippocrates administered it to treat many illnesses, including wounds, lung ailments, and depression. In the Middle Ages it was used as a tea to exorcise the demons and witches who were believed to control the soul of a depressed individual.

An ancient poem tells us how to harness the wort's power against witches (see how helpful I can be)? The poem is repeated in Dr. Steven Bratman's excellent book, *Beat Depression with St. John's Wort* (Prima Publishing, 1997):

> St. John's Wort doth charm the witches away,
> If gathered at midnight on the saint's holy day.
> And devils and witches have no power to harm
> Those that do gather the plant for charm.

—Christopher Hobbs, *HerbalGram* no. 18/19,
pp. 25–26, 1989

How is the "witch killer" made? The leaves and flowers are harvested and then dried, and alcohol is used to extract the medically useful chemicals from the plant. The powder is then shaped into a pill, coated, dried, and packaged. Then it's shipped to the stores and placed on the shelves, ready to be bought!

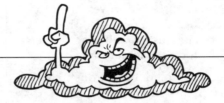

Funk-y Facts

You know alternative medicine is becoming more mainstream when medical therapies like acupuncture begin to be covered by some health insurance companies. Many traditional scientists are turning to Eastern sources for help in curing diseases. In fact, in 1998, the National Institute of Health's Office of Alternative Medicine and several other agencies gave $4.3 million to Duke University Medical Center to do a three-year study on the effectiveness of Hypericum. I can't wait to see the results of this research because there's still so much we need to know about why and how the wort works.

Three Worts a Day Keep the Blues Away

According to Dr. Harold Bloomfield, coauthor of *Hypericum and Depression* (Prelude Press, 1996) as well as other books on this topic, medical studies show that St. John's Wort is typically most effective when people take a 300 mg tablet or capsule three times a day. It may be easier to take one at each meal, but you could take two in the morning and one at night or some other combination. I found that I felt too sleepy in the afternoon if I took two tablets before mid-afternoon, so I take two at night and one in the morning. It really helps me sleep better and more easily.

If you're feeling depressed because things are not going well with your job, your kids, your spouse, and your life—and this misery has gone on for longer than two weeks—don't expect to take St. John's Wort for one day and be in a great mood the next. Nature's Prozac doesn't work right away and isn't appropriate for any bad feeling that has gone on for over two weeks.

Dr. Bloomfield suggests that you give St. John's Wort at least four to six weeks (taking 900 mg daily) before you decide whether you're benefiting from the treatment. It takes longer to reach its full effectiveness than do prescription antidepressants, perhaps because it's gentler on our systems and takes longer to naturally unfold and work its magic. The plus side of this time delay is that our systems are less challenged and we have few if any side effects during this time of adjustment.

St. John's Wort has an excellent safety record, Dr. Bloomfield assures us. Of the 20 million people who use the herb in Germany now—as well as those who've used it for the past 2,400 years— no one has reported any serious drug interaction problems or even toxicity after an accidental overdose. In a study of 3,250 patients taking St. John's Wort, only 2.4 percent experienced any side effects at all—consisting of mild cases of an allergic reaction, gastrointestinal irritation, tiredness, and restlessness—and most of these side effects disappeared over time.

Caution: When You're Already Taking Something...

St. John's Wort is so accessible, relatively inexpensive, and easy to use that people who aren't depressed may want to try it just to see if they could feel even better. But there's sobering news for you: You won't get a cheap high from this weed. There is no evidence showing that St. John's Wort makes people who feel just fine any more balanced, so if I were you I would use my money for something more useful (like an extra game of golf or a new workout outfit).

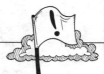

Blues Flag

The side effects you may experience when you first start taking St. John's Wort will probably go away by themselves once your body gets adjusted to the herb. But if they don't, stop taking it and call your doctor. All symptoms should fade altogether within a few days after you stop. However, a few people who take St. John's Wort report reduced sexual drive, adverse interaction with alcohol or drugs, dry mouth, headaches, or nausea—side effects typically associated with taking antidepressant drugs. But these self-reports of any significant side effects are few and far between.

Dr. Ellen Says

If your child seems depressed, check with your doctor or psychologist about trying an herbal remedy. Many physicians won't prescribe antidepressants for kids, but herbal experts say that kids respond well to some herbal medicines. This is a controversial area, however, so again check with your health-care professional before trying any of these solutions on your kids. Usually psychotherapy and parent counseling make a far greater difference in helping a child resolve his depression than *any* natural or prescribed substance.

But I do have many clients who are on antidepressants and wonder whether they should get off the hard stuff and join the Wort-heads. My advice to you if you are in this boat is: If you're taking something that works for you and you aren't having any side effects, why change? But if you are having trouble with your prescription antidepressants, you may want to look into trying St. John's Wort or, when your depression has lifted, you may wish to try it to cope more effectively with the everyday blues.

But *be careful!* Always check with your doctor before you stop taking any prescription medication or before you switch from one medicine to another—be it herbal or prescription (for more on prescription antidepressants mentioned in this chapter, see Chapter 23, "Better Living Through Chemistry"). There is no medical research that has looked at the effects of switching, but here are some rough guidelines, based on the experience of my clients:

➤ DO NOT just stop taking antidepressants cold turkey. Talk to your doctor about reducing the dosage gradually until you're off the medication altogether.

➤ DO NOT take St. John's Wort if you suffer from severe depression. If you aren't sure whether you are clinically depressed or just have a case of the blues, go back to Chapter 2 and take the quiz, or consult a psychologist or psychiatrist. Research shows that St. John's Wort works effectively to treat the blues or mild to moderate depression—but *not* major depression.

➤ DO NOT take St. John's Wort while taking Nardil or Parnate—both antidepressants that are in the family of Monoamine Oxidase Inhibitors (MAOIs). St. John's Wort seems to work something like a Selective Serotonin Reuptake Inhibitor (SSRI) because it increases the amount of serotonin production in your brain. Combining an SSRI with a MAOI can produce a dangerous rise in blood pressure. If you are taking a MAOI and you want to switch to St. John's Wort, experts suggest that you wait four weeks before taking any SSRIs—be it prescription or herbal.

➤ According to Dr. Bloomfield, if you're taking an SSRI such as Prozac, Paxil, or Zoloft, you may want to reduce the prescription SSRIs as you gradually introduce St. John's Wort. Remember, St. John's Wort takes longer to reach its full effect than prescription drugs. According to Dr. Bloomfield, this may indicate that you need to have a gradual building up of St. John's Wort over four to six weeks as you significantly reduce the dosage of the prescription antidepressant.

➤ Other clients with mild to moderate depressions have successfully weaned off their antidepressants in about a week by moving to smaller daily

Blues Flag

If you're severely depressed, don't get off Prozac without first talking to your doctor! The prescription drugs that you are taking may be saving your life. But if you think your depression is mild or moderate and you want to try St. John's Wort, talk to your doctor about the best way to get off the prescription drugs. Make sure you aren't taking any other drugs that may interfere with the herbal medicine.

doses and then to every other day to every few days taking their antidepressants. When they have completely stopped the antidepressant, they start on St. John's Wort and report continuing to feel better, even with the switch.

Be careful you don't load up your brain with too much serotonin because if that happens, you could end up with another bunch of unpleasant symptoms—confusion, agitation, lethargy, muscle jerks, and sometimes violent or suicidal feelings. If you get any of these symptoms, call your doctor right away.

There Are Other Herbs in the Forest

While St. John's Wort has been in the limelight of herbal treatments, it hasn't stolen the show of alternative medicines. Botanists have found many other herbal cures to today's maladies. And it's a good thing that they never could tell the forest from the trees because their tunnel vision and focus on specific plants is yielding many new herbal remedies.

The four top-selling herbs to hit the market, according to the *Nutrition Business Journal*, are: ginseng, garlic, ginkgo biloba, and St. John's Wort.

Let's look at some popular herbs more closely:

➤ *Ginseng.* This herb is used to boost mental and physical resistance to stress. It seems to increase oxygen and blood sugar metabolism and boost the immune system. Its powers have been known since ancient times for "quieting the spirit...stopping agitation...brightening the eyes...increasing wisdom," according to Chinese herbalist Tao Hung-Ching in A.D. 500.

➤ *Ginkgo biloba.* Enhances memory and has been found to improve cognitive functions in patients with Alzheimer's. It seems to increase blood flow to the brain and help heal the nervous system and is growing daily in its usage. "Over 120,000 physicians worldwide write over 10 million prescriptions for ginkgo each year," according to Dr. Bloomfield in his new book, *Healing Anxiety with Herbs* (HarperCollins, 1998).

The Chinese have used ginkgo for thousands of years to live longer, increase sexual endurance, and improve well-being. Over the past 10 years, the extract of ginkgo has become one of Europe's most widely prescribed drugs—and now the U.S. is on to it as well. The first double-blind study done in this country on the effects of this herb showed that it had a measurable effect on dementia. *But don't overinflate the findings.* Experts aren't suggesting that this herb will cure dementia or prevent Alzheimer's, but they do say that if Alzheimer's is treated early enough the patient's symptoms may be postponed.

➤ *Kava kava.* The latest herbal darling, kava comes from a pepper tree found in the South Pacific islands. (Can you hear the sounds of "Bali Hi" in the background?)

319

Often called "nature's tranquilizer," it's used to fight mild to moderate anxiety. Unlike St. John's Wort, however, which can be used for prolonged periods of time, kava is not recommended for use longer than four to six months. But while in use, it's reported to be a very helpful stress buster.

➤ *Black cohosh.* Relieves symptoms of menopause, including hot flashes, depression, nervousness, and more.

Don't worry if you can't memorize all these names—and believe me, there'll be a lot more names popping up as new herbal cures are found. It's exciting to see how many options we have today to treat the blues that weren't available to previous generations. So, if you're in a funk and need a pick-me-up, get a boost from Mother Nature and go botanical!

The Least You Need to Know

➤ The herbal business is booming, with sales of dietary supplements (which includes herbal products, vitamins, minerals, and amino acids) estimated to be $11.8 billion in 1997.

➤ The *Journal of the American Medical Association* (JAMA) reports that 40 percent of Americans now use alternative medicine.

➤ St. John's Wort (Hypericum) has received world-wide attention because it has been medically proven to treat mild to moderate depression as effectively as prescription drugs like Prozac but without the side effects.

➤ For St. John's Wort to be effective, it is typically reported that you take three pills of 300 mg each, for a period of at least four to six weeks.

➤ You can taper off an SSRI like Prozac while you begin to take St. John's Wort but do this only under the supervision of your physician.

➤ Other medicinal herbs on the market treat anxiety, enhance memory, and improve well-being. They include ginseng, ginkgo biloba, kava kava, and black cohosh.

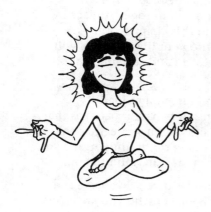

Chapter 25

Blues Immunization— Long-Term Protection for Your Mind, Body, and Soul

In This Chapter

➤ Make a PACT with yourself to conquer your blues

➤ People really do need people

➤ Don't just sit there, get moving!

➤ The luck of the draw: arts-and-letters therapy

➤ When to ride out the blues

➤ The healing Ps to the rescue

➤ Now you're the company; how's your stock?

Congratulations! One way or another, you've made it to the end of this book and moved up through the grades of emotional education. Now you've earned a place in the "Beat the Blues Graduate School." Of course to get here, we know you've read this book cover to cover and have done every action strategy religiously so that you've now got a great relationship with your parents and children, a good sex life with your partner, a great job and a respectable understanding with your boss, and of course, a fit, trim body to boot—now that you're perfect, should you really bother reading this chapter?

YES! Otherwise, you may have to read our sequel: *Return of the Blues*. Most of the chapters in this book have addressed what you can do to beat the blues when they strike. But you can prevent the blues from crashing down on you in the first place by following the long-term immunization strategies outlined in this chapter. Some of these exercises will take time to implement and integrate into your life, but they will help you keep your mental health in shape so you don't weaken and succumb to the blues as often.

These action strategies are the hardest to do because they require you to identify, analyze, and even change certain beliefs, attitudes, reactions, or behavior patterns that make you susceptible to the blues in first place. While the short-term strategies help you get through the hard times, they won't cure you in the long run if underneath you still feel self-destructive and continue to engage in behavior that is harmful to you.

Remember, you can make big changes in behavior and attitudes if you do a little at a time. And what you're changing is not the real you—the essence of who you are is just fine. You're changing the *bad habits* you've developed in the way you think, feel, and relate to others. These bad habits are often what are making you blue in the first place. To change your bad habits, practice the following long-term blues immunization strategies as much and as often as you can. You'll be strengthening yourself for a lifetime of successful blues management!

Make a PACT with Yourself

To beat the blues in the long run, you need to stay connected to yourself and what you really need. Don't be dependent on others to read or meet your needs or you'll stay blue and disappointed. Take responsibility for yourself and learn what you need. Then figure out a way to get it without hurting yourself or others. Commit to be the leader in the wonderful parade of your life and direct your production down the streets you want to travel. But if the blues threaten to rain on your parade, make a *PACT* with yourself to keep things sunny. PACT stands for People, Action, Creativity, and Time. Each letter represents a blues-busting action you can take. So every time you start to feel down, remember your PACT with yourself and you'll know that you're not going to stay down.

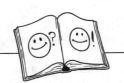

Terms of Encheerment

PACT stands for People, Action, Creativity, and Time and summarizes the major categories of action strategies you can use to keep the blues away in the short term and over the long haul.

I came up with the PACT strategy this summer while trying to figure out a way to calm my son's anxiety about going away to camp. Normally, going away to camp had been no problem for him. But last summer, at a new camp in the northern woods of Canada, he had a terrible experience of feeling and being out of control. So this summer, he was quite anxious about going off to another camp. One day after school, he came to my study where I was writing this book and flopped down on the couch in that world-is-ending style that only adolescents can master. He forlornly asked me what he could do to cope with blood-sucker mosquitoes, haunting homesickness, gripping insecurity about his athletic skills (which are actually more than fine), and in general, the summer-camp blues.

I felt good he asked, but bad that I didn't have the answer. So, buying time, I asked him to tell me more about what he was worried about. As he spoke, I speedily searched my memory files for a quick beat-the-blues strategy that was easy to use and that he wouldn't forget. Then it came to me: He needed to make a pact with himself that whenever he felt blue, he would use one of the PACT action strategies. We reviewed the PACT a number of times before he left, and he felt confident that he could cope when he said good-bye.

When he returned from camp, he joyously reported: "IT WORKED!" Whenever he felt that awful, stomach-churning, raw anxiety that made him want to hop on the next plane and head back to New York, he reached out to friends or the counselors, became active to take his mind off his mood (usually sports), did something creative (wrote and made some great drawings in his journal and made rubber stamps for his parents), and gave himself time to let the bad feelings pass, which they always did because they were the blues and not depression.

The "P" in PACT: People

"People who need people": Think about the Streisand song and as soon as you feel blue, connect with other people. The last thing you need to do is withdraw or take off by yourself, because the isolation will make you obsess over your mood even more as your mind rehashes the same thought over and over again. These ruminations are a waste of time. They take away your energy and don't solve your problems. Connecting with people will also distract you from your problems because you'll be able to focus on the other person instead of on yourself. You can connect in different ways:

➤ Get in touch with friends and family via phone, e-mail, or letter.

➤ Go out with coworkers after work to get some nachos or pizza.

➤ Go on a bus tour with a group.

➤ Plan to meet friends for coffee after you put the kids to bed.

Like me, you probably have only a few really close friends or relatives but tons of acquaintances (including colleagues, neighbors, people I know through school, and others). When I feel down I usually try to connect with my closest, most intimate friends first, including my husband—the people I love and trust the most. These are the relationships I've invested most of my energy in developing and maintaining.

Who are your closest friends or relatives? Where and with whom can you make the best investment of your time and energy?

To answer those questions, do a Relationship Inventory. Draw a circle with a bull's eye in the middle, and two more concentric circles around the bull's eye (see the following

Dr. Ellen Says

If you don't have a core group of people in your life whom you trust, feel close to, respect, and rely on, I urge you to develop a family of choice made up of people you select, and invest in them as if they were your family of origin. I've needed to create and invest in two families of choice, one in New York and one in California, and my children now have two sets of godparents. One family shares my commitment to psychology, personal growth, and intimate family gatherings with fabulous home-cooked meals. The other family prefers constant activity, excitement, large gatherings, and making things happen in the world. Both families serve different but equally important needs, and their diversity adds an incomparable richness to my and my family's lives.

A Relationship Inventory.

illustration). In the center circle, the bull's eye, write **Family of Choice**—these are the people you love and trust the most, the ones you can turn to when you are in trouble, whether they are blood-related or not. These are the people who will stick with you through thick and thin. Figure out who they are (they may or may not include family of origin and spouses) and put their names in the center circle of your Relationship Inventory.

In the second circle, write **Friends: Most Family of Origin**. This is where you can include aunts, uncles, cousins, and others. Good friends whom you may invite to a party and socialize with occasionally but whom you wouldn't pour your heart out to would go in this circle. These are people that can be there for you and do care, but not consistently.

In the third circle, write **Acquaintances**. Here you can list the most distant friends and people who don't fit into the other circles. These are people who come and go in your life depending on circumstances and mutual practical needs.

Now make a list of the people you know from work and your personal life and fill in their names in the appropriate circle. Keep the circle handy and refer to it when the blues hit you and you need to figure out whom you should call. If it's a serious problem that's causing the blues, you probably want to pick out a name from the first circle (family of choice). By consulting your Relationship Inventory circles, you'll clear up confusion about where to invest your time and energy for maximum return in relationships.

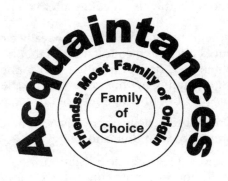

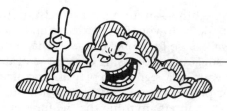

Funk-y Facts

People do need people! Feeling lonely and being isolated can kill your spirit. In *Love & Survival: The Scientific Basis for the Healing Power of Intimacy* (HarperCollins, 1998), Dr. Dean Ornish quotes Dr. Robert F. Lehman, the president of the Fetzer Institute, as saying that people who feel lonely and isolated are more likely to get sick because they are cut off from their spirit. All ancient traditions connect the spirit with healing through love—and spirit is another word for life. "That can be taken in a psychological way," Dr. Lehman continues, "but why not a physical way too? If there is a mind–body unity, then logic has it that when spirit is absent psychologically, then life is absent or depleted from the body as well."

Dr. Lehman quotes findings from a recent survey revealing that the number of people who say spiritual growth has become a big part of their life has gone up from 52 percent to 76 percent; while those who say that belonging to a religious institution is important has dropped from 78 percent to 50 percent. The reason the new spiritual movement is growing by leaps and bounds is that people are searching for a more integrated mind/body approach to happiness and well-being.

The "A" in PACT: Action

When you're feeling blue, don't just sit around till you're gray and grizzled! Get up and get moving! I know that doing even the smallest thing seems like a big ordeal because the blues drag you down and make you feel like someone's piled boulders on your shoulders. Everything about the blues makes you want to be inactive—you just want to sit, think, vegetate, be left alone, eat (or starve), drink, smoke. But to beat the blues, you've got to beat the Couch-Potato Syndrome. It may help to remember that you're supposed to eat vegetables, not act like them!

To combat the this syndrome, memorize the formula we mentioned in Chapter 6, "Quick Strategies for You to Beat the Blues" (you know, the one that reminded you of the chemistry class you flunked in college): Action = Energy = Power! That formula basically means that once you get up and do something, almost anything, you'll feel better because you'll have more energy. Over time, your energy builds and puts you in a better position to go after what you want and fight the negative thoughts that drain your energy.

So get up and do something—anything. Make a list of the three action strategies from this book that most appeal to you. Practice them and use them whenever you feel blue. Take a 10-minute walk or go for a bike ride (see Chapter 8, "Beating the Blues: Let's Get Physical," for more suggestions on using exercise to beat the blues), get out of bed, take a shower and wash your hair, sign up to play an organized sport, go to the bookstore to get a book about the problem you're struggling with, surf the Net to find people to commiserate with—just about anything that requires energy other than biting your nails will do!

The "C" in PACT: Creativity

Another part of PACT that contributes to your well-being is an exercise I call arts-and-letters therapy—therapy without the therapist. This strategy would keep me unemployed if more people would use it! But I don't have to hit the unemployment lines yet, because we've been taught so many hang-ups from third grade about our creative work not being good enough that many people avoid creative writing and drawing as adults.

Too bad, because this is a great action strategy to beat the blues. Creative action is what arts-and-letters therapy is all about. Writing and drawing about your feelings is an action strategy that you can use whenever you want and you don't have to rely on anyone else. Your defense mechanisms will less likely undermine your efforts, which gives you an opportunity not only to creatively identify and communicate what you're feeling, but also to view your life more objectively. When we put our feelings down on paper through words or drawings, they become real and are much more difficult to ignore or avoid. We begin to gain control over them as soon as we get the feelings out of our head and onto paper where we can see them more objectively.

Here is an example of how arts-and-letters therapy works.

One of my coaching clients stuck in a crummy job learned to take five-minute breaks from work to write about and draw her feelings when she felt burned out and mad. One day, she drew two quick sketches: One showed her punching a coworker with red blood flowing all over the office. It represented the anger she felt toward the coworker whose incompetence and complete disregard for others caused my client to work extra hours at night.

The other drawing expressed how much she missed her kids by showing two crying children calling "Mommy"

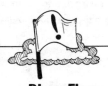

Blues Flag

One of the best ways to beat the blues is to write about your feelings regarding an incident that upset you. Recent research shows that people who go through a traumatic experience and write about their *feelings* involving the incident—not the details of the incident itself—recover more quickly. In one study, a group of middle-aged men who were fired from their jobs were asked to write about what it felt like to be fired. Those who expressed their painful feelings felt stronger and more confident more quickly.

and no one was there. The drawings helped her identify what she was feeling and cleared her head. She knew what she had to do: Tell the coworker to get her act together because my client didn't want to pick up after her anymore; and commit to leaving by 5:30 every night to spend more time with her family. My client would work after the kids were in bed or go in earlier if she had to; but she vowed to be there for those kids at night when they needed her most.

By trying to work out our feelings with arts-and-letters therapy we can gain a much clearer sense of how to solve our problems. Through arts-and-letters therapy we can focus on our own needs, rather than everybody else's, without being overwhelmed by them. Learning to integrate this form of expression into your life will save you pain and therapy expenses because you can do it on your own.

You're probably thinking: Draw? Give me a break. I can't even sketch a stick figure! But the beauty of this exercise is that you don't need a master's degree in graphic design or fine arts to do it! But, beware, there may be little demon voices inside your head clamoring for your attention every time you pick up a pen or pencil, hollering: "You can't draw, who do you think you are?" or "You've always been a lousy writer." Okay, so you are no Picasso. But you're still entitled to express your blues just like he did during his blue period! It's all right if your drawings look like chicken scratches and your writing resembles the "creative spelling" your daughter is learning in kindergarten. All that matters is that whatever you do represents what you feel!

You can express any violent feelings you have in any way you wish as long as the feelings *stay symbolic* and are not translated into reality. You must remind yourself that you cannot express destructive feelings in real behavior. Any *feeling* is fine, but destructive *behavior* is not. So try it out and commit yourself to doing arts-and-letters therapy for at least one week.

Just throw into your purse or briefcase several blank pages or index cards and some colored pens or markers. You can stick the paper in a binder later if you want a visual diary of your emotional life. Jot down words (they don't even have to be full sentences) to describe how you feel when you're down. Always include the time, place, and situation when you experienced these feelings—this way you can look back and trace any patterns showing you are more vulnerable to the blues at certain times or on certain days.

Here's an example excerpted from a client's journal:

> *August 4, 1998 (12:30 p.m.—at my desk during lunch while everybody is gone): I can't believe my birthday is here, I don't know exactly how I feel about it but I know it's BAD! What's there to celebrate anyhow, I'm tired and overwhelmed and don't feel like doing anything. I just want to sleep. I wish I did want to celebrate it somehow, I remember having parties when I was younger, how I looked forward to them. But now, who cares?*

Then under the words she drew a gray blob dripping over the edges of a desk with two half-closed eyes forming a face. The blob uttered one word: "HELLLLLP!"

Guiltless Pleasures

As you do the long-term exercises to reduce stress, increase confidence, and lessen the likelihood of getting the blues, praise yourself over and over again. It takes courage to admit that you feel down and need help. It takes faith to change the way you think, feel, and behave. And it takes spirit to hang in there for the long haul knowing that, in the end, you'll like yourself a lot more and enjoy a sense of freedom you've never imagined. Being good to yourself and complimenting yourself is part of the healing and keeping the blues at bay for the long term.

Through writing and drawing in her journal, the client discovered that she wasn't feeling very special these days—and for a good reason, because she was overworked, underpaid, and had no time for anything else. But she prevented the blues from turning to black by taking action: She realized she needed to do something for herself. So after work, she headed to the shopping mall to buy a new outfit, made plans to meet a friend for dinner, wrote a warm letter to her mother—and wound up having a wonderful birthday. The next drawing she did at work still showed a cage as her office, but this time, instead of a blob, there was a lioness inside waiting to spring to action at the next opportunity for freedom.

When the words won't come, switch to drawing. The great thing about arts-and-letters therapy is that you can go back and forth between the media if you get blocked on one side of your brain. Often an answer will spring out from the other side of the brain when you least expect it. And the best part is that you create the answer yourself from your own creative resources and don't have to depend on anyone else. The kind of freedom and self-reliance you achieve from your own creative activity provides a real blues-buster.

The "T" in PACT: Time

It's all in the timing: Surf the blue feelings until the wave breaks and the feeling weakens. When you feel really rotten, you're often tempted to do stupid, self-destructive things—like pigging out on greasy food, calling up old an boyfriend or girlfriend who dumped you and begging to be taken back, or taking illicit drugs or drinking too much. But research shows that you may be able to stop yourself from losing control if you just wait the 4–12 minutes when the impulse is most intense and ride out the urge to do something bad to yourself or others (see Chapter 7, "The Moody Food Blues: Caving in to Cravings," for more about using the 4–12–minute test to fight food cravings).

Even if the 12 minutes are up and you still feel like punching anyone who comes along, chances are your anger will be less intense and much more manageable. So when you feel out of control, remember that you have a 4–12–minute window. And since we're throwing in some numbers, let me add another reminder. If the angry, sad, or mad feelings go on every day for 12 to 14 days, even after you've tried to ride out the blues, then it's likely that you have a clinical depression and need help. Review Chapter 2 and take the "Are You Blue or Are You Depressed?" quiz. If you believe you're depressed, get professional help immediately!

The Healing Ps: Plants, Pets, and People

Making a PACT with yourself will put you in touch with your feelings so you can get a grip on your grief and feel more connected with people. The focus of these exercises is on giving yourself strength. Another way to beat the blues is to take care of plants, pets, and people—the Healing Ps Solution. Why not? They all need tender loving care to grow, just like you!

➤ *Plants.* Research conducted by Dr. Ellen Langer, a psychologist on the faculty at Harvard University, revealed that nursing-homes residents who took care of plants had fewer physical and emotional complaints than those who didn't. So whether your thumb is green or brown, plant and care for some herbs, flowers, or plants to keep that thumb of yours from turning blue.

➤ *Pets.* Pets are also good blues-busters. In *Love & Survival: The Scientific Basis for the Healing Power of Intimacy* (HarperCollins, 1998), Dr. Dean Ornish quotes findings from a study of patients recovering from heart disease. The study found that after one year, only 6 percent of the pet owners died, compared with 28 percent of the patients who did not own pets. Just remember: A mutt, kitty cat, or any other kind of pet may massage your heart toward health!

➤ *People power.* Reaching out and giving to somebody else also makes you feel more powerful and healthy. Dr. Dean Ornish cites research that showed those who volunteered to help others at least once a week were *two and a half times* less likely to die during the study as those who never volunteered. So get behind a food line to slap some mush on a plate, put on your overalls and help build houses, or go to the your local hospital to help reduce the hospital blues of those who must reside there. Giving to others can prolong your own life.

Check Your Blues Medication Daily (Not the Prescription Kind)

Are you smoking cigarettes, watching too much TV, eating too many Whoppers, doing drugs, or drinking too much as a means of beating the blues? Because if you are, get ready to dive into the depths of your blue soul. The next stop is the black hole. The Georgetown University Medical Center recently released a study revealing that people who are depressed are more likely to start smoking because they think it improves their mood and they're less able to stop if they're depressed. So what can you do if you're using some destructive substance or activity as a medication to chase away the blues? Here are some strategies to try.

When smoking is the blues medication: Join a structured program for quitting and kicking the habit. Don't try to do it alone, because the nicotine addiction may be too powerful as a blues medication. Find out information about Smoke Enders and other programs at the local hospitals and choose a program or coach to help you quit.

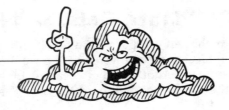

Funk-y Facts

What are your family values and beliefs? If your children are clear about what your family stands for they'll have a better sense of what's right and wrong—and may be less susceptible to getting the blues. Stephen R. Covey, author of *The 7 Habits of Highly Effective Families* (Franklin Covey Company, 1997) suggests each family should develop a mission statement that spells out what the family is all about and the principles underlying the rules governing family life. Here are his suggestions on the best way to go about it:

First step: Get everyone's feelings and ideas on the table. Children love to be included in this process. Make sure everyone has a chance to give input, repeat what each person is saying to make sure everyone understands, and ask someone in the family to write down ideas.

Second step: Based on the ideas thrown on the table, draft the family mission statement so that the family members can look at it, think about it, and discuss it. Write out the statement everyone agrees to and make sure all family members have a copy.

Third step: Use the statement to keep on track during the following months. Covey emphasizes that a mission statement doesn't have to be a formal document; it could be a word, phrase, or image that represents your family values. To get some ideas on how to approach writing a mission statement, take a look at the worksheets for developing such documents provided on the Internet at http://www.franklincovey.com.

When TV is the blues medication: If you are like most average Americans who watch three to four hours of TV a day, you're probably feeling pretty bleary-eyed, belly full but soul empty. TV is a primary avoidance tool in our culture, which means we are often watching it as an excuse to not do other things or to tune out a world we find too difficult and painful. Cut back on TV an hour at a time, a week at a time, until you get to a comfortable point with it and you're not watching more than an hour a day. Use the extra time to be with people, work on creative projects, or take your dog Millie for a walk.

When food is the blues medication: Our whole economy is geared up to medicate our stressed moods through food. The Golden Arches is the greatest dispenser of antidepressants in our culture. Drive thru and leave with a Big Mac, large fries, and a Coke: guaranteed to fill you with so much fat and sugar you feel temporarily distracted from your woes. One reason there is such an explosive growth in fast food is that we are starved for time and for good moods. Instead of overeating fast food, keep a mood journal to record your feelings whenever you want to eat food that you know isn't good for you and develop healthy satisfying substitutes. Or allow yourself a treat a day as a reward for doing well, not to medicate your blue feelings.

When drugs and drinking are the blues medication: Look at the link between your mood and the drugs that you are taking. Alcohol is the most common antidepressant we use; although, ironically, drinking too much makes people depressed. If you suspect you drink or take drugs when you feel bad, or friends and family have said you're in trouble with either drugs or alcohol, then take the warning seriously and get professional help or attend AA (Alcoholics Anonymous) or NA (Narcotics Anonymous) meetings. Drink and drugs only deepen the blues and grow your addiction until both slip out of your control and you drop into the black pit.

You're the Most Important Company: Take Stock of Your Stock

You've worked hard to develop a good attitude, to change self-defeating thoughts and habits that kept you from being the best you can be and leading a more meaningful life. Now, the key is maintenance. How do you keep your life in check so that you continue feeling good about yourself?

Think of yourself as a very important company that performs many different services and produces important goods. Do an annual, semiannual, or quarterly evaluation of the company's well-being. Think of this exercise as an end-of-the-year report. You are taking an assessment of your company's growth potential, liabilities, and goals. The original idea for this approach was described several years ago in an article in *The Wall Street Journal* and it seemed so useful, I adopted it as a strategy to beat the blues.

Under growth potential, write down areas you'd like to see change. Under liabilities, spell out what is getting in the way of your success. And finally, include three or more goals as strategies for overcoming the barriers and getting what you want. The following table may give you some ideas to get started.

Growth potential	You've got a loving wife who feels distant from you but loves you.
Liabilities	You are never home because you work late and travel a lot.
Goals	1) Structure your time so you're home earlier when you're in town. 2) Make sure you plan quality time vacation with her. 3) Send her flowers or call more while you're traveling. 4) If you don't already have one, buy a computer and stay in touch by e-mail.
Growth potential	You hate your current marketing job but have always been interested in financing.
Liabilities	It's hard to change directions, especially when you are in your 40s. Plus, you may have to take a pay cut.
Goals	1) Take courses in financing. 2) Talk to five people who are doing what you want to do. 3) Go to a career counselor to help you think it through. 4) Read several books about careers in finance.
Growth potential	Your kid is a budding basketball star, but you don't spend much time shooting hoops with him in spite of his repeated requests for your companionship.
Liabilities	Working so hard, it's difficult to find time to be with him.
Goals	1) Set aside Saturday mornings to play. 2) Sign him up for basketball clinic. 3) Take him to basketball games. 4) Check in with him daily by phone or in person about how it's going.

What is the state of your most important asset, your company, which includes all parts of your mind, body, and soul? Make a list of what you want to change in your life. Let your mind flow and include everything you can think of, from relationships with family members to cleaning up your office. Then select three areas you'd like to take action on immediately and follow the format of the previous examples to do an assessment of your growth potential, liabilities, and goals. When you constantly take stock of the stock in your company and take action to correct problems, your long-term blues immunization program will ensure you'll beat the blues. Good luck and enjoy the new strength and health of your company!

The Least You Need to Know

➤ Whenever you feel down, make a PACT with yourself—connect with People, take Action, use your Creativity to get to the heart of your blues, and take Time to weaken destructive impulses.

➤ To find out who your "family of choice" is, do a Relationship Inventory. Then reach out to those people whenever you feel down.

➤ Drawing or writing will help you figure out why you are upset and what you can do about it.

➤ If you've got the blues, watch out for destructive habits. Quit smoking, watch less TV, avoid junk foods, don't take illegal drugs (or legal drugs unwisely), and monitor your use of alcohol and drugs.

➤ To find out what types of changes you want to make in your life, be your own CEO and do a reading of your company's stock. Develop goals to decrease liabilities and increase strengths for the following year.

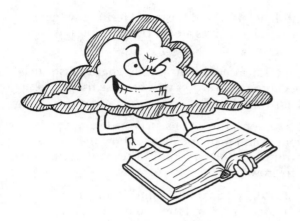

Glossary

Age-Rage Blues   The healthy dose of lousy feelings men and women experience because they are growing older in a society that values youth and sees old age as something to dread, postpone, and, if possible, avoid.

Alexithymia   An ancient term resurrected by Ronald Levant, author of *Masculinity Reconstructed*, that means "words without emotions." It's a condition that many men suffer from because they can't express what they feel.

Bad-Boss Blues   The frustrating, disturbing, and vulnerable feelings we get when our bosses treat us badly and disrespectfully, and we feel too powerless to do anything about it.

Bedroom Blues   The sad, mad, and bad feelings all of us have when we feel disappointed, frustrated, empty, or conflicted in our relationships with our spouses.

behavioral therapy   A type of short-term psychological treatment that zeroes in on changing specific behaviors.

biofeedback   A technique of monitoring the physiological system so a person can regulate certain body sensations. Through this technique, people can learn to, for instance, tighten the muscles of their bladder so they can better control impaired bladder function.

Body-Image Blues   The negative feelings of shame, contempt, and disappointment in our bodies that most women and many men experience as they try to meet the unrealistic cultural standards of physical perfection, beauty, sex appeal, youth, and fashion.

Burnout Blues   The bad feelings we experience from being constantly tired, overwhelmed, stressed, and drained by the increasing demands and role conflicts confronting men and women today.

Cancer Blues   The anxious, fearful, helpless, and frustrated feelings we get when we are told we have cancer, or that someone we love has cancer.

Cardiovascular Blues   The anxious, fearful, helpless, and frustrated feelings we get when we are told we have heart disease and that our lives are on the line unless we take drastic steps to change the way we live, think, and behave.

cognitive therapy   Short-term psychological treatment that seeks to change distorted thinking that often contributes to feeling depressed. It works well because the quickest way to change how you feel is to change how you think.

cultural conscience   A person's core of traditions, the set of sanctioned values and thinking that exists deep within every woman and man and dictates how they must behave and what roles are "right" and "wrong" for them to fulfill. These values are taught to children as soon as they begin to grow.

Decoronation Blues   The frustrated, confused, and anxious feelings many men experience as they are forced to redefine "masculinity" and their changing role in society.

deep breathing   A technique used to release tension.

eating disorders   These include anorexia, bulimia, and compulsive eating. Victims of anorexia starve and exercise excessively to get well below their recommended weight. Those with bulimia repeatedly binge on food and purge through vomiting or laxatives. Compulsive eaters stuff themselves with food even when they're not hungry.

everyday blues   Realistic feelings of pain, sadness, and disappointment that stem from life's negative experiences, including normal losses, unfair treatment, and unresolved past sadness triggered by a current event. People who have the everyday blues can still function, although usually not as well as they would like.

family of choice   A core group of people who function like members of a healthy family. They support and encourage you when you need them during an emotional, physical, or financial crisis.

Home-Alone Blues   The sad, frustrated, desperate feelings we get when we want to find somebody to share our lives but we either don't have the skills to develop and maintain a relationship or the pickings are slim so we can't find anyone we like.

Hypericum (St. John's Wort)   An herb that has been proven to be an effective treatment for mild to moderate depression. Hypericum is the most extensively researched and used herbal antidepressant known.

meditation   A form of relaxation that helps your muscles relax and slows down your breathing so you feel peaceful, restful.

Monoamine Oxidase Inhibitors (MAOIs)   A class of antidepressants that stop the enzyme monoamine oxidase from breaking down, thereby boosting the levels of norepinephrine, serotonin, and dopamine in the brain and improving mood.

Monday-Morning Blues   The dreadful, disheartened, and demoralizing feelings we experience when we are unhappy with our working arrangement—because we don't like our jobs, we don't get along with our work mates, we don't feel valued by our bosses, or we fear we'll lose our jobs.

Moody Food Blues   The frustrated, anxious, bad, and mad feelings we get when we promise ourselves that we'll stick to our diets "this time," but then go off them big time as we take "just one bite" of our favorite food and then pig out on everything else because we feel we've already "blown it" anyhow.

My Fair Lady Blues   The frustrated, exhausted, and upset feelings women get as they struggle to balance their traditional and modern roles.

neurotransmitters   Chemicals in the brain and nervous system that carry messages across the gaps between neurons. The three main neurotransmitters involved in the development of depression are dopamine, norepinephrine, and serotonin.

Parent Approval Blues   The angry, frustrated, and hurt feelings we get when our parents dislike what we do, disapprove of how we feel, and criticize the way we think— or at least we think they disapprove.

Pooped-Parent Blues   The sad, bad, frustrating, exhausted, and guilty feelings we get when we do what we think is right for our children but they don't react the way we expect them to and we don't know what to do about it.

psychopharmacologists   Medical specialists who study the effects of antidepressants on the behavior of depressed people and examine how the naturally occurring substances within the brain affect the part of the brain that deals with emotions and regulates moods.

psychotherapy   A proven form of treatment that is based on resolving emotional and mental conflicts by talking about the problem and trying new behaviors to solve the problems.

Seasonal Affective Disorder (SAD)   A form of clinical depression that usually starts in the autumn and lasts until spring, typically affecting people on gloomy winter days.

Seasonal Blues   The sad, gloomy feelings we get in response to the changing seasons or to an anniversary like a birthday, Mother's Day, or Father's Day.

Selective Serotonin Reuptake Inhibitors (SSRIs)   One of the newest classes of antidepressants—including Prozac, Zoloft, and Paxil—that improve mood by blocking the reabsorption of serotonin in the brain that causes depression.

serotonin   A chemical in your brain that is related to good and bad moods. If you don't have enough of it in your brain, you'll feel bad. You lose serotonin under prolonged stress.

tricyclics   A class of traditional drugs that treat depression by blocking the reabsorption of several different neurotransmitters, which allows brain to use them to produce positive moods.

visualization/imagery   A mental process in which patients envision positive situations so they can improve their moods, attitudes, behaviors, and even physiological responses.

Working-Parents Blues   The frustrated, angry, guilty, upset feelings we get when we try to do what's best for our children and our jobs, but long hours at work, chores, and responsibilities get in the way of our spending quality time with the kids.

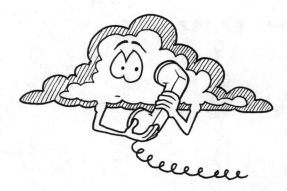

Resources

Self-Help Organizations

Al-Anon, Alateen and Adult Children of Alcoholics
Al-Anon Family Group Headquarters, Inc.
1600 Corporate Landing Highway
Virginia Beach, VA 23454
(800) 344-2666
http://www.solar.rtd.utk.edu/~al-non

Alcoholics Anonymous
P.O. Box 459
Grand Central Station
New York, NY 10163
(212) 870-3400
http://www.aa.org.com

National Clearinghouse for Alcohol and Drug Information
National Institute on Drug Abuse (NIDA)
5600 Fishers Lane, Room 15C-05
Rockville, MD 20807
(800) 729-6686 or (301) 468-2600
http://www.nida.gov/

National Mental Health Consumer Self-Help Clearinghouse
311 South Jupiter Street, Room 902
Philadelphia, PA 19107
(215) 735-6367
http://www.med.upenn.edu/~cmhpsr/mhlinks.html

Depression/Mental Health Organizations

American Psychiatric Association
1400 K Street, N.W.
Washington, DC 20005
(202) 682-6124
http://www.psych.org

American Psychological Association
1200 17th Street, N.W.
Washington, DC 20056
(202) 336-5500

Anxiety Disorders Association of America
6000 Executive Boulevard, Suite 515
Rockville, MD 20852
(301) 231-9350

Center for Mental Health Services (CMHS)
Office of External Liaison
5600 Fishers Lane, Room 13-103
Rockville, MD 20807
(301) 443-2792
http://www.mentalhealth.org/mhlinks/index.htm

Depression Awareness, Recognition, Treatment (D/ART) Program
National Institute of Mental Health
5600 Fishers Lane
Rockville, MD 20807
(800) 421-4211

National Alliance for the Mentally Ill
200 N. Glebe Road, Suite 1015
Arlington, VA 22203-3754
(800) 950-6264
http://www.nami.org

National Anxiety Foundation
3135 Custer Drive
Lexington, KY 40517
(606) 272-7166

National Foundation for Depressive Illness (NFDI)
P.O. Box 2257
New York, NY 10016
(800) 248-4344

Alternative Medicine Organizations

American Association of Acupuncture and Oriental Medicine
433 Front Street
Catasaqua, PA 18032
(610) 264-2768

Herb Research Foundation
1007 Pearl Street, Suite 200
Boulder, CO 80302
(303) 449-2265
http://www.herbs.org

Society for Light Treatment and Biological Rhythms
Light Therapy Unit
New York Psychiatric Institute
Box 50
722 W. 168th Street
New York, NY 10032

Seniors

American Association of Retired Persons (AARP)
1909 K. Street, N.W.
Washington, DC 20024
(202) 872-4700
http://www.aarp.org

National Council on the Aging
409 3rd Street, S.W., 2nd Floor
Washington, DC 20024
(202) 479-1200

National Institute on Aging
Information Office
Federal Building 6C12
Bethesda, MD 20892
(800) 222-2225

Ethnic

National Asian Women's Health Organization
250 Montgomery Street, Suite 410
San Francisco, CA 94104
(415) 989-9747

National Black Women's Health Project
1237 Ralph David Abernathy Boulevard, S.W.
Atlanta, GA 30310
(404) 758-9590

National Latina Health Organization
P.O. Box 7567
Oakland, CA 94601
(510) 534-1362

Body Image

Overeaters Anonymous
4025 Spencer Street, Suite 203
Torrance, CA 43229
(310) 618-8835
http://www.hiwaay.net/recovery

Health-Related Organizations

American Cancer Society (all aspects of cancer)
1599 Clifton Road, N.E.
Atlanta, GA 30329
(404) 320-3333
http://www.cancer.org

Depression After Delivery
P.O. Box 1282
Morrisville, PA 19067
(800) 944-4PPD

National Cancer Institute (all aspects of cancer)
Office of Cancer Communications
Building 31, Room 10A24
Bethesda, MD 20892
(800) 4-CANCER (800-422-6237)

Internet Resources

American Botanical Council
http://www.herbalgram.org./abcmission.html

American Heart Association
http://www.amhrt.org/

American Mental Health Alliance
http://www.psych.org

Ask Dr. Weil
http://www.drweil.com

Attention Deficit Hyperactivity Disorder Page
http://www.healthguide.com/ADHD

Herb Research Foundation
http://www.herbs.org

Hypericum (St. John's Wort)
http://www.hypericum.com

Mental Health Net
http://www.cmhc.com/

National Institute of Mental Health
http://www.nimh.nih.gov

Office of Alternative Medicine
http://altmed.od.nih.gov

Office of Dietary Supplements
http://dietarysupplements.info.nih.gov

Stress Release
http://www.stressrelease.com/strssbus.html

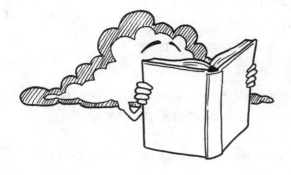

Suggested Reading

Bloomfield. Harold. *How to Heal Depression* (Prelude Press, 1996)

Bloomfield. Harold. *Hypericum and Depression* (Prelude Press, 1996)

Bruce, Debra Fulghum and Harris H. McIlwain. *The Unofficial Guide to Alternative Medicine* (Alpha Books, 1998)

Buff, Sheila and Alan Pressman. *The Complete Idiot's Guide to Alternative Medicine* (Alpha Books, 1998)

Burns, David. *The Feeling Good Handbook* (Penguin Group, 1989)

Carlson, Richard. *You Can Be Happy No Matter What* (Richard Carlson, 1997)

Cooper, Robert. *The Performance Edge* (Houghton Mifflin, 1991)

Emery, Gary. *Getting Un-Depressed* (Simon & Schuster, 1988)

Fisher, Roger and William Ury. *Getting to YES* (Penguin Books, 1991)

Friedan, Betty. *The Fountain of Age* (Simon & Schuster, 1993)

Gray, John. *Men Are From Mars, Women Are From Venus* (HarperCollins, 1992)

Gullo, Stephen. *Thin Tastes Better* (Food Control Center, 1995)

Haber, Sandra and Barbara Rubin Wainrib. *Prostate Cancer: A Guide for Women and the Men They Love* (Dell, 1996)

Halpern, Howard. *How to Break Your Addiction to a Person* (MJF Books, 1982)

Kaplan, Eliot. *Making the Prozac Decision* (Lowell House, 1997)

Korda, Michael. *Man to Man: Surviving Prostate Cancer* (Random House, 1996)

Kramer, Peter. *Listening to Prozac* (Penguin, 1997)

Kuriansky, Judy. *The Complete Idiot's Guide to a Healthy Relationship* (Alpha Books, 1998)

Kuriansky, Judy. *The Complete Idiot's Guide to Dating* (Alpha Books, 1998)

Levant, Ronald. *Masculinity Reconstructed* (Penguin, 1995)

Levine, James. *Working Fathers* (Addison Wesley, 1997)

Lunden, Joan. *Joan Lunden's Healthy Living* (Crown Publishers, 1997)

McGrath, Ellen. *When Feeling Bad Is Good* (Henry Holt, 1992)

Nolen-Hoeksma, Susan. *Sex Differences In Depression* (Stanford University Press, 1990)

Ornish, Dean. *Love and Survival: The Scientific Basis for the Healing Power of Intimacy* (HarperCollins, 1998)

Price, Susan Crites and Tom Price. *The Working Parents Help Book* (Peterson's, 1996)

Rosenthal, Norman. *Winter Blues* (Guilford Press, 1993)

Russell, Bertrand. *The Conquest of Happiness* (Liverlight, 1971)

Sheehy, Gail. *New Passages* (Ballantine, 1995)

Sheehy, Gail. *Understanding Men's Passages: Discovering the New Map of Men's Lives* (Random House, 1998)

Siegel, Bernie. *Love, Medicine and Miracles* (Harper Perennial, 1990)

Styron, William. *Darkness Visible: A Memoir of Madness* (Vintage Books, 1992)

Turecki, Stanley. *The Difficult Child* (Bantam, 1985)

Turkington, Carol. *Making the Prozac Decision* (RGA Publishing Group, Inc., 1995)

Waterhouse, Debra. *Why Women Need Chocolate* (Hyperion, 1995)

Williams, Redford. *The Trusting Heart: Great News About Type A Behavior* (NY Times Books, 1989)

Bridge Ventures: Executive Coaching Systems

Assessment ➤ Feedback ➤ Coaching

For executives and staff in corporations, small businesses, entrepreneurial ventures, and family businesses to achieve the following goals as the bridge to their success:

➤ Remove obstacles to success for maximum personal and professional growth

➤ Increase strengths/decrease problem areas to fulfill company performance goals

➤ Improve communication skills and relationship management skills

➤ Assess potential new hires for company fit and fitness to produce

➤ Leadership team development for increased productivity and job satisfaction

➤ Help executives and their families cope with health crises to recover ASAP

Assessment	Customized, unique 360 feedback questionnaires developed to meet company needs; instruments assess variables associated with employee *retention*, *productivity*, and *potential*; test executives and employees for strength and problem areas to obtain objective performance profile
Feedback	Feedback to all participants delivered by experienced psychologists trained in conflict resolution and constructive behavioral change; written action plans are developed to enhance strengths for future professional growth and for problems to be improved or resolved by next evaluation
Coaching	Individual and group coaching on skill development in areas critical for business and personal success; help in solving personal problems *if* they interfere with professional performance; coaching sessions typically range from two sessions to two years; the average falls between three to six months
Director	Ellen McGrath, Ph.D., President and Founder; 25 years experience as clinical psychologist and executive coach; psychology expert for *ABC/Good Morning America*; voted Outstanding Psychologist of the Year (1997)—APA; named top coach/therapist by three national magazines

Dear Reader,

Over the years, I've received many requests for support material to better manage the blues, depression, stress, cardiac recovery, and cancer problems for clients and their families. I'm delighted to now be able to respond to your requests. If you think any of the following would be helpful in your quest to beat the blues, please fill out the form below and mail it to the address at the end. We'll make every effort to respond to your requests. **Remember, we're in this together!**

Name: _____

Address: _____

City: _____ State: _____ ZIP: _____

Country: _____

Telephone: _____ Fax: _____

_____ Single   _____ Married   _____ Divorced   _____ Widowed   _____ Live with

_____ Female   _____ Male   Age _____

Occupation: _____

Please:

_____ Put me on the mailing list.

_____ Mail the items checked below.

_____ Contact me about being a business or executive coach.

_____ Contact me about coming to speak to your organization.

Check the items you wish to receive:

Audiotapes ($12.00 each):

_____ (A1) *When Feeling Bad Is Good*: 10 Proven Action Strategies To Convert Negative Feelings Into New Energy And Power

_____ (A2) New Mental Fitness Techniques: Blues Action Strategies For The Car, Walking, Or Exercise

_____ (A3) Women In Business: Coaching Yourself To Success In Your Professional And Personal Lives

_____ (A4) Men In Business: Coaching Yourself To Success In Your Professional And Personal Lives

Videotapes ($25.00 each):

_____ (V1) A sample of Dr. Ellen's appearances on *ABC News, Oprah, Nightline, Good Morning America, Fox On Psychology*, and *Your Mind and Body* regarding trauma, stress, and depression management topics.

Photos (5×7 black and white for $5.00 or 8×10 color for $10.00):

_____ (P1) Autographed photo of Dr. Ellen which says: "Don't forget… We're in this together!"

_____ Merchandise total

_____ Sales tax (New York residents pay 8.25%)

_____ Shipping and Handling (use following table)

_____ **Total**

Shipping and Handling Charges	
Up to $20	$4.75
$20.01 to $30	$5.75
$30.01 to $40	$6.98
$40.01 to $50	$7.98
$50.01 to $75	$10.75
$75.01 to $100	$12.75
$100.01 to $150	$14.98
Over $150	$15.98

Send this form, along with a check or money order, to:

Bridge Ventures
P.O. Box 022250
Brooklyn, New York 11202

Index

H-I-J

$30 < 50$

$45 > 42$

$30 > 50$